Surgical
RECALL

SIXTH EDITION

Lorne H. Blackbourne

BOOKMARK

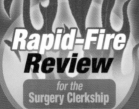

Rapid-Fire Review
for the
Surgery Clerkship

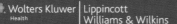

Wolters Kluwer | Lippincott
Health | Williams & Wilkins

OP NOTE
Remember the acronym PPP SAFE DISC:

Preop dx
Postop dx
Procedure

Surgeon (and assistants)
Anesthesia
Fluids
Estimated blood loss (EBL)

Drains
IV fluids
Specimen
Complications

Surgical Knot Tying Anchor Bookmark

Use this bookmark to practice tying surgical knots!

1. Find a piece of suture.
2. Place the bookmark in back of the book with the hole showing underneath.
3. Open the book to Chapter 8—Surgical Knot Tying (p. 65).
4. Use the anchor to practice tying surgical knots by placing the suture through the hole.

Visit Lippincott Williams & Wilkins
on the Internet:
LWW.com/medstudent

Wolters Kluwer | Lippincott
Health | Williams & Wilkins

SURGICAL RECALL
6th Edition

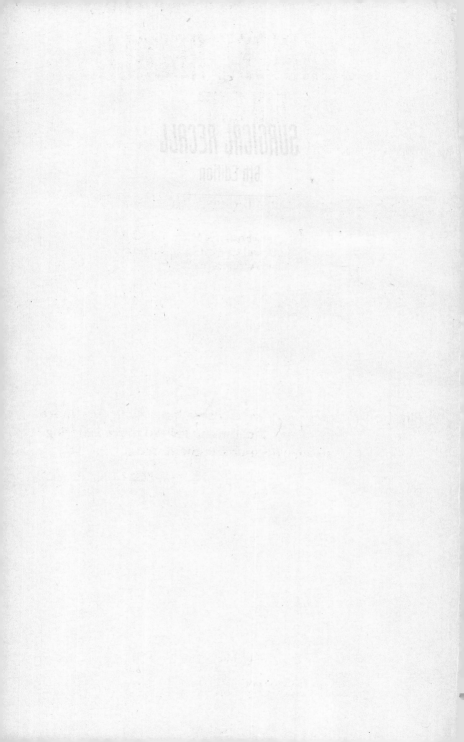

SURGICAL RECALL
6th Edition

RECALL SERIES EDITOR AND SENIOR EDITOR

Lorne H. Blackbourne, M.D., F.A.C.S.
Trauma, Burn, and Critical Care Surgeon
San Antonio, Texas

"In the operating room we can save more lives, cure more cancer, restore more function, and relieve more suffering than anywhere else in the hospital."

—R. SCOTT JONES, M.D.

Wolters Kluwer | Lippincott Williams & Wilkins
Health
Philadelphia · Baltimore · New York · London
Buenos Aires · Hong Kong · Sydney · Tokyo

Acquisitions Editor: Susan Rhyner
Product Manager: Joyce Murphy
Marketing Manager: Joy Fisher-Williams
Manufacturing Manager: Margie Orzech
Design Coordinator: Holly Reid McLaughlin
Compositor: Aptara, Inc.

Sixth Edition

Copyright © 2012, 2009, 2006, 2002, 1998, 1994 Lippincott Williams & Wilkins, a Wolters Kluwer business.

351 West Camden Street   Two Commerce Square, 2001 Market Street
Baltimore, MD 21201   Philadelphia, PA 19103

Printed in China

9 8 7 6 5 4 3 2

Library of Congress Cataloging-in-Publication Data

Available upon request

DISCLAIMER

Care has been taken to confirm the accuracy of the information present and to describe generally
accepted practices. However, the authors, editors, and publisher are not responsible for errors or omissions
or for any consequences from application of the information in this book and make no warranty, expressed
or implied, with respect to the currency, completeness, or accuracy of the contents of the publication. Application of this information in a particular situation remains the professional responsibility of the practitioner;
the clinical treatments described and recommended may not be considered absolute and universal recommendations.

The authors, editors, and publisher have exerted every effort to ensure that drug selection and dosage
set forth in this text are in accordance with the current recommendations and practice at the time of publication. However, in view of ongoing research, changes in government regulations, and the constant flow of
information relating to drug therapy and drug reactions, the reader is urged to check the package insert for
each drug for any change in indications and dosage and for added warnings and precautions. This is particularly important when the recommended agent is a new or infrequently employed drug.

Some drugs and medical devices presented in this publication have Food and Drug Administration (FDA)
clearance for limited use in restricted research settings. It is the responsibility of the health care provider to
ascertain the FDA status of each drug or device planned for use in their clinical practice.

To purchase additional copies of this book, call our customer service department at **(800) 638-3030** or fax
orders to **(301) 223-2320.** International customers should call **(301) 223-2300.**

Visit Lippincott Williams & Wilkins on the Internet: http://www.lww.com. Lippincott Williams & Wilkins
customer service representatives are available from 8:30 am to 6:00 pm, EST.

Dedication

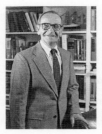

This book is dedicated to the memory of Leslie E. Rudolf, Professor of Surgery and Vice-Chairman of the Department of Surgery at the University of Virginia. Dr. Rudolf was born on November 12, 1927, in New Rochelle, New York. He served in the U.S. Army Counter-Intelligence Corps in Europe after World War II.

He graduated from Union College in 1951 and attended Cornell Medical College, where he graduated in 1955. He then entered his surgical residency at Peter Brigham Hospital in Boston, Massachusetts, and completed his residency there, serving as Chief Resident Surgeon in 1961.

Dr. Rudolf came to Charlottesville, Virginia as an Assistant Professor of Surgery in 1963. He rapidly rose through the ranks, becoming Professor of Surgery and Vice-Chairman of the Department in 1974 and a Markle Scholar in Academic Medicine from 1966 until 1971. His research interests included organ and tissue transplantation and preservation. Dr. Rudolf was instrumental in initiating the Kidney Transplant Program at the University of Virginia Health Sciences Center. His active involvement in service to the Charlottesville community is particularly exemplified by his early work with the Charlottesville/Albemarle Rescue Squad, and he received the Governor's Citation for the Commonwealth of Virginia Emergency Medical Services in 1980.

His colleagues at the University of Virginia Health Sciences Center, including faculty and residents, recognized his keen interests in teaching medical students, evaluating and teaching residents, and helping the young surgical faculty. He took a serious interest in medical student education, and he would have strongly approved of this teaching manual, affectionately known as the "Rudolf" guide, as an extension of ward rounds and textbook reading.

In addition to his distinguished academic accomplishments, Dr. Rudolf was a talented person with many diverse scholarly pursuits and hobbies. His advice and counsel on topics ranging from Chinese cooking to orchid raising were sought by a wide spectrum of friends and admirers.

This book is a logical extension of Dr. Rudolf's interests in teaching. No one book, operation, or set of rounds can begin to answer all questions of surgical disease processes; however, in a constellation of learning endeavors, this effort would certainly have pleased him.

John B. Hanks, M.D.
Professor of Surgery
University of Virginia
Charlottesville, Virginia

Editors and Contributors

ADVISOR:

Curtis G. Tribble, M.D.
Professor of Surgery
University of Mississippi
Jackson, Mississippi

PAST EDITORS AND CONTRIBUTORS:

Bruce Crookes, M.D.

C. Suzanne Cutter, M.D.

Alfa O. Diallo, M.D.

Matthew Edwards, M.D.

Ara J. Fienstein, M.D.

E. William Johnson, M.D.

Peter Lopez, M.D.

Martin I. Newman, M.D.

Carl Schulman, M.D.

David Shatz, M.D.

Nicholas R. Alverez, B.S.

Jos Amortequi, M.D.

Joshua I. Bleier, M.D.

Andrew Cameron, M.D.

Diane Diesen, M.D.

Gladys L. Giron, M.D.

Lawerence V. Gulotta, M.D.

Fahim Habib, M.D.

Jennifer Hall, M.D.

David King, M.D.

Joseph Michaels V, M.D.

Rupen G. Modi, M.B.A.

Paymann Moin, B.S.

Todd M. Morgan, M.D.

Andrew Newman, B.S.

Louis Pizano, M.D.

Dimitris G. Placantonakis, M.D. Ph.D.

Justin Yovino, M.D.

Esteban Ambrad-Chalela, M.D.

David Chessin, M.D.

Owen Johnson, B.S.

Peter T. Kennealy, M.D.

Geoffery Lam, M.D.

Garrett Nash, M.D.

Inderpal Sarkaria, M.D.

Alysandra Schwarz, M.D.

Ali Vafa, M.D.

Nabil Wasif, M.D.

INTERNATIONAL EDITORS:

Mohammad Azfar, M.B.B.S., F.R.C.S.
General Surgeon
Abu Dhabi, United Arab Emirates

Gwinyai Masukume, M.B.Ch.B.
University of Zimbabwe
College of Health Sciences
Harare, Zimbabwe

Foreword

Surgical Recall represents the culmination of several years' effort by Lorne Blackbourne and his friends, who began the project when they were third-year medical students. Lorne, who completed his residency in General Surgery at the University of Virginia, has involved other surgical residents and medical students to provide annual updates and revisions.

This reflects the interest, enthusiasm, and true dedication to learning and teaching that permeates the medical school classes and surgical residencies in our institution. It is an honor, privilege, and a continuing stimulus to work in the midst of this group of dedicated young people. I congratulate all the students and residents involved in this project and also acknowledge the leadership of the surgical faculty. The professor's ultimate satisfaction occurs when all the learners assume ownership of learning and teaching.

This book encompasses the essential information in general surgery and surgical specialties usually imparted to students in our surgical clerkship and reviewed and developed further in electives. Developed from the learner's standpoint, the text includes fundamental information such as a description of the diseases, signs, symptoms, essentials of pathophysiology, treatments, and possible outcomes. The unique format of this study guide uses the Socratic method by employing a list of questions or problems posed along the left side of the page with answers or responses on the right. In addition, the guide includes numerous practical tips for students and junior residents to facilitate comprehensive and effective management of patients. This material is essential for students in the core course of surgery and for those taking senior electives.

R. Scott Jones, M.D.
University of Virginia
Charlottesville, Virginia

Preface

Surgical Recall began as a source of surgical facts during my Surgery Clerkship when I was a third-year medical student at the University of Virginia. My goal has been to provide concise information that every third-year surgical student should know in a "rapid fire," two-column format.

The format of *Surgical Recall* is conducive to the recall of basic surgical facts because it relies on repetition and positive feedback. As one repeats the question-and-answer format, one gains success.

We have dedicated our work to the living memory of Professor Leslie Rudolf. It is our hope that those who knew Dr. Rudolf will remember him and those who did not will ask.

Lorne H. Blackbourne, M.D., F.A.C.S
Trauma, Burn, and Critical Care Surgeon
San Antonio, Texas

P.S. We would like to hear from you if you have any corrections, acronyms, and classic ward or operating room questions (all contributors will be credited). You can reach me via e-mail in care of Lippincott Williams & Wilkins at book_comments@lww.com.

Contents

SECTION I
OVERVIEW AND BACKGROUND SURGICAL INFORMATION

SECTION III
SUBSPECIALTY SURGERY

Section I

Overview and Background Surgical Information

Chapter 1

Introduction

PREPARING FOR THE SURGERY CLERKSHIP

USING THE STUDY GUIDE

This study guide was written to accompany the surgical clerkship. It has evolved over the years through student feedback and continued updating. In this regard, we welcome any feedback (both positive and negative) or suggestions for improvement. The objective of the guide is to provide a rapid overview of common surgical topics. The guide is organized in a self-study/quiz format. By covering the information/answers on the right with the bookmark, you can attempt to answer the questions on the left to assess your understanding of the information. Keep the guide with you at all times, and when you have even a few spare minutes (e.g., between cases) hammer out a page or at least a few questions. Many students read this book as a primer before the clerkship even begins!

Your study objectives in surgery should include the following four points:
1. O.R. question-and-answer periods
2. Ward questioning
3. Oral exam
4. Written exam

The optimal plan of action would include daily reading in a text, anatomy review prior to each O.R. case, and *Surgical Recall*. But remember, this guide helps you recall basic facts about surgical topics. Reading should be done daily! The advanced student should read *Advanced Surgical Recall*.

To facilitate learning a surgical topic, first break down each topic into the following categories and, in turn, master each category:
1. What is it?
2. Incidence
3. Risk factors

4. Signs and symptoms
5. Laboratory and radiologic tests
6. Diagnostic criteria
7. Differential diagnoses
8. Medical and surgical treatment
9. Postoperative care
10. Complications
11. Stages and prognosis

Granted, it is hard to read after a full day in the O.R. For a change, go to sleep right away and wake up a few hours early the next day and read **before** going to the hospital. It sounds crazy, but it does work.

Remember—REPETITION is the key to learning for most adults.

APPEARANCE

Why is your appearance so important?	The patient sees only the wound dressing, the skin closure, and you. You can wear whatever you want, **but you must look clean. Do not wear religious or political buttons because this is not fair to your patients with different beliefs!**

WHAT THE PERFECT SURGICAL STUDENT CARRIES IN HER LAB COAT

Stethoscope
Penlight
Scissors
Minibook on medications (e.g., trade names, doses)
Tape/4 × 4s
Sutures to practice tying
Pen/notepad/small notebook to write down pearls
Notebook or clipboard with patient's data (always write down chores with a box next to them so you can check off the box when the chore is completed)
Small calculator
List of commonly used telephone numbers (e.g., radiology)
(Oh, and of course, *Surgical Recall*!)

THE PERFECT PREPARATION FOR ROUNDS

Interview your patient (e.g., problems, pain, wishes)
Talk with your patient's nurse (e.g., "Were there any events during the last shift?")
Examine patient (e.g., cor/pulm/abd/**wound**)

Record vital signs (e.g., T_{max})
Record input (e.g., IVF, PO)
Record output (e.g., urine, drains)
Check labs
Check microbiology (e.g., culture reports, Gram stains)
Check x-rays
Check pathology reports.
Know the patient's allergies
Check allied health updates (e.g., PT, OT)
Read chart
Check medication (don't forget H_2 blocker in hyperalimentation)
Check nutrition
Always check with the intern for chores, updates, or insider information
 before rounds

PRESENTING ON ROUNDS

Your presentation on rounds should be like an iceberg. State important points about your patient (the tip of the iceberg visible above the ocean), but know **everything** else about your patient that your chief might ask about (that part of the iceberg under the ocean). Always include:

Name
Postoperative day s/p-procedure
Concise overall assessment of how the patient is doing
Vital signs/temp status/antibiotics day
Input/output-urine, drains, PO intake, IVF
Change in physical examination
Any complaints (not yours—the patient's)
Plan

Your presentation should be concise, with good eye contact (you should not simply read from a clipboard). The intangible element of confidence cannot be overemphasized; if you do not know the answer to a question about a patient, however, the correct response should be "I do not know, but I will find out." Never lie or hedge on an answer because it will only serve to make the remainder of your surgical rotation less than desirable. Furthermore, do your best to be enthusiastic and motivated. **Never, ever whine.** And remember to be a **team player.** Never make your fellow students look bad! Residents pick up on this immediately and will slam you.

THE PERFECT SURGERY STUDENT

Never whines
Never pimps his residents or fellow students (or attendings)
Never complains
Is never hungry, thirsty, or tired

Is always enthusiastic

Loves to do scut work and can never get enough

Never makes a fellow student look bad

Is always clean (a patient sees only you and the wound dressing)

Is never late

Smiles a lot and has a good sense of humor

Makes things happen

Is not a "know-it-all"

Never corrects anyone **during** rounds unless it will affect patient care

Makes the intern/resident/chief look good at all times, if at all possible

Knows more about her patients than anyone else

Loves the O.R.

Never wants to leave the hospital

Takes correction, direction, and instruction very well

Says "Sir" and "Ma'am" to the scrub nurses (and to the attending, unless corrected)

Never asks questions he can look up for himself

Knows the patient's disease, surgery, indication for surgery, and the anatomy before going to the O.R.

Is the first one to arrive at clinic and the last one to leave

Always places x-rays up in the O.R.

Reads from a surgery text **every day**

Is a team player

Asks for feedback

Never has a chip on her shoulder

Loves to suture

Is honest and always admits fault and errors

Knows when his patient is going to the O.R. (e.g., by calling)

Is confident but **not** cocky

Has a **"Can-Do"** attitude and can figure out things on her own

Is not afraid to get help when needed

Never says **"No"** or **"Maybe"** to involvement in patient care

Treats everyone (e.g., nurses, fellow students) with respect

Always respects patients' modesty (e.g., covers groin with a sheet as soon as possible in the trauma bay)

Follows the chain of command

Praises others when appropriate

Checks with the intern beforehand for information for rounds (test results/ surprises)

RUNS for materials, lab values, test results, etc., during rounds before any house officer

Gives credit where credit is due

Dresses and undresses wounds on rounds

Has a steel bladder, a cast-iron stomach, and a heart of gold

Always writes the OP note without question
Always checks with the intern after rounds for chores
Always makes sure there is a medical student in every case
Always follows the patient to the recovery room
In the O.R., always asks permission to ask a question
Always reviews anatomy prior to going to the O.R.
Does what the intern asks (i.e., the chief will get feedback from the intern)
Is a high-speed, low-drag, hardcore **HAMMERHEAD**

Define HAMMERHEAD.   A hammerhead is an individual who places his head to the ground and **hammers** through any and all obstacles to get a job done and then asks for more work. One who gives 110% and never complains. One who **desires** work.

OPERATING ROOM

Your job in the O.R. will be to retract (water-skiing) and answer questions posed by the attending physicians and residents. Retracting is basically idiot-proof. Many students emphasize anticipating the surgeon's next move, but stick to following the surgeon's request. More than 75% of the questions asked in the O.R. deal with anatomy; therefore, read about the anatomy and pathophysiology of the case, which will reduce the "I don't knows."

Never argue with the scrub nurses—they are always right. They are the selfless warriors of the operating suite's sterile field, and arguing with one will only **make matters worse.**

Never touch or take instruments from the Mayo tray (tray with instruments on it over the patient's feet) unless given explicit permission to do so. Each day as you approach the O.R. suite door, **STOP** and ask yourself if you have on scrubs, shoe covers, a cap, and a mask to avoid the embarrassing situation of being yelled at by the O.R. staff (a.k.a. the 3 strikes test: strike 1 = no mask, strike 2 = no headcover, strike 3 = no shoe covers . . . any strikes and you are outta here—place a mental stop sign outside of the O.R. with the 3 strikes rule on it)! Always wear eye protection. When entering the O.R., first introduce yourself to the scrub nurse and ask if you can get your gloves or gown. If you have questions in the O.R., first **ask** if you can ask a question because it may be a bad time and this way it will not appear as though you are pimping the resident/attending.

Other thoughts on the O.R.:

If you feel faint, ask if you can sit down (try to eat prior to going to the O.R.). If your feet swell in the O.R., try wearing support hose socks. If your back hurts, try taking some ibuprofen (with a meal) **prior** to the case. Also, sit-ups or abdominal crunches help to relieve back pain by strengthening the abdominal muscles. At the end of the case, ask the scrub nurse for some leftover ties (clean ones) to practice tying knots with and, if there is time, start writing your OP note.

OPERATING ROOM FAQS

What if I have to sneeze?	Back up STRAIGHT back; do not turn your head, as the sneeze exits through the sides of your mask!
What if I feel faint?	Do not be a hero—say, "I feel faint. May I sit down?" This is no big deal and is very common (**Note:** It helps to always eat before going to the O.R.)
What should I say when I first enter the O.R.?	Introduce yourself as a student; state that you have been invited to scrub and ask if you need to get out your gloves and/or gown
Should I wear my ID tag into the O.R.?	Yes
Can I wear nail polish?	Yes, as long as it is not chipped
Can I wear my rings and my watch when scrubbed in the O.R.?	No
Can I wear earrings?	No
When scrubbed, is my back sterile?	No
When in the surgical gown, are my underarms sterile?	No; do not put your hands under your arms
How far down my gown is considered part of the sterile field?	Just to your waist
How far up my gown is considered sterile?	Up to the nipples

How do I stand if I am waiting for the case to start?

Hands together in front above your waist

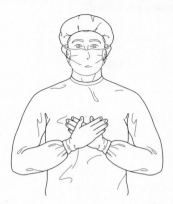

Can I button up a surgical gown (when I am not scrubbed!) with bare hands?

Yes (***Remember:*** the back of the gown is NOT sterile)

How many pairs of gloves should I wear when scrubbed?

2 (2 layers)

What is the normal order of sizes of gloves: small pair, then larger pair?

No; usually the order is a larger size followed by a smaller size (e.g., men commonly wear a size #8 covered by a size #7.5; women commonly wear a size #7 covered by a size #6.5)

What is a "scrub nurse" versus a "circulating nurse"?

The scrub nurse is "scrubbed" and hands the surgeon sutures, instruments, and so forth; this person is often an Operating Room Technician (a.k.a. "Scrub Tech")

The circulating nurse "circulates" and gets everything needed before and during the procedure

What items comprise the sterile field in the operating room?

The instrument table, the Mayo tray, and the anterior drapes on the patient

What is the tray with the instruments called?

Mayo tray

Can I grab things off the Mayo tray?

No; ask the scrub nurse/tech for permission

How do you remove blood with a laparotomy pad ("lap pad")?

Dab; do not wipe, because wiping removes platelet plugs

Can you grab the skin with DeBakey pickups?

NO; pickups for the skin must have teeth (e.g., Adson, rat-tooth) because it is "better to cut the skin than crush it"

How should you cut the sutures after tying a knot?

1. Rest the cutting hand on the noncutting hand
2. Slip the scissors down to the knot and then cant the scissors at a 45-degree angle so you do not cut the knot itself

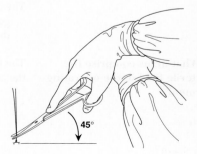

What should you do when you are scrubbed and someone is tying a suture?	Ask the scrub nurse for a pair of suture scissors, so you are ready if you are asked to cut the sutures
Why always wipe the Betadine® (povidone-iodine) off your patient at the end of the procedure?	Betadine® can become very irritating and itchy

SURGICAL NOTES

HISTORY AND PHYSICAL REPORT

The history and physical examination report, better known as the H & P, can make the difference between life and death. You should take this responsibility very **seriously.** Fatal errors can be made in the H & P, including the incorrect diagnosis, the wrong side, the wrong medications, the wrong allergies, and the wrong past surgical history. Operative reports of the patient's past surgical procedures are invaluable! The surgical H & P needs to be both accurate and **concise.** To save space, use − for a negative sign/symptom and + for a positive sign/symptom.

What are the two words most commonly misspelled in a surgical history note?	1. Guaiac 2. Abscess

Favorite Trick Questions

What is the most common intra-operative bladder "tumor"?	Foley catheter
Describe a stool with melena.	Melenic—not melanotic
Is amylase part of Ranson's criteria?	Amylase is NOT part of Ranson's criteria!
Can a patient in shock have "STABLE" vital signs?	Yes—stable vital signs are any vital signs that are not changing! Always say "normal" vital signs, not "stable!"
What is the most commonly pimped, yet the rarest, cause of pancreatitis?	Pancreatitis from a scorpion bite (scorpion found on island of Trinidad)
Where can you go to obtain an abdominal CT scan on a 600-pound, morbidly obese patient?	The ZOO (used in the past, but now rare due to liability)

Example H & P (very brief—for illustrative purposes only—see below or next section for abbreviation key):

Mr. Smith is a 22-year-old African American man who was in his normal state of excellent health until he noted the onset of periumbilical pain 1 day prior to admission. This pain was followed ≈4 hours later by pain in his right lower quadrant that any movement exacerbated. + vomiting, anorexia. − fever, urinary tract symptoms, change in bowel habits, constipation, BRBPR, hematemesis, or diarrhea.

Medications:	ibuprofen prn headaches
Allergies:	NKDA
PMH:	none
PSH:	none
SH:	EtOH, tobacco
FH:	−CA
ROS:	−resp disease, −cardiac disease, −renal disease
Physical Exam:	V/S 120/80 85 12 T 37° C
	HEENT ncat, tms clear
	cor nsr, −m, r, g
	pulm clear b/l
	abd nondistended, +bs, +tender RLQ, +rebound RLQ
	rectal guaiac −nl tone, −mass
	ext nt, −c, c, e
	neuro wnl
LABS:	urinalysis (ua) normal, chem 7, PT/PTT, CBC pending
X-RAYS:	none
ASSESSMENT:	22 y.o. m with Hx and physical findings of right lower quadrant peritoneal signs consistent with (c/w) appendicitis
Plan:	NPO
	Consent
	IVF with Lactated Ringer's
	IV cefoxitin
	To O.R. for appendectomy

Wilson Tyler cc III/

NKDA = no known drug allergies; PMH = past medical history; PSH = past surgical history; SH = social history; FH = family history; ROS = review of systems; V/S = vital signs; ncat = normocephalic atraumatic; tms = tympanic membranes; cor = heart; m, r, g = murmur, rub, gallop; NSR = normal sinus rhythm; b/l = bilateral; bs = bowel sounds; ext = extremity; nt = nontender; c, c, e = cyanosis, clubbing, or erythema; wnl = within normal limits; cc III = clinical clerk, third year

PREOP NOTE

The preop note is written in the progress notes the day before the operation

Example:

Preop Dx:	colon CA
Labs:	CBC, chem 7, PT/PTT
CXR:	−infiltrate
Blood:	T & C × 2 units
EKG:	NSR, wnl
Anesthesia:	preop completed
Consent:	signed and on front of chart
Orders:	1. Void OCTOR
	2. 1 gm cefoxitin OCTOR
	3. Hibiclens scrub this p.m.
	4. Bowel prep today
	5. NPO p̄ MN

NPO = nothing by mouth; OCTOR = on call to O.R.; p̄ = after; MN = midnight

OP NOTE

The OP note is written in the progress note section of the chart in the O.R. before the patient is in the PACU (or recovery room).

Example:

Preop Dx:	acute appendicitis
Postop Dx:	same
Procedure:	appendectomy
Surgeon:	Halsted
Assistants:	Cushing, Tribble
OP findings:	no perforation
Anesthesia:	GET
°I/O:	1000 mL LR/uo 600 mL
°EBL:	50 mL
Specimen:	appendix to pathology
Drains:	none
Complications:	none (***Note:*** If there are complications, ask what you should write.)

To PACU in stable condition

GET = general endotracheal; I/O = ins and outs; uo = urine output; EBL = estimated blood loss; PACU = postanesthesia care unit
°Ask the anesthesiologist or Certified Registered Nurse Anesthetist (CRNA) for this information.

How do I remember what is in the OP note when I am in the O.R.?	Remember the acronym **"PPP SAFE DISC"**:
	Preop Dx
	Postop Dx
	Procedure
	Surgeon (and assistants)
	Anesthesia
	Fluids
	Estimated blood loss (EBL)
	Drains
	IV Fluids
	Specimen
	Complications

POSTOP NOTE

The postop note is written on the day of the operation in the progress notes
Example:

Procedure:	appendectomy
Neuro:	A&O $\times$ 3
V/S:	wnl/afebrile
I/O:	1 L LR/uo 600 mL
Labs:	postop Hct: 36
PE:	cor RRR
	pulm CTA
	abd drsg dry and intact
Drains:	JP 30 mL serosanguinous fluid
Assess:	stable postop
Plan:	1. IV hydration
	2. 1 g cefoxitin q 8 hr

A&O $\times$ 3 = alert and oriented times 3; V/S = vital signs; uo = urine output; Hct = hematocrit; RRR = regular rhythm and rate; JP = Jackson-Pratt; wnl = within normal limits

ADMISSION ORDERS

The admission orders are written in the physician orders section of the patient's chart on admission, transfer, or postop
Example:

Admit to 5E Dr. DeBakey

Dx:	AAA
Condition:	stable
V/S:	q 4 hr or q shift; if postop, q 15 min $\times$ 2 hr, then q 1 hr $\times$ 4, then q 4 hr
Allergies:	NKDA

Activity:	bedrest or OOB to chair
Nursing:	daily wgt; I/O; change drsg q shift
Call HO for:	temp >38.5
	UO <30 mL/hr
	SBP >180 <90
	DBP >100
	HR <60 >110
Diet:	NPO
IVF:	D5 1/2 NS c̄ 20 KCL
Drugs:	ANCEF
Labs:	CBC

OOB = out of bed; I/O = ins and outs; HO = House Officer; SBP = systolic blood pressure; DBP = diastolic blood pressure; HR = heart rate; KCL = potassium chloride

ADMISSION ORDERS/POSTOP ORDERS

"AC/DC AVA PAIN DUD":

Admit to 5E
Care Provider
Diagnosis
Condition

Allergies
Vitals
Activity

Pain meds
Antibiotics
IVF/Incentive Spirometry
Nursing (Drains, etc.)

DVT prophylaxis
Ulcer prophylaxis
Diet

DAILY NOTE—PROGRESS NOTE

Basically a SOAP note, but it is not necessary to write out SOAP; for many reasons, make your notes very OBJECTIVE and, as a student, do not mention discharge because this leads to confusion
Example:
10/1/90 Blue Surgery
POD #4 s/p appendectomy
Day #5 cefoxitin
Pt without c/o

V/S: 120/80 76 12 afebrile (T_{max} 38)
I/O: 1000/600
Drains: JP #1 60 last shift
PE: cor RRR—no m, g, r
    pulm CTA
    abd +BS, +flatus, −rigidity
    ext nt, −cyanosis, −erythema
ASSESS: Stable POD #4 on IV antibiotics
PLAN:
   1. Increase PO intake
   2. Increase ambulation
   3. Follow cultures
Grayson Stuart, cc III/
Important: Always date, time, and sign your notes and leave space for them to be cosigned!

POD = Postop day (***Note:*** The day after operation is POD #1. The day of operation is the operative day. ***But:*** Antibiotic day #1 is the day the antibiotics were started.); c/o = complains of; nt = nontender; cc III = clinical clerk, third year

The following is an acronym for what should be checked on your patient daily before rounding with the surgical team: **"AVOID WTE":**
    Appearance—any subjective complaints
    Vital signs
    Output—urine/drains
    Intake—IV/PO
    Drains—# of/output/character

    Wound/dressing/weight
    Temperature
    Exam—cor, pulm, abd, etc.

INTENSIVE CARE NOTE

This note is by systems:
Neurologic (GCS, MAE)
Pulmonary (vent settings, etc.)
CVS (pressors, swann numbers, etc.)
Heme (CBC)
FEN (Chem 10, nutrition, etc.)
Renal (urine output, BUN, Cr, etc.)
I & D (T_{max}, WBC, antibiotics, etc.)
Assessment
Plan

CVS = current vital signs; FEN = fluids, electrolytes, nutrition; BUN = blood urea nitrogen; Cr = creatinine; I & D = incision and drainage (**Note:** PE, labs, radiology studies, etc. are included in each section. This is also an excellent way to write progress notes for the very complicated floor patient.)

CLINIC NOTE

Often the clinic note is a letter to the referring doctor. It should always include:
1. Patient name, history #, date
2. Brief Hx, current complaints/symptoms
3. PE, labs, x-rays
4. Assessment
5. Plan

**How is a medication
prescription written?**

Tylenol® 500 mg tablet
Disp (dispense): 100 tablets
sig: 1–2 PO q 4 hrs PRN pain

COMMON ABBREVIATIONS YOU SHOULD KNOW

(Check with *your* hospital for approved abbreviations!)

ā	Before
AAA	Abdominal aortic aneurysm; "triple A"
ABD	Army battle dressing
ABG	Arterial blood gas
ABI	Ankle to brachial index
AKA	Above the knee amputation
a.k.a.	Also known as
Ao	Aorta
APR	Abdominoperineal resection
ARDS	Acute respiratory distress syndrome
ASA	Aspirin
AXR	Abdominal x-ray
B1	Billroth 1 gastroduodenostomy
B2	Billroth 2 gastrojejunostomy
BCP	Birth control pill
BE	Barium enema
BIH	Bilateral inguinal hernia
BKA	Below the knee amputation
BRBPR	Bright red blood per rectum
BS	Bowel sounds; Breath sounds; Blood sugar
BSE	Breast self-examination
c̄	With
CA	Cancer
CABG	Coronary artery bypass graft ("CABBAGE")
CBC	Complete blood cell count

CBD	Common bile duct
c/o	Complains of
COPD	Chronic obstructive pulmonary disease
CP	Chest pain
CTA	Clear to auscultation; CT angiogram
CVA	Cerebral vascular accident
CVAT	Costovertebral angle tenderness
CVP	Central venous pressure
CXR	Chest x-ray
Dx	Diagnosis
DDx	Differential diagnosis
DI	Diabetes insipidus
DP	Dorsalis pedalis
DPL	Diagnostic peritoneal lavage
DPC	Delayed primary closure
DT	Delirium tremens
DVT	Deep venous thrombosis
EBL	Estimated blood loss
ECMO	Extracorporeal membrane oxygenation
EGD	Esophagogastroduodenoscopy (UGI scope)
EKG	Electrocardiogram (also ECG)
ELAP	Exploratory laparotomy
EOMI	Extraocular muscles intact
ERCP	Endoscopic retrograde cholangiopancreatography
EtOH	Alcohol
EUA	Exam under anesthesia
EX LAP	Exploratory laparotomy
FAP	Familial adenomatous polyposis
FAST	Focused abdominal sonogram for trauma
FEN	Fluids, electrolytes, nutrition
FNA	Fine needle aspiration
FOBT	Fecal occult blood test
GCS	Glasgow Coma Scale
GERD	Gastroesophageal reflux disease
GET(A)	General endotracheal (anesthesia)
GU	Genitourinary
HCT	Hematocrit
HEENT	Head, eyes, ears, nose, and throat
HO	House officer
Hx	History
IABP	Intra-aortic balloon pump
IBD	Inflammatory bowel disease
ICU	Intensive care unit
I & D	Incision and drainage
I & O	Ins and outs, in and out
IMV	Intermittent mandatory ventilation

IVC	Inferior vena cava
IVF	Intravenous fluids
IVP	Intravenous pyelography
IVPB	Intravenous piggyback
JVD	Jugular venous distention
Ⓛ	Left
LE	Lower extremity
LES	Lower esophageal sphincter
LIH	Left inguinal hernia
LLQ	Left lower quadrant
LR	Lactated Ringer's
LUQ	Left upper quadrant
MAE	Moving all extremities
MAST	Military antishock trousers
MEN	Multiple endocrine neoplasia
MI	Myocardial infarction
MSO4	Morphine sulfate
NGT	Nasogastric tube
NPO	Nothing per os
NS	Normal saline
OBR	Ortho bowel routine
OCTOR	On call to O.R.
OOB	Out of bed
ORIF	Open reduction internal fixation
p̄	After
PCWP	Pulmonary capillary wedge pressure
PE	Pulmonary embolism; Physical examination
PEEP	Positive end-expiratory pressure
PEG	Percutaneous endoscopic gastrostomy (via EGD and skin incision)
PERRL	Pupils equal and react to light
PFT	Pulmonary function tests
PICC	Peripherally inserted central catheter
PGV	Proximal gastric vagotomy (i.e., leaves fibers to pylorus intact to preserve emptying)
PID	Pelvic inflammatory disease
PO	Per os (by mouth)
POD	Postoperative day
PR	Per rectum
PRN	As needed, literally, *pro re nata*
PT	Physical therapy; Patient; Posterior tibial; Prothrombin time
PTC	Percutaneous transhepatic cholangiogram (dye injected via a catheter through skin and into dilated intrahepatic bile duct)
PTCA	Percutaneous transluminal coronary angioplasty
PTX	pneumothorax

$\overline{q}$ or **q**	Every
®	Right
RIH	Right inguinal hernia
RLQ	Right lower quadrant
Rx	Treatment
RTC	Return to clinic
s̄	Without
SBO	Small bowel obstruction
SCD	Sequential compression device
SIADH	Syndrome of inappropriate antidiuretic hormone
SICU	Surgical intensive care unit
SOAP	Subjective, objective, assessment, and plan
S/P	Status post
STSG	Split thickness skin graft
SVC	Superior vena cava
Sx	Symptoms
TEE	Transesophageal echocardiography
T & C	Type and cross
T & S	Type and screen
T$_{max}$	Maximal temperature
TPN	Total parenteral nutrition
TURP	Transurethral resection of the prostate
UE	Upper extremity
UGI	Upper gastrointestinal
UO	Urine output
U/S	Ultrasound
UTI	Urinary tract infection
VAD	Ventricular assist device
VOCTOR	Void on call to O.R.
W→D	Wet-to-dry dressing
XRT	X-ray therapy
−	No; negative
+	Yes; positive
↑	Increase; more
↓	Decrease; less
<	Less than
>	Greater than
≈	Approximately

GLOSSARY OF SURGICAL TERMS YOU SHOULD KNOW

Abscess	Localized collection of pus anywhere in the body, surrounded and walled off by damaged and inflamed tissues

Achlorhydria	Absence of hydrochloric acid in the stomach
Acholic stool	Light-colored stool as a result of decreased bile content
Adeno-	Prefix denoting gland or glands
Adhesion	Union of two normally separate surfaces
Adnexa	Adjoining parts; usually means ovary/ fallopian tube
Adventitia	Outer coat of the wall of a vein or artery (composed of loose connective tissue)
Afferent	Toward
-algia	Suffix denoting pain
Amaurosis fugax	Transient visual loss in one eye
Ampulla	Enlarged or dilated ending of a tube or canal
Analgesic	Drug that prevents pain
Anastomosis	Connection between two tubular organs or parts
Angio-	Prefix denoting blood or lymph vessels
Anomaly	Any deviation from the normal (i.e., congenital or developmental defect)
Apnea	Cessation of breathing
Atelectasis	Collapse of alveoli
Bariatric	Weight reduction; bariatric surgery is performed on morbidly obese patients to effect weight loss
Bifurcation	Point at which division into two branches occurs

Bile salts   Alkaline salts of bile necessary for the emulsification of fats

Bili-   Prefix denoting bile

Boil   Tender inflamed area of the skin containing pus

Bovie   Electrocautery

Calculus   Stone

Carbuncle   Collection of boils (furuncles) with multiple drainage channels (CARbuncle = car = big)

Cauterization   Destruction of tissue by direct application of heat

Celiotomy   Surgical incision into the peritoneal cavity (laparotomy = celiotomy)

Cephal-   Prefix denoting the head

Chole-   Prefix denoting bile

Cholecyst-   Prefix denoting gallbladder

Choledocho-   Prefix denoting the common bile duct

Cleido-   Prefix denoting the clavicle

Colic   Intermittent abdominal pain usually indicating pathology in a tubular organ (e.g., small bowel)

Colloid   Fluid with large particles (e.g., albumin)

Colonoscopy   Endoscopic examination of the colon

Colostomy   Surgical operation in which part of the colon is brought through the abdominal wall

Constipation   Infrequent or difficult passage of stool

Cor pulmonale	Enlargement of the right ventricle caused by lung disease and resultant pulmonary hypertension
Curettage	Scraping of the internal surface of an organ or body cavity by means of a spoon-shaped instrument
Cyst	Abnormal sac or closed cavity lined with epithelium and filled with fluid or semisolid material
Direct bilirubin	Conjugated bilirubin (indirect = unconjugated)
-dynia	Suffix denoting pain
Dys-	Prefix: difficult/painful/abnormal
Dyspareunia	Painful sexual intercourse
Dysphagia	Difficulty in swallowing
Ecchymosis	Bruise
-ectomy	Suffix denoting the surgical removal of a part or all of an organ (e.g., gastrectomy)
Efferent	Away from
Endarterectomy	Surgical removal of an atheroma and the inner part of the vessel wall to relieve an obstruction (carotid endarterectomy = CEA)
Enteritis	Inflammation of the small intestine, usually causing diarrhea
Enterolysis	Lysis of peritoneal adhesions; not to be confused with enteroclysis, which is a contrast study of the small bowel
Eschar	Scab produced by the action of heat or a corrosive substance on the skin

Excisional biopsy	Biopsy with removal of entire tumor (Think: Excisional = Entire removal)
Fascia	Sheet of strong connective tissue
Fistula	Abnormal communication between two hollow, epithelialized organs or between a hollow organ and the exterior (skin)
Foley	Bladder catheter
Frequency	Abnormally increased frequency (e.g., urinary frequency)
Furuncle	Boil, small subcutaneous staphylococcal infection of follicle (Think: Furuncle = follicle < car = carbuncle)
Gastropexy	Surgical attachment of the stomach to the abdominal wall
Hemangioma	Benign tumor of blood vessels
Hematemesis	Vomiting of blood
Hematoma	Accumulation of blood within the tissues, which clots to form a solid swelling
Hemoptysis	Coughing up blood
Hemothorax	Blood in the pleural cavity
Hepato-	Prefix denoting the liver
Herniorrhaphy	Surgical repair of a hernia
Hesitancy	Difficulty in initiating urination
Hiatus	Opening or aperture
Hidradenitis	Inflammation of the apocrine glands, usually caused by blockage of the glands
Icterus	Jaundice

Ileostomy	Surgical connection between the lumen of the ileum and the skin of the abdominal wall
Ileus	Abnormal intestinal motility (usually paralytic)
Incisional biopsy	Biopsy with only a "slice" of tumor removed
Induration	Abnormal hardening of a tissue or organ
Inspissated	Hard
Intussusception	Telescoping of one part of the bowel into another
-itis	Suffix denoting inflammation of an organ, tissue, etc. (e.g., gastritis)
Lap appy	Appendectomy via laparoscopy
Laparoscopy	Visualization of the peritoneal cavity via a laparoscope
Laparotomy	Surgical incision into the abdominal cavity (laparotomy = celiotomy)
Lap chole	Cholecystectomy via laparoscopy
Leiomyoma	Benign tumor of smooth muscle
Leiomyosarcoma	Malignant tumor of smooth muscle
Lieno-	Denoting the spleen
Melena	Black tarry stool (melenic, not melanotic stools)
Necrotic	Dead
Obstipation	Failure to pass flatus or stool
Odynophagia	Painful swallowing
-orraphy	Surgical repair (e.g., herniorrhaphy)

-ostomy

General term referring to any operation in which an artificial opening is created between two hollow organs or between one viscera and the abdominal wall for drainage purposes (e.g., colostomy) or for feeding (e.g., gastrostomy)

-otomy

Suffix denoting surgical incision into an organ

Percutaneous

Performed through the skin

-pexy

Suffix denoting fixation

Phleb-

Prefix denoting vein or relating to veins

Phlebolith

Calcification in a vein—a vein stone

Phlegmon

Diffuse inflammation of soft tissue, resulting in a swollen mass of tissue (most commonly seen with pancreatic tissue)

Plica

Fold or ridge

Plicae circulares

Circular (complete circles) folds in the lumen of the small intestine (a.k.a. valvulae conniventes)

Plicae semilunares

Folds (semicircular) into lumen of the large intestine

Pneumaturia

Passage of urine containing air

Pneumothorax

Collapse of lung with air in pleural space

Pseudocyst

Fluid-filled cavity resembling a true cyst, but **not** lined with epithelium

Pus

Liquid product of inflammation, consisting of dying leukocytes and other fluids from the inflammatory response

Rubor   Redness; a classic sign of inflammation

Steatorrhea   Fatty stools as a result of decreased fat absorption

Stenosis   Abnormal narrowing of a passage or opening

Sterile field   Area covered by sterile drapes or prepped in sterile fashion using antiseptics (e.g., Betadine®)

Succus   Fluid (e.g., succus entericus is fluid from the bowel lumen)

Tenesmus   Urge to defecate with ineffectual straining

Thoracotomy   Surgical opening of the chest cavity

Transect   To divide transversely (to cut in half)

Trendelenburg   Patient posture with pelvis higher than the head, inclined about 45° (a.k.a. "headdownenburg")

Urgency   Sudden strong urge to urinate; often seen with a UTI

Wet-to-dry dressing   Damp gauze dressing placed on a wound and removed after the dressing dries to the wound, providing microdébridement

SURGERY SIGNS, TRIADS, ETC. YOU SHOULD KNOW

What are the ABCDs of melanoma?

Signs of melanoma:
    Asymmetric
    Border irregularities
    Color variation
    Diameter >0.6 cm and **D**ark color

What is the Allen's test?

Test for patency of ulnar artery prior to placing a radial arterial line or performing an ABG: Examiner occludes both ulnar and radial arteries with fingers as patient makes fist; patient opens fist while examiner releases ulnar artery occlusion to assess blood flow to hand

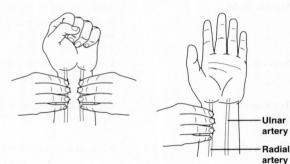

Ulnar artery

Radial artery

Define the following terms:

Ballance's sign

Constant dullness to percussion in the left flank/LUQ and resonance to percussion in the right flank seen with splenic rupture/hematoma

Barrett's esophagus

Columnar metaplasia of the distal esophagus (GERD related)

Battle's sign

Ecchymosis over the mastoid process in patients with basilar skull fractures

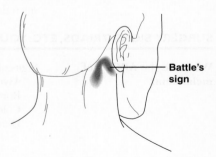

Battle's sign

Beck's triad

Seen in patients with cardiac tamponade:
1. JVD
2. Decreased or muffled heart sounds
3. Decreased blood pressure

Bergman's triad

Seen with fat emboli syndrome:
1. Mental status changes
2. Petechiae (often in the axilla/thorax)
3. Dyspnea

Blumer's shelf

Metastatic disease to the rectouterine (pouch of Douglas) or rectovesical pouch creating a "shelf" that is palpable on rectal examination

Boas' sign

Right subscapular pain resulting from cholelithiasis

Borchardt's triad

Seen with gastric volvulus:
1. Emesis followed by retching
2. Epigastric distention
3. Failure to pass an NGT

Carcinoid triad

Seen with carcinoid syndrome (Think: **"FDR"**):
1. **F**lushing
2. **D**iarrhea
3. **R**ight-sided heart failure

Charcot's triad

Seen with cholangitis:
1. Fever (chills)
2. Jaundice
3. Right upper quadrant pain
(Pronounced "char-cohs")

Chvostek's sign

Twitching of facial muscles upon tapping the facial nerve in patients with hypocalcemia (Think: **CH**vostek's = **CH**eek)

Courvoisier's law

Enlarged nontender gallbladder seen with obstruction of the common bile duct, most commonly with pancreatic cancer *Note:* not seen with gallstone obstruction because the gallbladder is scarred secondary to chronic cholelithiasis (Pronounced "koor-vwah-ze-ay")

Cullen's sign   Bluish discoloration of the periumbilical area due to retroperitoneal hemorrhage tracking around to the anterior abdominal wall through fascial planes (e.g., acute hemorrhagic pancreatitis)

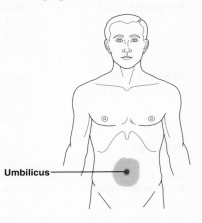

Umbilicus

Cushing's triad   Signs of increased intracranial pressure:
1. Hypertension
2. Bradycardia
3. Irregular respirations

Dance's sign   Empty right lower quadrant in children with ileocecal intussusception

Fothergill's sign   Used to differentiate an intra-abdominal mass from one in the abdominal wall; if mass is felt while there is tension on the musculature, then it is in the wall (i.e., sitting halfway upright)

Fox's sign   Ecchymosis of inguinal ligament seen with retroperitoneal bleeding

Goodsall's rule   Anal fistulae course in a straight path anteriorly and a curved path posteriorly from midline (Think of a dog with a straight anterior nose and a curved posterior tail)

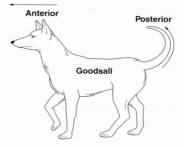

Grey Turner's sign	Ecchymosis or discoloration of the flank in patients with retroperitoneal hemorrhage as a result of dissecting blood from the retroperitoneum (Think: **TURN**er's = **TURN** side-to-side = flank)
Hamman's sign/crunch	Crunching sound on auscultation of the heart resulting from emphysematous mediastinum; seen with Boerhaave's syndrome, pneumomediastinum, etc.
Homans' sign	Calf pain on forced dorsiflexion of the foot in patients with DVT
Howship-Romberg sign	Pain along the inner aspect of the thigh; seen with an obturator hernia as the result of nerve compression
Kehr's sign	Severe left shoulder pain in patients with splenic rupture (as a result of referred pain from diaphragmatic irritation)
Kelly's sign	Visible peristalsis of the ureter in response to squeezing or retraction; used to identify the ureter during surgery
Krukenberg tumor	Metastatic tumor to the ovary (classically from gastric cancer)
Laplace's law	Wall tension = pressure × radius (thus, the colon perforates preferentially at the cecum because of the increased radius and resultant increased wall tension)

McBurney's point	One third the distance from the anterior iliac spine to the umbilicus on a line connecting the two
McBurney's sign	Tenderness at McBurney's point in patients with appendicitis
Meckel's diverticulum rule of 2s	2% of the population have a Meckel's diverticulum, 2% of those are symptomatic, and they occur within ≈2 feet of the ileocecal valve
Mittelschmerz	Lower quadrant pain due to ovulation
Murphy's sign	Cessation of inspiration while palpating under the right costal margin; the patient cannot continue to inspire deeply because it brings an inflamed gallbladder under pressure (seen in acute cholecystitis)
Obturator sign	Pain upon internal rotation of the leg with the hip and knee flexed; seen in patients with appendicitis/pelvic abscess

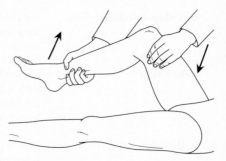

Pheochromocytoma SYMPTOMS triad	Think of the first three letters in the word pheochromocytoma—**"P-H-E"**: **P**alpitations **H**eadache **E**pisodic diaphoresis
Pheochromocytoma rule of 10s	10% bilateral, 10% malignant, 10% in children, 10% extra-adrenal, 10% have multiple tumors

Psoas sign

Pain elicited by extending the hip with the knee in full extension, seen with appendicitis and psoas inflammation

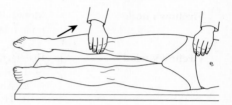

Raccoon eyes

Bilateral black eyes as a result of basilar skull fracture

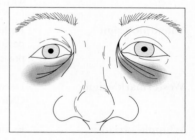

Reynold's pentad

1. Fever
2. Jaundice
3. Right upper quadrant pain
4. Mental status changes
5. Shock/sepsis

Thus, Charcot's triad plus #4 and #5; seen in patients with **suppurative** cholangitis

Rovsing's sign

Palpation of the left lower quadrant resulting in pain in the right lower quadrant; seen in appendicitis

Saint's triad

1. Cholelithiasis
2. Hiatal hernia
3. Diverticular disease

Silk glove sign

Indirect hernia sac in the pediatric patient; the sac feels like a finger of a silk glove when rolled under the examining finger

Sister Mary Joseph's sign (a.k.a. Sister Mary Joseph's node)	Metastatic tumor to umbilical lymph node(s)
Virchow's node	Metastatic tumor to left supraclavicular node (classically due to gastric cancer)
Virchow's triad	Risk factors for thrombosis: 1. Stasis 2. Abnormal endothelium 3. Hypercoagulability
Trousseau's sign	Carpal spasm after occlusion of blood to the forearm with a BP cuff in patients with hypocalcemia
Valentino's sign	Right lower quadrant pain from a perforated peptic ulcer due to succus/pus draining into the RLQ
Westermark's sign	Decreased pulmonary vascular markings on CXR in a patient with pulmonary embolus
Whipple's triad	Evidence for insulinoma: 1. Hypoglycemia (<50) 2. CNS and vasomotor symptoms (e.g., syncope, diaphoresis) 3. Relief of symptoms with administration of glucose

---

Chapter 2

Surgical Syndromes

What is afferent loop syndrome?	Obstruction of the afferent loop of a Billroth II gastrojejunostomy
What does ARDS stand for?	**A**cute **R**espiratory **D**istress **S**yndrome (poor oxygenation caused by leaky capillaries)

What is blind loop syndrome?	Bacterial overgrowth of intestine caused by stasis
What is Boerhaave's syndrome?	Esophageal perforation
What is Budd-Chiari syndrome?	Thrombosis of hepatic veins
What is carcinoid syndrome?	Syndrome of **"B FDR"**: **B**ronchospasm **F**lushing **D**iarrhea **R**ight-sided heart failure (caused by factors released by carcinoid tumor)
What is compartment syndrome?	Compartmental hypertension caused by edema, resulting in muscle necrosis of the lower extremity, often seen in the calf; patient may have a distal pulse
What is Cushing's syndrome?	Excessive cortisol production
What is dumping syndrome?	Delivery of a large amount of hyperosmolar chyme into the small bowel, usually after vagotomy and a gastric drainage procedure (pyloroplasty/gastrojejunostomy); results in autonomic instability, abdominal pain, and diarrhea
What is Fitz-Hugh-Curtis syndrome?	Perihepatic gonorrhea infection
What is Gardner's syndrome?	GI polyps and associated findings of **S**ebaceous cysts, **O**steomas, and **D**esmoid tumors (**SOD**); polyps have high malignancy potential (Think: A **Gardner** plants **SOD**)
What is HITT syndrome?	**H**eparin-**I**nduced **T**hrombocytopenic **T**hrombosis syndrome: Heparin-induced platelet antibodies cause platelets to thrombose vessels, often resulting in loss of limb or life

What is Leriche's syndrome?
Claudication of buttocks and thighs, **I**mpotence, **A**trophy of legs (seen with iliac occlusive disease) (Think: **CIA**)

What is Mallory-Weiss syndrome?
Post-emesis/-retching tears in the gastric mucosa (near gastroesophageal junction)

What is Mendelson's syndrome?
Chemical pneumonitis after aspiration of gastric contents

What is Mirizzi's syndrome?
Extrinsic obstruction of the common hepatic bile duct from a gallstone in the gallbladder or cystic duct

What is Munchausen syndrome?
Self-induced illness

What is Ogilvie's syndrome?
Massive **nonobstructive** colonic dilatation

What is Peutz-Jeghers syndrome?
Benign GI polyps and buccal pigmentation (Think: **P**eutz = **P**igmentation)

What is Plummer-Vinson syndrome?
Syndrome of:
1. Esophageal web
2. Iron-deficiency anemia
3. Dysphagia
4. Spoon-shaped nails
5. Atrophic oral and tongue mucosa
Typically occurs in elderly women; 10% develop squamous cell carcinoma

What is RED reaction syndrome?
Syndrome of rapid vancomycin infusion, resulting in skin erythema

What is refeeding syndrome?
Hypokalemia, hypomagnesemia, and hypophosphatemia after refeeding a starved patient

What is Rendu-Osler-Weber (ROW) syndrome?
Syndrome of GI tract telangiectasia/A-V malformations

What is short-gut syndrome?
Malnutrition resulting from <200 cm of viable small bowel

What is SIADH?	Syndrome of **I**nappropriate **A**nti**D**iuretic **H**ormone (Think: **I**nappropriately **I**ncreased ADH)
What is another name for Sipple's syndrome?	MEN II
What is superior vena cava (SVC) syndrome?	Obstruction of the SVC (e.g., by tumor, thrombosis)
What is thoracic outlet syndrome?	Compression of the structures exiting from the thoracic outlet
What is Tietze's syndrome?	Costochondritis of rib cartilage; aseptic (treat with NSAIDs)
What is toxic shock syndrome?	*Staphylococcus aureus* toxin-induced syndrome marked by fever, hypotension, organ failure, and **rash** (desquamation— especially palms and soles)
What is Trousseau's syndrome?	Syndrome of deep venous thrombosis (DVT) associated with carcinoma
What is another name for Wermer's syndrome?	MEN I
What is Zollinger-Ellison syndrome?	Gastrinoma and PUD

Chapter 3

Surgical Most Commons

What is the most common: Indication for surgery with Crohn's disease?	Small bowel obstruction (SBO)
Type of melanoma?	Superficial spreading
Type of breast cancer?	Infiltrating ductal

Site of breast cancer?	Upper outer quadrant
Vessel involved with a bleeding duodenal ulcer?	Gastroduodenal artery
Cause of common bile duct obstruction?	Choledocholithiasis
Cause of cholangitis?	Bile duct obstruction resulting from choledocholithiasis
Cause of pancreatitis?	EtOH
Bacteria in stool?	*Bacteroides fragilis* ("B. frag")
Cause of SBO in adults in the United States?	Postop peritoneal adhesions
Cause of SBO in children?	Hernias
Cause of emergency abdominal surgery in the United States?	Acute appendicitis
Site of GI carcinoids?	Appendix
Abdominal x-ray (AXR) finding with SBO?	Air-fluid levels
Electrolyte deficiency causing ileus?	Hypokalemia
Cause of transfusion hemolysis?	Clerical error
Cause of blood transfusion resulting in death?	Clerical error (wrong blood types)
Site of distant metastasis of sarcoma?	Lungs
Cause of shock in a surgical patient?	Hypovolemia
Position of anal fissure?	Posterior

Cause of large bowel obstruction?	Colon cancer
Type of colonic volvulus?	Sigmoid volvulus
Cause of fever <48 post-operative hours?	Atelectasis
Bacterial cause of urinary tract infection (UTI)?	*Escherichia coli*
Chest x-ray (CXR) finding with traumatic thoracic aortic injury?	Widened mediastinum
Abdominal organ injured in blunt abdominal trauma?	Liver (not the spleen, as noted in recent studies!)
Abdominal organ injured in penetrating abdominal trauma?	Small bowel
Benign tumor of the liver?	Hemangioma
Malignancy of the liver?	Metastasis
Pneumonia in the ICU?	Gram-negative bacteria
Cause of epidural hematoma?	Middle meningeal artery injury
Cause of lower GI bleeding?	Upper GI bleeding
Hernia?	Inguinal hernia (right more than left)
Cause of esophageal perforation?	Iatrogenic instrumentation (e.g., EGD)
Cancer in females?	Lung cancer
Cancer in males?	Prostate cancer

Type of cancer causing DEATH in males and females?	LUNG cancer
Cause of free peritoneal air?	Perforated PUD
Symptom with gastric cancer?	Weight loss
Site of colon cancer hematogenous metastasis?	Liver
Cause of death ages 1–44?	TRAUMA

Chapter 4

Surgical Percentages

What percentage of people in the United States will develop acute appendicitis?	≈7%
What is the acceptable percentage of normal appendices removed with the preoperative diagnosis of appendicitis?	Up to 20%; it is better to remove some normal appendices than to miss a case of acute appendicitis, which could result in a ruptured appendix
In what percentage of cases can ultrasound diagnose cholelithiasis?	98%
In what percentage of cases does a lower GI bleed stop spontaneously?	≈90%
In what percentage of cases does a UGI bleed stop spontaneously?	≈80%

What percentage of patients undergoing laparotomy develop a postoperative small bowel obstruction at some time later?	≈5%
What percentage of American women develop breast cancer?	10%
What percentage of patients with acute appendicitis will have a radiopaque fecalith on abdominal x-ray (AXR)?	Only about 5%
What percentage of patients with gallstones will have radiopaque gallstones on AXR?	≈10%
What percentage of kidney stones are radiopaque on AXR?	≈90%
At 6 weeks, wounds have achieved what percentage of their total tensile strength?	≈90%
What percentage of patients with ARDS will die?	≈40%
What percentage of the population have a Meckel's diverticulum?	2%
What is the risk of appendiceal rupture 24 hours after the onset of symptoms?	≈25%
What percentage of colonic villous adenomas contain cancer?	≈40% (Think: **VILL**ous = **VILL**ain)
One unit of packed RBCs increases the hematocrit by how much?	3%

Additional 1 liter by nasal cannula increases FIO$_2$ by how much?	3%
What percentage of porcelain gallbladders will contain cancer?	≈50%
What percentage of patients with gastric ulcers have cancer on biopsy?	10%

Chapter 5   **Surgical History**

Identify the following:

First to use antiseptic (carbolic acid)	Lister (British surgeon)
First to advocate surgical gloves	Halsted (made by GOODYEAR®)
Father of antiseptic surgery	Lister (1827–1912)
Father of American neurosurgery	Harvey Cushing
Developer of vascular grafts	DeBakey (he hand-sewed them!)
Developed electrocautery for surgery with Dr. Cushing	Bovie (1928)
The Mayo Brothers' scrub nurse	Sister Joseph (of St. Mary's hospital)

Developed the cardio-pulmonary bypass	Gibbon

Identify the year the follow-ing procedures were first performed and the physician who performed them:

Renal transplant	1954; Murray
CABG	1962; Sabiston
CEA	1953; DeBakey
Heart transplant	1967; Barnard
Artificial heart valve	1960; Starr
Liver transplant	1963; Starzl
Total parenteral nutrition (TPN)	1968; Rhoades
Vascular anastomosis	1902; Carrel
Lung transplant	1964; Hardy
Pancreatic transplant	1966; Najarian
Heart-lung transplant	1982; Reitz
AAA Rx	1951; Dubost
First lap chole	1987; Mouret and Dubois in France
First appendectomy	1848; Hancock
First gastric resection	1881; Billroth
First lap appy	1983; Semm (GYN DOCTOR!)
Who was the only surgeon to win the Pulitzer Prize?	Cushing (for his biography on Osler)

Which surgeons have won the Nobel Prize? (9)

Kocher 1909 (thyroid surgery)
Gullstrand 1911 (ophthalmology)
Carrel 1912 (transplantation/vascular anastomosis)
Bárány 1914 (inner ear disease/vestibular disease)
Banting 1922 (insulin)
Hess 1949 (brain physiology)
Forssman 1956 (cardiac catheterization)
Huggins 1966 (oncology)
Murray 1990 (kidney transplant)

When was the Dakin solution developed?

World War I; Dakin developed the solution to treat dirty combat wounds

---

Chapter 6

Surgical Instruments

How should a pair of scissors/needle-driver/clamp be held?

With the thumb and **fourth** finger, using the index finger to steady

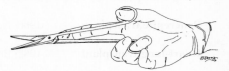

Is it better to hold the skin with a DeBakey or an Adson, or toothed, forcep?

Better to use an Adson, or toothed, pickup because it is better to cut the skin rather than crush it!

What helps steady the scissor- or Bovie-hand?

Resting it on the opposite hand

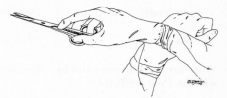

What can be done to guarantee that you do not cut the knot when cutting sutures?

Slide the scissors down to the knot, then turn the scissors at a 45° angle, and cut

How should a pair of forceps be held?

Like a pencil

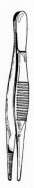

What are forceps also known as?

"Pickups"

Identify the following instruments:

Forcep

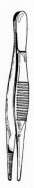

DeBakey pickup

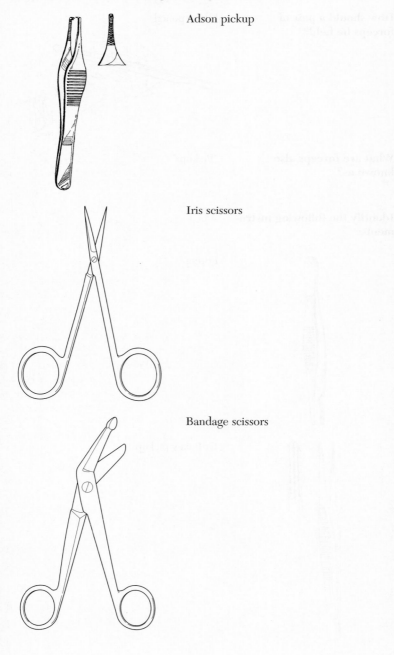

Adson pickup

Iris scissors

Bandage scissors

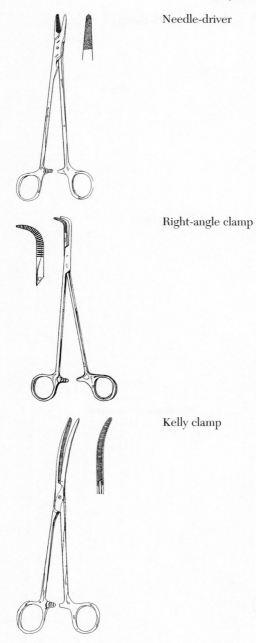

Needle-driver

Right-angle clamp

Kelly clamp

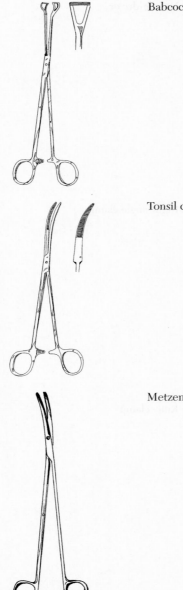

Babcock clamp

Tonsil clamp

Metzenbaum scissors

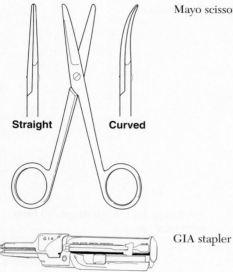

Mayo scissors (heavy scissors)

Straight   **Curved**

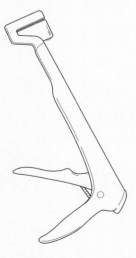

GIA stapler

What does "GIA" stand for? **G**astro**I**ntestinal **A**nastomosis

TA stapler

What does "TA" stand for? **T**horaco**A**bdominal

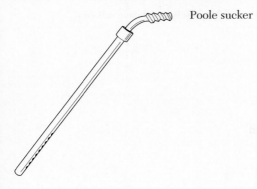

Poole sucker

What is the Poole sucker used for?

Suctioning fluid (often irrigation) from peritoneal cavity

Gigli saw

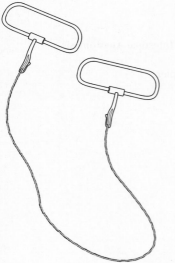

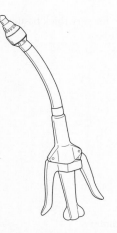

EEA stapler

What does "EEA" stand for? End-to-End Anastomosis

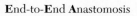

Pott's scissors

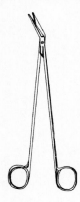

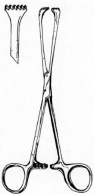

Allis clamp

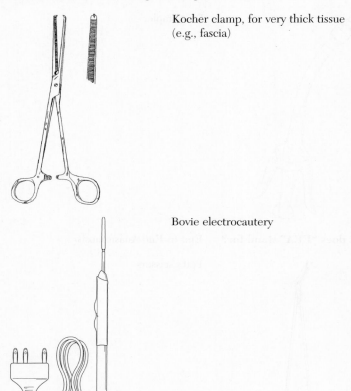

Kocher clamp, for very thick tissue (e.g., fascia)

Bovie electrocautery

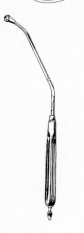

Yankauer suction (sucker)

Define the following scalpel blades:

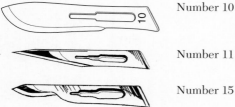

Number 10

Number 11

Number 15

RETRACTORS (YOU WILL GET TO KNOW THEM WELL!)

What does it mean to "toe in" the retractor?

To angle the tip of the retractor in by angling the retractor handle up

Identify the following retractors:

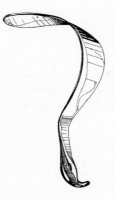

Deaver retractor

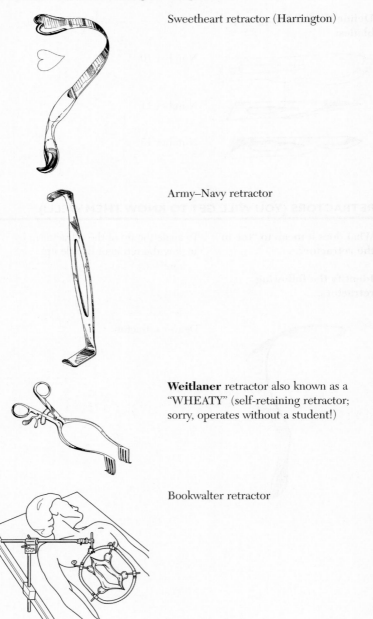

Sweetheart retractor (Harrington)

Army–Navy retractor

Weitlaner retractor also known as a "WHEATY" (self-retaining retractor; sorry, operates without a student!)

Bookwalter retractor

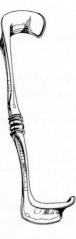

Richardson retractor, also known as a "RICH"

What is a "malleable" retractor?

Metal retractor that can be bent to customize to the situation at hand

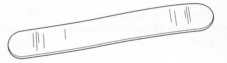

Chapter 7

Sutures and Stitches

SUTURE MATERIALS

GENERAL INFORMATION

What is a suture?

Any strand of material used to ligate blood vessels or to approximate tissues

How are sutures sized?

By diameter; stated as a number of O's: the higher the number of O's, the smaller the diameter (e.g., 2-O suture has a larger diameter than 5-O suture)

Which is thicker, 1-O suture or 3-O suture?

1-O suture (pronounced "one oh")

CLASSIFICATION

What are the two most basic suture types?	Absorbable and nonabsorbable
What is an absorbable suture?	Suture that is completely broken down by the body (dissolving suture)
What is a nonabsorbable suture?	Suture is not broken down (permanent suture)

SUTURES

Catgut

What are "catgut" sutures made of?	Purified collagen fibers from the intestines of healthy cows or sheep (sorry, no cats)
What are the two types of gut sutures?	Plain and chromic
What is the difference between plain and chromic gut?	Chromic gut is treated with chromium salts (chromium trioxide), which results in more collagen crosslinks, making the suture more resistant to breakdown by the body

Vicryl® Suture

What is it?	Absorbable, braided, multifilamentous copolymer of lactide and glycoside
How long does it retain its strength?	60% at 2 weeks, 8% at 4 weeks
Should you ever use PURPLE-colored Vicryl® for skin closure?	NO—it may cause purple tattooing

PDS®

What is it?	Absorbable, monofilament polymer of polydioxanone (absorbable fishing line)
How long does it maintain its tensile strength?	70% to 74% at 2 weeks, 50% to 58% at 4 weeks, 25% to 41% at 6 weeks
How long does it take to complete absorption?	180 days (6 months)

What is silk?

Braided protein filaments spun by the silkworm larva; known as a nonabsorbable suture

What is Prolene?

Nonabsorbable suture (used for vascular anastomoses, hernias, abdominal fascial closure)

What is nylon?

Nonabsorbable "fishing line"

What is monocryl?

Absorbable monofilament

What kind of suture should be used for the biliary tract or the urinary tract?

ABSORBABLE—otherwise the suture will end up as a nidus for stone formation!

WOUND CLOSURE

GENERAL INFORMATION

What is the purpose of a suture closure?

To approximate divided tissues to enhance wound healing

What are the three types of wound healing?

1. Primary closure (intention)
2. Secondary intention
3. Tertiary intention (**D**elayed **P**rimary **C**losure = **DPC**)

What is primary intention?

When the edges of a clean wound are closed in some manner immediately (e.g., suture, Steri-Strips®, staples)

What is secondary intention?

When a wound is allowed to remain open and heal by granulation, epithelization, and contraction—used for dirty wounds, otherwise an abscess can form

What is tertiary intention?

When a wound is allowed to remain open for a time and then closed, allowing for débridement and other wound care to reduce bacterial counts prior to closure (i.e., delayed primary closure)

What is another term for tertiary intention?

DPC = **D**elayed **P**rimary **C**losure

Classic time to wait before closing an open abdominal wound by DPC?	5 days
What rule is constantly told to medical students about wound closure?	"Approximate, don't strangulate!" Translation: If sutures are pulled too tight, then the tissue becomes ischemic because the blood supply is decreased, possibly resulting in necrosis, infection, and/or scar

SUTURE TECHNIQUES

What is a taper-point needle?	Round body, leaves a round hole in tissue (spreads without cutting tissue)

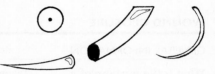

What is it used for?	Suturing of soft tissues other than skin (e.g., GI tract, muscle, nerve, peritoneum, fascia)
What is a conventional cutting needle?	Triangular body with the sharp edge toward the inner circumference; leaves a triangular hole in tissue

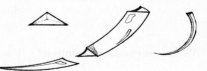

What are its uses?	Suturing of **skin**
What is a simple interrupted stitch?	

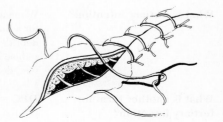

What is a vertical mattress stitch?

Simple stitch is made, the needle is reversed, and a small bite is taken from each wound edge; the knot ends up on one side of the wound

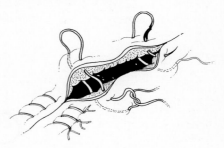

What is the vertical mattress stitch also known as?

Far-far, near-near stitch—oriented perpendicular to wound

What is it used for?

Difficult-to-approximate skin edges; everts tissue well

What is a horizontal mattress stitch?

Simple stitch is made, the needle is reversed, and the same size bite is taken again—oriented parallel to wound

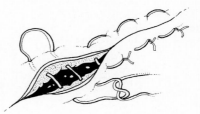

What is a simple running (continuous) stitch?

Stitches made in succession without knotting each stitch

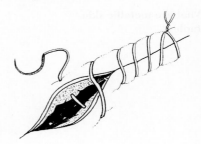

What is a subcuticular stitch?

Stitch (usually running) placed just underneath the epidermis, can be either absorbable or nonabsorbable (pull-out stitch if nonabsorbable)

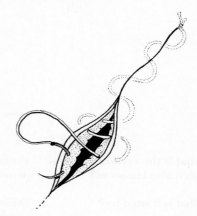

What is a pursestring suture?

Stitch that encircles a tube perforating a hollow viscus (e.g., gastrostomy tube), allowing the hole to be drawn tight and thus preventing leakage

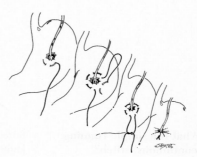

What are metallic skin staples?

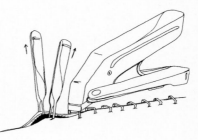

What is a staple removal device?

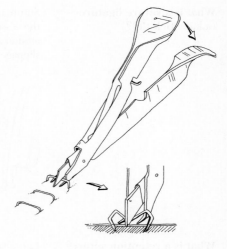

What is a gastrointestinal anastomosis (GIA) device?

Stapling device that lays two rows of small staples in a hemostatic row and **automatically cuts** in between them

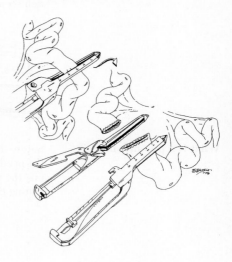

What is a suture ligature (a.k.a. stick tie)?

Suture is anchored by passing it through the vessel **on a needle** before wrapping it around and occluding the vessel; prevents slippage of knot-use on larger vessels

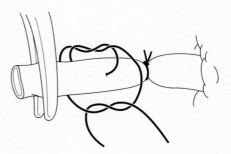

What is a retention suture?

Large suture (#2) that is full thickness through the entire abdominal wall except the peritoneum; used to buttress an abdominal wound at risk for dehiscence

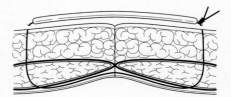

What is a pop-off suture?

Suture that is not permanently swaged to the needle, allowing the surgeon to "pop off" the needle from the suture without cutting the suture

Chapter 8

Surgical Knot Tying

KNOTS AND EARS

What is the basic surgical knot?

Square knot

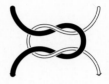

What is the first knot that should be mastered?

Instrument knot

What is a "surgeon's knot"?

Double-wrap throw followed by single square knot throws

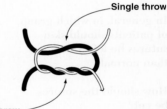

Single throw

Double throw

How many (correct) throws are necessary to ensure that your knots do not slip?

As many as the attending surgeon wants

What are the guidelines for the number of minimal throws needed?

Depends on the suture material
   Silk—3
   Gut—4
   Vicryl®, Dexon®, other braided synthetics—4
   Nylon, polyester, polypropylene, PDS, Maxon—6

How long should the ears of the knot be cut?	Some guidelines are: **Silk vessel ties**—1 to 2 mm **Abdominal fascia closure**—5 mm **Skin sutures, drain sutures**—5 to 10 mm (makes them easier to find and remove)
When should skin sutures be removed?	As soon as the wound has healed enough to withstand expected mechanical trauma Any stitch left in more than ≈10 days will leave a scar Guidelines are: **Face**—3 to 5 days **Extremities**—10 days **Joints**—10–14 days **Back**—14 days **Abdomen**—7 days
How can strength be added to an incision during and after suture removal?	With Steri-Strips®
In general, in which group of patients should skin sutures be left in longer than normal?	Patients on steroids
How should the sutures be cut?	Use the tips of the scissors to avoid cutting other tissues Try to remove the cut ends (less foreign material decreases risk of infection) Rest the scissor-hand on the non–scissor-hand to steady
How is an instrument knot tied?	Always start with a double wrap, known as a "surgeon's knot," and then use a single wrap, pulling the suture in the opposite directions after every "throw"
Does a student need to know a one-hand tie?	No! Master the two-hand tie and the instrument tie

INSTRUMENT TIE

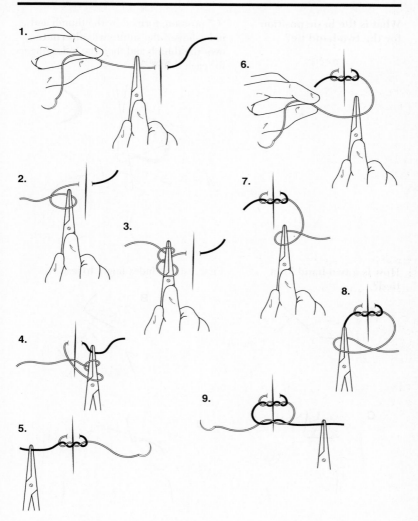

1.

2.

3.

4.

5.

6.

7.

8.

9.

Then continue with single throws

TWO-HAND TIE

What is the basic position for the two-hand tie?

"C" position, formed by the thumb and index finger; the suture will **alternate** over the thumb and then the index finger for each throw

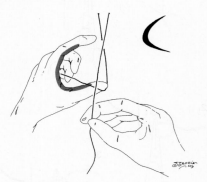

How is a two-hand knot tied?

First, use the index finger to lead

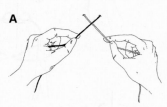
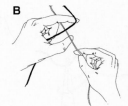

A
B

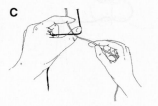
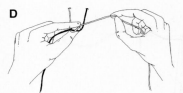

C
D

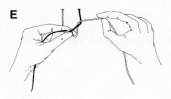
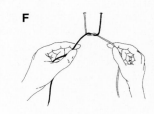

E
F

Then use thumb to lead:

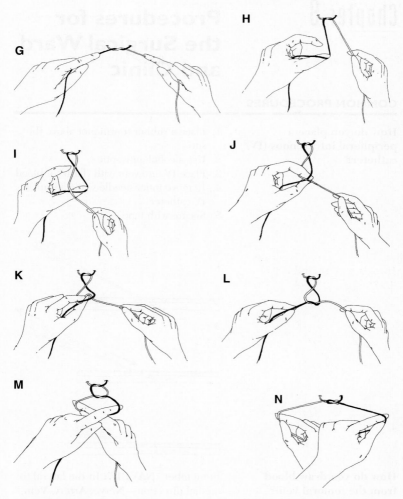

Ask a resident or intern to help you after you have tried for a while.

Open book to this page for guidance.

Place the *Surgical Recall* bookmark at back of book to use as a suture anchor.

Chapter 9

Procedures for the Surgical Ward and Clinic

COMMON PROCEDURES

How do you place a peripheral intravenous (IV) catheter?

1. Place a rubber tourniquet above the site
2. Use alcohol antiseptic
3. Place IV into vein with "flash" of blood
4. Remove inner needle while advancing IV catheter
5. Secure with tape

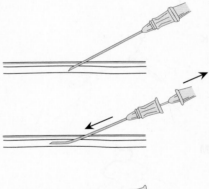

How do you draw blood from the femoral vein?

Remember "**NAVEL**": In the lateral to medial direction—**N**erve, **A**rtery, **V**ein, **E**mpty space, **L**ymphatics—and thus place needle medial to the femoral pulse

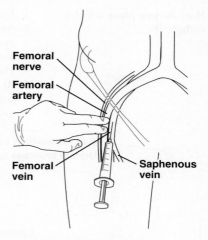

How do you remove staples?

Use a staple remover (see Chapter 7), then place Steri-Strips®

How do you remove stitches?

1. Cut the suture next to the knot
2. Pull end of suture out by holding onto the knot
3. Place Steri-Strips®

How do you place Steri-Strips®?

1. Dry the skin edges of the wound
2. Place adhesive (e.g., benzoin)
3. With the Adson pickup or with your fingers, place strips to gently appose epidermis (**Note:** Avoid any tension or blisters will appear!)

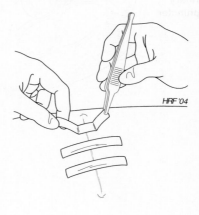

How do you place a Foley catheter?

1. Stay sterile
2. Apply Betadine® to the urethral opening (meatus)
3. Lubricate the catheter
4. Place catheter into urethra
5. As soon as urine returns, inflate balloon with saline (balloon size is given in cc on the catheter)

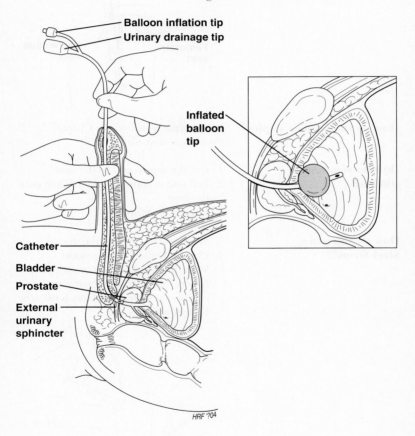

Balloon inflation tip
Urinary drainage tip
Inflated balloon tip
Catheter
Bladder
Prostate
External urinary sphincter

HRF '04

How do you find the urethra in females?

First find the clitoris and clitoral hood: The urethra is just below these structures; wiping a Betadine®-soaked sponge over this area will often result in having the urethra "wink" open

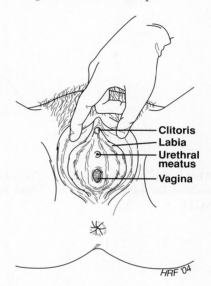

Can you inflate the Foley balloon before you get urine return?

No, you might blow up a balloon in the urethra!

NASOGASTRIC TUBE (NGT) PROCEDURES

How do you determine how much of the NGT should be advanced into the body for the correct position?

Rough guide: from nose, around ear, to 5 cm below the xiphoid

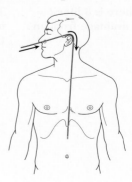

How do you place the NGT in a nare?

First place lubrication (e.g., Surgilube®) then place NGT straight back—not up or down!

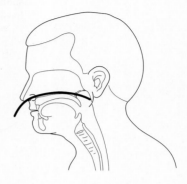

What is the best neck position for advancing the NGT?

Neck FLEXED! Also have the patient drink some water (using a straw)

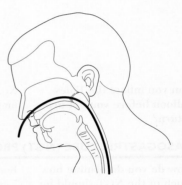

What if there is 3 liters/ 24 hours drainage from an NGT?

Think DUODENUM—the NGT may be in the duodenum and not the stomach! Check an x-ray

How can you clinically confirm that an NGT is in the stomach?

Use a Toomey syringe to "inject" air while listening over the stomach with a stethoscope; you will hear the "swish" if the NGT is in place

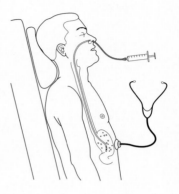

How do you tape an NGT?

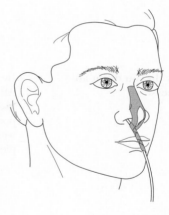

What MUST you obtain and examine before using an NGT for feeding?

LOWER chest/upper abdominal x-ray to absolutely verify placement into the stomach and NOT the LUNG—patients have died from pulmonary tube feeding!

How do you draw a radial arterial blood gas (ABG)?

Feel for the pulse and advance directly into the artery; ABG syringes do not have to have the plunger withdrawn manually

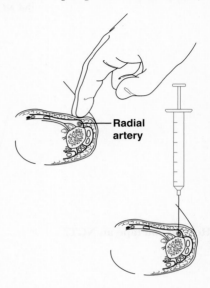

Radial artery

How do you drain an abscess?

By incision and drainage (or "I & D"): After using local anesthetic, use a #11 blade to incise and then open the abscess pocket; large abscesses are best drained with a cruciate incision or removal of a piece of skin; pack the open wound

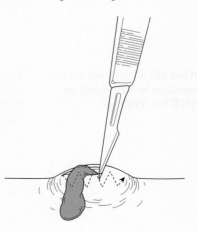

How do you remove an epidermal cyst or sebaceous cyst?

1. Administer local anesthetic
2. Remove the ellipse of skin overlying the cyst, including the pore
3. Remove the cyst with the encompassing sac lining

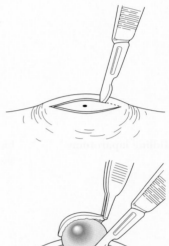

Chapter 10

Incisions

If a patient has an old incision, is it best to make a subsequent incision next to or through the old incision?

Through the old incision, or excise the old incision, because it has scar tissue that limits the amount of collaterals that would be needed to heal an incision placed next to it

What is used to incise the epidermis?

Scalpel blade

What is used to incise the dermis?

Scalpel or electrocautery

Describe the following incisions:

Kocher

Right subcostal incision for open cholecystectomy:

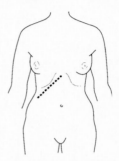

Midline laparotomy

Incision down the middle of abdomen along and through the linea alba:

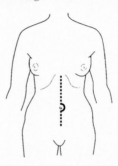

McBurney's

Small, oblique right lower quadrant incision for an appendectomy through McBurney's point (one third from the anterior superior iliac spine to the umbilicus):

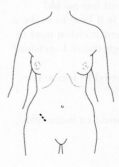

Rocky-Davis

Like a McBurney's incision except transverse (straight across):

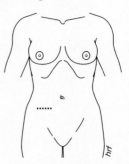

Pfannenstiel ("fan-en-steel")

Low transverse abdominal incision with retraction of the rectus muscles laterally; most often used for gynecologic procedures:

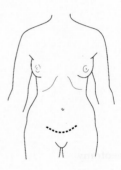

Kidney transplant

Lower quadrant; kidney placed extraperitoneally:

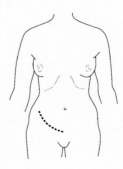

Liver transplant

Chevron or Mercedes-Benz® incision in the upper abdomen:

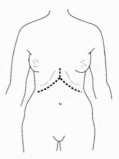

Median sternotomy

Midline sternotomy incision for heart procedures; less painful than a lateral thoracotomy:

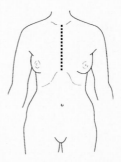

Thoracotomy

Usually through the fourth or fifth intercostal space; may be anterior or posterior lateral incisions
Very painful, but many are performed with muscle sparing (muscle retraction and not muscle transection):

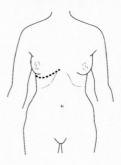

CEA (carotid endarterectomy)

Incision down anterior border of the sternocleidomastoid muscle to expose the carotid:

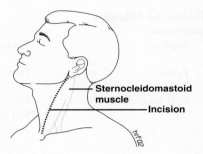

Inguinal hernia repair (open)

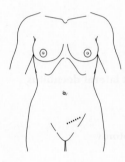

Laparoscopic cholecystectomy

Four trocar incisions:

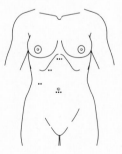

Chapter 11

Surgical Positions

Define the following positions:

Supine

Patient lying flat, face up

Prone

Patient lying flat, face down

Left lateral decubitus

Patient lying down on his left side (Think: **left** lateral decubitus = **left** side down)

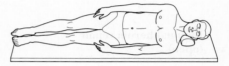

Right lateral decubitus

Patient lying down on his right side (Think: **right** lateral decubitus = **right** side down)

Lithotomy

Patient lying supine with legs spread

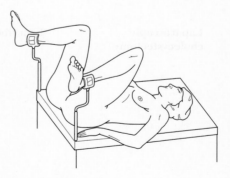

Trendelenburg	Patient supine with head lowered (a.k.a. "headdownenburg"—used during placement of a subclavian vein catheter as the veins distend with blood from gravity flow)

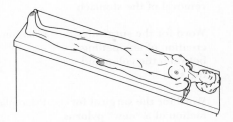

Reverse Trendelenburg	Patient supine with head elevated (usual position for laparoscopic cholecystectomy to make the intestines fall away from the operative field)
What is the best position for a pregnant patient?	Left side down to take gravid uterus off of the IVC

Chapter 12   Surgical Speak

The language of surgery is quite simple if you master a few suffixes.

Define the suffix:

-ectomy	To surgically **remove** part of or an entire structure/organ
-orraphy	Surgical **repair**
-otomy	Surgical **incision into** an organ
-ostomy	Surgically created **opening** between two organs, or organ and skin
-plasty	Surgical "shaping" or formation

Now test your knowledge of surgical speak:

Word for the surgical repair of a hernia	Herniorrhaphy
Word for the surgical removal of the stomach	Gastrectomy
Word for the surgical creation of an opening between the colon and the skin	Colostomy
Word for the surgical formation of a "new" pylorus	Pyloroplasty
Word for the surgical opening of the stomach	Gastrotomy
Surgical creation of an opening (anastomosis) between the common bile duct and jejunum	Choledochojejunostomy
Surgical creation of an opening (anastomosis) between the stomach and jejunum	Gastrojejunostomy

---

Chapter 13

Preoperative 101

When can a patient eat prior to major surgery?	Patient should be NPO after midnight the night before or for at least 8 hours before surgery
What risks should be discussed with all patients and documented on the consent form for a surgical procedure?	Bleeding, infection, anesthesia, scar; other risks are specific to the individual procedure (also MI, CVA, and death if cardiovascular disease is present)
If a patient is on antihypertensive medications, should the patient take them on the day of the procedure?	Yes, (remember clonidine "rebound")

If a patient is on an oral hypoglycemic agent (OHA), should the patient take the OHA on the day of surgery?	Not if the patient is to be NPO on the day of surgery
If a patient is taking insulin, should the patient take it on the day of surgery?	No, only half of a long-acting insulin (e.g., lente) and start D5 NS IV; check glucose levels often preoperatively, operatively, and postoperatively
Should a patient who smokes cigarettes stop before an operation?	Yes, improvement is seen in just 2 to 4 weeks after smoking cessation
What laboratory test must all women of childbearing age have before entering the O.R.?	β-HCG and CBC because of the possibility of pregnancy and anemia from menses
What is a preop colon surgery "bowel prep"?	Bowel prep with colon cathartic (e.g., GoLYTELY), oral antibiotics (neomycin and erythromycin base), and IV antibiotic before incision
Has a preop bowel prep been shown conclusively to decrease postop infections in colon surgery?	No, there is no data to support its use
What preoperative medication can decrease postoperative cardiac events and death?	β-blockers!
What must you always order preoperatively for your patient undergoing a major operation?	1. NPO/IVF 2. Preoperative antibiotics 3. Type and cross blood (PRBCs)
What electrolyte must you check preoperatively if a patient is on hemodialysis?	Potassium
Who gets a preoperative ECG?	Patients older than 40 years of age

Chapter 14

Surgical Operations You Should Know

Define the following procedures:

    Billroth I

Antrectomy with gastroduodenostomy

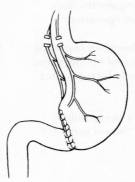

    Billroth II

Antrectomy with gastrojejunostomy

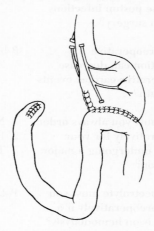

How can the difference between a Billroth I and a Billroth II be remembered?

Billroth 1 has one limb; Billroth 2 has two limbs

Describe the following procedures:

Roux-en-Y limb

Jejunojejunostomy forming a Y-shaped figure of small bowel; the free end can then be anastomosed to a second hollow structure (e.g., esophagojejunostomy)

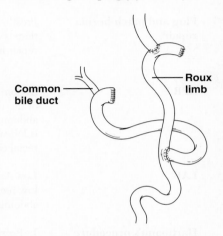

Brooke ileostomy

Standard ileostomy that is **folded on itself** to protrude from the abdomen ≈2 cm to allow easy appliance placement and collection of succus

CEA

Carotid **E**nd**A**rterectomy; removal of atherosclerotic plaque from a carotid artery

Bassini herniorrhaphy

Repair of inguinal hernia by approximating transversus abdominis aponeurosis and the conjoint tendon to the reflection of **Poupart's** (inguinal) ligament

McVay herniorrhaphy

Repair of inguinal hernia by approximating the transversus abdominis aponeurosis and the conjoint tendon to **Cooper's** ligament (which is basically the superior pubic bone periosteum)

Lichtenstein herniorrhaphy

"Tension-free" inguinal hernia repair using mesh (**synthetic** graft material)

Shouldice herniorrhaphy

Repair of inguinal hernia by **imbrication** of the transversalis fascia, transversus abdominis aponeurosis, and the conjoint tendon and approximation of the transversus abdominis aponeurosis and the conjoint tendon to the inguinal ligament

Plug and patch hernia repair

Prosthetic plug pushes hernia sac in and then is covered with a prosthetic patch to repair inguinal hernias

APR

Abdomino**P**erineal **R**esection; removal of the rectum and sigmoid colon through abdominal and perineal incisions (patient is left with a colostomy); used for low rectal cancers <8 cm from the anal verge

LAR

Low **A**nterior **R**esection; **resection** of **low** rectal tumors through an **anterior** abdominal incision

Hartmann's procedure

1. Proximal colostomy
2. Distal stapled-off colon or rectum that is left in peritoneal cavity

Mucous fistula

Distal end of the colon is brought to the abdominal skin as a stoma (proximal end is brought up to skin as an end colostomy)

Kocher ("koh-ker") maneuver

Dissection of the duodenum from the right-sided peritoneal attachment to allow mobilization and visualization of the back of the duodenum/pancreas

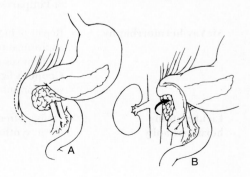

Seldinger technique   Placement of a central line by first placing
                                 a wire in the vein, followed by placing the
                                 catheter over the wire

Cricothyroidotomy   Emergent surgical airway through the
                                 cricoid membrane

Hepaticojejunostomy   Anastomosis between a jejunal roux limb
                                 and the hepatic ducts

Puestow procedure   Side-to-side anastomosis of the pancreas
                                 and jejunum (pancreatic duct is filleted
                                 open)

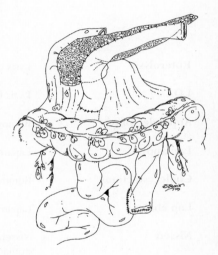

Stamm gastrostomy   Gastrostomy placed by open surgical
                                 incision and tacked to the abdominal
                                 wall

Highly selective vagotomy

Transection of vagal fibers to the body of the stomach without interruption of fibers to the pylorus (does not need pyloroplasty or other drainage procedure because the pylorus should still function)

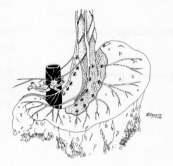

Enterolysis

Lysis of peritoneal adhesions

LOA

Lysis **O**f **A**dhesions (enterolysis)

Appendectomy

Removal of the appendix

Lap appy

Laparoscopic removal of the appendix

Cholecystectomy

Removal of the gallbladder

Lap chole

Laparoscopic removal of the gallbladder

Nissen

Nissen fundoplication; 360° wrap of the stomach by the fundus of the stomach around the distal esophagus to prevent reflux

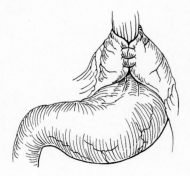

Lap Nissen   Nissen fundoplication with laparoscopy

Simple mastectomy   Removal of breast and nipple without
                                  removal of nodes

Choledochojejunostomy   Anastomosis of the common bile duct to
                                  the jejunum (end to side)

Graham patch   Placement of omentum with stitches over
                                  a gastric or duodenal perforation (i.e.,
                                  omentum is used to plug the hole)

Heineke-Mikulicz   Longitudinal incision through all layers of
pyloroplasty   the pylorus, sewing closed in a transverse
                                  direction to make the pylorus nonfunctional
                                  (used after truncal vagotomy)

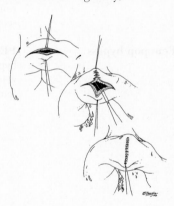

Pringle maneuver   Temporary occlusion of the porta hepatis
                                  (for temporary control of liver blood flow
                                  when liver parenchyma is actively bleeding)

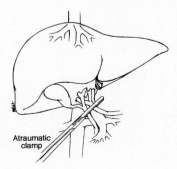

Atraumatic
clamp

Modified radical mastectomy — Removal of the breast, nipple, **and axillary lymph nodes** (no muscle is removed)

Lumpectomy and radiation — Removal of breast mass and axillary lymph nodes; normal surrounding breast tissue is spared; patient then undergoes postoperative radiation treatments

I & D — **I**ncision and **D**rainage of pus; the wound is then packed open

Exploratory laparotomy — Laparotomy to explore the peritoneal cavity looking for the cause of pain, peritoneal signs, obstruction, hemorrhage, etc.

TURP — **T**rans**U**rethral **R**esection of the **P**rostate; removal of obstructing prostatic tissue via scope in the urethral lumen

Fem pop bypass — **FEM**oral artery to **POP**liteal artery bypass using synthetic graft or saphenous vein; used to bypass blockage in the femoral artery

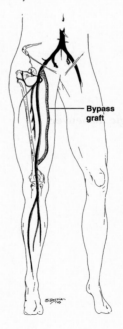

Bypass graft

Ax Fem

Long prosthetic graft tunneled under the skin placed from the **AX**illary artery to the **FEM**oral artery

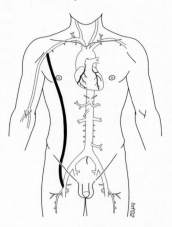

Triple A repair

Repair of an **AAA** (**A**bdominal **A**ortic **A**neurysm): Open aneurysm and place prosthetic graft; then close old aneurysm sac around graft

CABG

Coronary **A**rtery **B**ypass **G**rafting; via saphenous vein graft or internal mammary artery bypass grafts to coronary arteries from aorta (cardiac revascularization)

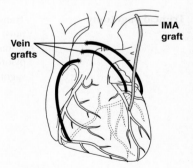

Hartmann's pouch

Oversewing of a rectal stump (or distal colonic stump) after resection of a colonic segment; patient is left with a proximal colostomy

PEG

Percutaneous **E**ndoscopic **G**astrostomy: Endoscope is placed in the stomach, which is then inflated with air; a needle is passed into the stomach percutaneously, wire is passed through the needle traversing the abdominal wall, and the gastrostomy is then placed by using the Seldinger technique over the wire

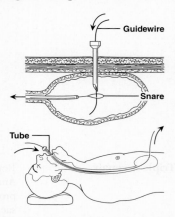

Ileoanal pull-through

Anastomosis of the ileum to the anus after total proctocolectomy

Hemicolectomy

Removal of a colonic segment (i.e., partial colectomy)

Truncal vagotomy

Transection of the vagus nerve trunks; must provide drainage procedure to stomach (e.g., gastrojejunostomy or pyloroplasty) because after truncal vagotomy, the **pylorus does not relax**

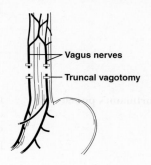

Antrectomy   Removal of stomach antrum

Whipple procedure   Pancreaticoduodenectomy:
                           Cholecystectomy
                           Truncal vagotomy
                           Pancreaticoduodenectomy—removal
                           of the head of the pancreas and
                           duodenum
                           Choledochojejunostomy
                           Pancreaticojejunostomy (anastomosis
                           of distal pancreas remnant to the
                           jejunum)
                           Gastrojejunostomy (anastomosis of
                           stomach to jejunum)

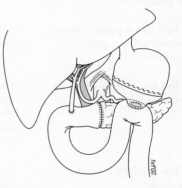

Excisional biopsy   Biopsy with complete excision of all
                           suspect tissue (mass)

Incisional biopsy   Biopsy with incomplete removal of
                           suspect tissue (incises tissue from mass)

Tracheostomy   Placement of airway tube into trachea
                           surgically or percutaneously

Chapter 15

Wounds

Define the following terms:
   Primary wound closure   Suture wound closes immediately (a.k.a.
                                "first intention")

Secondary wound closure	Wound is left open and heals over time **without sutures** (a.k.a. "secondary intention"); it heals by granulation, contraction, and epithelialization over weeks (leaves a larger scar)
Delayed primary closure (DPC)	Suture wound closes 3 to 5 days AFTER incision (classically 5 days)
How long until a sutured wound epithelializes?	24–48 hours
After a primary closure, when should the dressing be removed?	POD #2
When can a patient take a shower after a primary closure?	Anytime after POD #2 (after wound epithelializes)
What is a wet-to-dry dressing?	Damp (not wet) gauze dressing placed over a granulating wound and then allowed to dry to the wound; removal allows for "microdébridement" of the wound
What inhibits wound healing?	Infection, ischemia, diabetes mellitus, malnutrition, anemia, steroids, cancer, radiation, smoking
What reverses the deleterious effects of steroids on wound healing?	Vitamin A
What is an abdominal wound dehiscence?	Opening of the fascial closure (not skin); treat by returning to the O.R. for immediate fascial reclosure
What is Dakin solution?	Dilute sodium hypochlorite (**bleach**) used in contaminated wounds

Chapter 16

Drains and Tubes

What is the purpose of drains?

1. Withdrawal of fluids
2. Apposition of tissues to remove a potential space by suction

What is a Jackson-Pratt (JP) drain?

Closed drainage system attached to a suction bulb ("grenade")

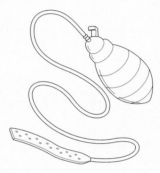

What are the "three S's" of Jackson-Pratt drain removal?

1. **S**titch removal
2. **S**uction discontinuation
3. **S**low, steady pull

What is a Penrose drain?

Open drainage system composed of a thin rubber hose; associated with increased infection rate in clean wounds

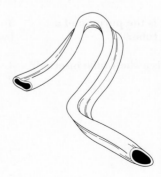

Define the following terms:
   G-tube

Gastrostomy tube; used for drainage or feeding

J-tube

Jejunostomy tube; used for feeding; may be a small-needle catheter (remember to flush after use or it will clog) or a large, red rubber catheter

Cholecystostomy tube

Tube placed surgically or percutaneously with ultrasound guidance to drain the gallbladder

T-tube

Tube placed in the common bile duct with an ascending and descending limb that forms a "T"

Drains percutaneously; placed after common bile duct exploration

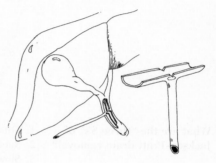

CHEST TUBES

What is a thoracostomy tube?   Chest tube

What is the purpose of a chest tube?

To appose the parietal and visceral pleura by draining blood, pus, fluid, chyle, or air

How is a chest tube inserted?

1. Administer local anesthetic
2. Incise skin in the fourth or fifth intercostal space between the mid- and anterior-axillary lines
3. Perform blunt Kelly-clamp dissection **over** the rib into the pleural space
4. Perform finger exploration to confirm intrapleural placement
5. Place tube posteriorly and superiorly

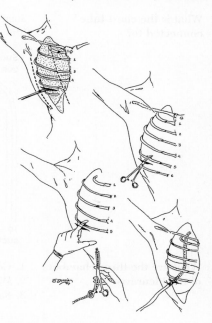

Is the chest tube placed under or over the rib?

Over to avoid the vessels and nerves

What are the goals of chest tube insertion?

Drain the pleural cavity
Appose parietal and visceral pleura to seal any visceral pleural holes

In most cases, where should the chest tube be positioned?

Posteriorly into the apex

How can you tell on CXR if the last hole on the chest tube is in the pleural cavity?

Last hole is cut through the radiopaque line in the chest tube and is seen on CXR as a break in the line, which should be within the pleural cavity

What are the cm measurements on a chest tube?

Centimeters from the last hole on the chest tube

What is the chest tube connected to?

Suction, waterseal, collection system (three-chambered box, e.g., Pleuravac®)

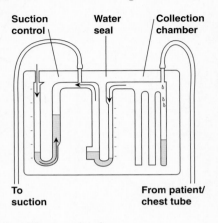

What are the three chambers of the Pleuravac®?

1. Collection chamber
2. Water seal
3. Suction control

Describe how each chamber of the Pleuravac® box works as the old three-bottle system:
Collection chamber

Collects fluid, pus, blood, or chyle and measures the amount; connects to the water seal bottle and to the chest tube

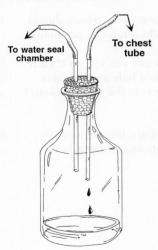

Water-seal chamber

One-way valve—allows air to be removed from the pleural space; does not allow air to enter pleural cavity; connects to the suction control bottle and to the collection chamber

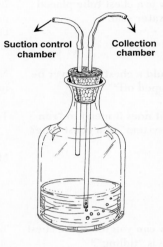

Suction control chamber

Collection chamber

Suction-control chamber

Controls the amount of suction by the height of the water column; sucking in room air releases excessive suction; connects to wall suction and to the water seal bottle

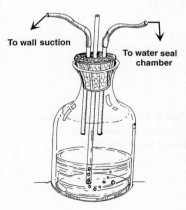

To wall suction

To water seal chamber

Give a good example of a water seal.

Place a straw in a cup of water—you can blow air out but if you suck in, the straw fills with water and thus forms a one-way valve for air just like the chest tube water seal

How is a chest tube placed on water seal?

By removing the suction; a tension pneumothorax (PTX) cannot form because the one-way valve (water seal) allows release of air buildup

Should a chest tube ever be clamped off?

No, except to "run the system" **momentarily**

What does it mean to "run the system" of a chest tube?

To see if the air leak is from a leak in the pleural cavity (e.g., hole in lung) or from a leak in the tubing
Momentarily occlude the chest tube and if the air leak is still present, it is from the tubing or tubing connection, not from the chest

How can you tell if the chest tube is "tidling"?

Take the Pleuravac® off of suction and look at the water seal chamber: Fluid should move with respiration/ventilation (called "tidling"); this decreases and ceases if the pleura seals off the chest tube

How can you check for an air leak?

Look at the water seal chamber on suction:
If bubbles pass through the water seal fluid, a large air leak (i.e., air leaking into chest tube) is present; if no air leak is evident on suction, remove suction and ask the patient to cough
If air bubbles through the water seal, a small air leak is present

What is the usual course for removing a chest tube placed for a PTX?

1. Suction until the PTX resolves and the air leak is gone
2. Water seal for 24 hours
3. Remove the chest tube if no PTX or air leak is present after 24 hours of water seal

How fast is a small, stable PTX absorbed?

$\approx 1\%$ daily; therefore, a 10% PTX by volume will absorb in ≈ 10 days

How should a chest tube be removed?

1. Cut the stitch
2. Ask the patient to exhale or inhale maximally
3. Rapidly remove the tube (split second) and at same time, place petroleum jelly gauze covered by 4 × 4's and then tape
4. Obtain a CXR

What is a Heimlich valve?

One-way flutter valve for a chest tube

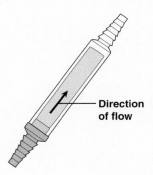

Direction of flow

NASOGASTRIC TUBES (NGT)

How should an NGT be placed?

1. Use lubrication and have suction up on the bed
2. Use anesthetic to numb nose
3. Place head in flexion
4. Ask patient to drink a small amount of water when the tube is in the back of the throat and to swallow the tube; if the patient can talk without difficulty and succus returns, the tube should be in the stomach (Get an x-ray if there is any question about position)

How should an NGT be removed?

Give patient a tissue, discontinue suction, untape nose, remove quickly, and tell patient to blow nose

What test should be performed before feeding via any tube?

High abdominal x-ray to confirm placement into the GI tract and NOT the lung!

How does an NGT work?

Sump pump, dual lumen tube—the large clear tube is hooked to suction and the small blue tube allows for air sump (i.e., circuit sump pump with air in the blue tube and air and succus sucked out through the large clear lumen)

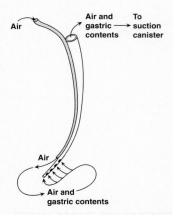

How can you check to see if the NGT is working?

Blue port will make a sucking noise; always keep the blue port opening above the stomach

Should an NGT be placed on continuous or intermittent suction?

Continuous low suction—side holes disengage if they are against mucosa because of the sump mechanism and multiple holes

What happens if the NGT is clogged?

Tube will not decompress the stomach and will keep the low esophageal sphincter (LES) open (i.e., a setup for aspiration)

How should an NGT be unclogged?

Saline-flush the clear port, reconnect to suction, and flush air down the blue sump port

What is a common cause of excessive NGT drainage?

Tip of the NGT is inadvertently placed in the duodenum and drains the pancreatic fluid and bile; an x-ray should be taken and the tube repositioned into the stomach

What is the difference between a feeding tube (Dobbhoff tube) and an NGT?

A feeding tube is a thin tube weighted at the end that is not a sump pump but a simple catheter; usually placed past the pylorus, which is facilitated by the weighted end and peristalsis

FOLEY CATHETER

What is a Foley catheter?

Catheter into the bladder, allowing accurate urine output determination

What is a coudé catheter?

Foley catheter with a small, curved tip to help maneuver around a large prostate

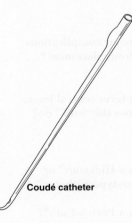

Coudé catheter

If a Foley catheter cannot be inserted, what are the next steps?

1. Anesthetize the urethra with a sterile local anesthetic (e.g., lidocaine jelly)
2. Try a **larger** Foley catheter

What if a patient has a urethral injury and a Foley cannot be placed?

A suprapubic catheter will need to be placed

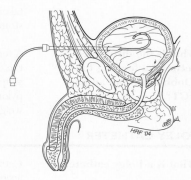

CENTRAL LINES

What are they?

Catheters placed into the major veins (central veins) via subclavian, internal jugular, or femoral vein approaches

What major complications result from placement?

PTX (always obtain postplacement CXR), bleeding, malposition (e.g., into the neck from subclavian approach), dysrhythmias

In long-term central lines, what does the "cuff" do?

Allows ingrowth of fibrous tissue, which:
  Holds the line in place
  Forms a barrier to the advance of bacteria

What is a Hickman® or Hickman-type catheter?

External central line tunneled under the skin with a "cuff"

What is a Port-A-Cath®?

Central line that has a port buried under the skin that must be accessed through the skin (percutaneously)

What is a "cordis"?

Large central line catheter; used for massive fluid resuscitation or for placing a Swan-Ganz catheter

If you try to place a subclavian central line unsuccessfully, what must you do before trying the other side?

Get a CXR—a bilateral pneumothorax can be fatal!

MISCELLANEOUS

How can diameter in mm be determined from a French measurement?	Divide the French size by π or 3.14 (e.g., a 15 French tube has a diameter of 5 mm)
How can needle-gauge size be determined?	14-gauge needle is 1/14 of an inch (Thus, a 14-gauge needle is larger than a 21-gauge needle)
What is a Tenckhoff catheter?	Catheter placed into the peritoneal cavity for peritoneal dialysis

Chapter 17

Surgical Anatomy Pearls

What is the drainage of the left testicular vein?	Left renal vein
What is the drainage of the right testicular vein?	IVC
What is Gerota's fascia?	Fascia surrounding the kidney
What are the prominent collateral circulations seen in portal hypertension?	Esophageal varices, hemorrhoids (inferior hemorrhoidal vein to internal iliac vein), patent umbilical vein (caput medusa), and retroperitoneal vein via lumbar tributaries
What parts of the GI tract are retroperitoneal?	Most of the duodenum, the ascending colon, the descending colon, and the pancreas
What is the gubernaculum?	Embryologic structure that adheres the testes to the scrotal sac; used to help manipulate the testes during indirect hernia repair

Which artery bleeds in bleeding duodenal ulcers?	Gastroduodenal artery
What is the name of the lymph nodes between the pectoralis minor and major muscles?	Rotter's lymph nodes
Is the left vagus nerve anterior or posterior?	Anterior; remember that the esophagus rotates during development
What is Morrison's pouch?	Hepatorenal recess; the most posterior cavity within the peritoneal cavity

Give the locations of the following structures:

Foregut	Mouth to ampulla of Vater
Midgut	Ampulla of Vater to distal third of transverse colon
Hindgut	Distal third of transverse colon to the anus
Where are the blood vessels on a rib?	Vein, Artery, and Nerve (**VAN**) are underneath the rib (thus, place chest tubes and thoracentesis needles above the rib!)
What is the order of the femoral vessels?	Femoral vein is medial to the femoral artery (Think: **"NAVEL"** for the order of the right femoral vessels—Nerve, Artery, Vein, Empty space, Lymphatics)
What is Hesselbach's triangle?	The area bordered by: 1. Inguinal ligament 2. Epigastric vessels 3. Lateral border of the rectus sheath
What nerve is located on top of the spermatic cord?	Ilioinguinal nerve
What is Calot's triangle?	The area bordered by: 1. Cystic duct 2. Common hepatic duct 3. Cystic artery (Pronounced "kal-ohs")

What is Calot's node? Lymph node found in Calot's triangle

What separates the right and left lobes of the liver? Cantle's line—a line drawn from the IVC to just left of the gallbladder fossa

What is the gastrinoma triangle? Triangle where >90% of gastrinomas are located, bordered by:
1. Junction of the second and third portions of the duodenum
2. Cystic duct
3. Pancreatic neck

Which artery is responsible for anterior spinal syndrome? Artery of Adamkiewicz

Where is McBurney's point? One third the distance from the anterior superior iliac spine to the umbilicus (estimate of the position of the appendix)

How can you find the appendix after you find the cecum? Trace the taeniae back as they converge on the origin of the appendix

Where is the space of Retzius? Preperitoneal space anterior to the bladder

What are the white lines of Toldt? Lateral peritoneal reflections of the ascending and descending colon

What is the strongest layer of the small bowel? Submucosa (*not* the serosa, think: **SU**bmucosa = **SU**perior)

Which parts of the GI tract do not have a serosa? Esophagus
Middle and distal rectum

What is the vein that overlies the pylorus? Vein of Mayo

What is the pouch of Douglas? Pouch between the rectum and bladder or uterus

What does the thoracic duct empty into? Left subclavian vein; left internal jugular vein junction

What is the coronary vein?   Left gastric vein

What is the hypogastric artery?   Internal iliac artery

Which is longer, the left or right renal vein?   Left

What are the layers of the abdominal wall?
1. Skin, then fat
2. Scarpa's fascia, then more fat
3. External oblique
4. Internal oblique
5. Transversus abdominis
6. Transversalis fascia
7. Preperitoneal fat
8. Peritoneum

What are the plicae circulares?   Plicae = folds, circulares = circular; thus, the circular folds of mucosa of the small bowel

What is another name for the plicae circulares?   Valvulae conniventes

What are the major structural differences between the jejunum and ileum?

Jejunum—long vasa rectae; large plicae circulares; thicker wall

Ileum—shorter vasa rectae; smaller plicae circulares; thinner wall (Think: **I**leum = **I**nferior vasa rectae, **I**nferior plicae circulares, and **I**nferior wall)

What are the major anatomic differences between the colon and the small bowel?   Colon has taeniae coli, haustra, and appendices epiploicae (fat appendages), whereas the small intestine is smooth

How far up does the diaphragm extend?   To the nipples in men (fourth intercostal space; thus, the abdomen extends to the level of the nipples)

What dermatome is at the umbilicus?   T10

What are the major layers of an artery?

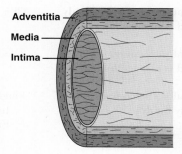

- Adventitia
- Media
- Intima

Chapter 18

Fluids and Electrolytes

What are the two major body fluid compartments?

1. Intracellular
2. Extracellular

What are the two subcompartments of extracellular fluid?

1. Interstitial fluid (in between cells)
2. Intravascular fluid (plasma)

What percentage of body weight is in fluid?

60%

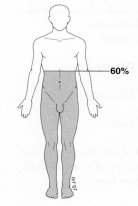

60%

What percentage of body fluid is intracellular?	66%
What percentage of body fluid is extracellular?	33%

What is the composition of body fluid?	Fluids = 60% total body weight:
	   Intracellular = 40% total body weight
	   Extracellular = 20% total body weight
	     (Think: 60, 40, 20)

How can body fluid distribution by weight be remembered?	"TIE":
	  T = **T**otal body fluid = 60% of body weight
	  I = **I**ntracellular = 40% of body weight
	  E = **E**xtracellular = 20% of body weight

On average, what percentage of body weight does blood account for in adults?	≈7%
How many liters of blood are in a 70-kg man?	$0.07 \times 70 = 5$ liters
What are the fluid requirements every 24 hours for each of the following substances:	
Water	≈30 to 35 mL/kg
Potassium	≈1 mEq/kg
Chloride	≈1.5 mEq/kg
Sodium	≈1–2 mEq/kg
What are the levels and sources of normal daily water loss?	Urine—1200 to 1500 mL (25–30 mL/kg) Sweat—200 to 400 mL Respiratory losses—500 to 700 mL Feces—100 to 200 mL
What are the levels and sources of normal daily electrolyte loss?	Sodium and potassium = 100 mEq Chloride = 150 mEq

What are the levels of sodium and chloride in sweat?	≈ 40 mEq/L
What is the major electrolyte in colonic feculent fluid?	Potassium—65 mEq/L
What is the physiologic response to hypovolemia?	Sodium/H_2O retention via renin $\rightarrow$ aldosterone, water retention via ADH, vasoconstriction via angiotensin II and sympathetics, low urine output and tachycardia (early), hypotension (late)

THIRD SPACING

What is it?	Fluid accumulation in the interstitium of tissues, as in edema, e.g., loss of fluid into the interstitium and lumen of a paralytic bowel following surgery (think of the intravascular and intracellular spaces as the first two spaces)
When does "third-spacing" occur postoperatively?	Third-spaced fluid tends to mobilize back into the intravascular space around POD #3 (**Note:** Beware of fluid overload once the fluid begins to return to the intravascular space); switch to hypotonic fluid and decrease IV rate
What are the classic signs of third spacing?	Tachycardia Decreased urine output
What is the treatment?	IV hydration with isotonic fluids
What are the surgical causes of the following conditions: Metabolic acidosis	Loss of bicarbonate: diarrhea, ileus, fistula, high-output ileostomy, carbonic anhydrase inhibitors Increase in acids: lactic acidosis (ischemia), ketoacidosis, renal failure, necrotic tissue
Hypochloremic alkalosis	NGT suction, loss of gastric HCl through vomiting/NGT

Metabolic alkalosis	Vomiting, NG suction, diuretics, alkali ingestion, mineralocorticoid excess
Respiratory acidosis	Hypoventilation (e.g., CNS depression), drugs (e.g., morphine), PTX, pleural effusion, parenchymal lung disease, acute airway obstruction
Respiratory alkalosis	Hyperventilation (e.g., anxiety, pain, fever, wrong ventilator settings)
What is the "classic" acid-base finding with significant vomiting or NGT suctioning?	Hypokalemic hypochloremic metabolic alkalosis
Why hypokalemia with NGT suctioning?	Loss in gastric fluid—loss of HCl causes alkalosis, driving K^+ into cells
What is the treatment for hypokalemic hypochloremic metabolic alkalosis?	IVF, Cl^-/K^+ replacement
What is paradoxic alkalotic aciduria?	Seen in severe hypokalemic, hypovolemic, hypochloremic metabolic alkalosis with paradoxic metabolic alkalosis of serum and acidic urine
How does paradoxic alkalotic aciduria occur?	H^+ is lost in the urine in exchange for Na^+ in an attempt to restore volume
With paradoxic alkalotic aciduria, why is H^+ preferentially lost?	H^+ is exchanged preferentially into the urine instead of K^+ because of the low concentration of K^+
What can be followed to assess fluid status?	Urine output, base deficit, lactic acid, vital signs, weight changes, skin turgor, jugular venous distention (JVD), mucosal membranes, rales (crackles), central venous pressure, PCWP, chest x-ray findings
With hypovolemia, what changes occur in vital signs?	Tachycardia, tachypnea, initial rise in diastolic blood pressure because of clamping down (peripheral vasoconstriction) with subsequent decrease in both systolic and diastolic blood pressures

What are the insensible fluid losses?

Loss of fluid not measured:
  Feces—100 to 200 mL/24 hours
  Breathing—500 to 700 mL/24 hours
    (*Note:* increases with fever and tachypnea)
  Skin—≈300 mL/24 hours, increased with fever; thus, insensible fluid loss is not directly measured

What are the quantities of daily secretions:

Bile

≈1000 mL/24 hours

Gastric

≈2000 mL/ 24 hours

Pancreatic

≈600 mL/ 24 hours

Small intestine

≈3000 mL/day

Saliva

≈1500 mL/24 hours
(*Note:* almost all secretions are reabsorbed)

How can the estimated levels of daily secretions from bile, gastric, and small-bowel sources be remembered?

Alphabetically and numerically: **BGS** and **123** or **B1, G2, S3**, because Bile, Gastric, and Small bowel produce roughly **1** L, **2** L, and **3** L, respectively!

COMMON IV REPLACEMENT FLUIDS (ALL VALUES ARE PER LITER)

What comprises normal saline (NS)?

154 mEq of Cl^-
154 mEq of Na^+

What comprises 1/2 NS?

77 mEq of Cl^-
77 mEq of Na^+

What comprises 1/4 NS?

39 mEq of Cl^-
39 mEq of Na^+

What comprises lactated Ringer's (LR)?

130 mEq Na^+
109 mEq Cl^-
28 mEq lactate
4 mEq K^+
3 mEq Ca^+

What comprises D5W?

5% dextrose (50 g) in H_2O

What accounts for tonicity?	Mainly electrolytes; thus, NS and LR are both isotonic, whereas 1/2 NS is hypotonic to serum
What happens to the lactate in LR in the body?	Converted into bicarbonate; thus, LR cannot be used as a maintenance fluid because patients would become alkalotic

IVF replacement by anatomic site:

Gastric (NGT)	D5 1/2 NS + 20 KCl
Biliary	LR+/−sodium bicarbonate
Pancreatic	LR+/−sodium bicarbonate
Small bowel (ileostomy)	LR
Colonic (diarrhea)	LR+/−sodium bicarbonate

CALCULATION OF MAINTENANCE FLUIDS

What is the 100/50/20 rule?	Maintenance IV fluids for a 24-hour period: **100** mL/kg for the first 10 kg **50** mL/kg for the next 10 kg **20** mL/kg for every kg over 20 (divide by 24 for hourly rate)
What is the 4/2/1 rule?	Maintenance IV fluids for hourly rate: **4** mL/kg for the first 10 kg **2** mL/kg for the next 10 kg **1** mL/kg for every kg over 20
What is the maintenance for a 70-kg man?	Using 100/50/20: 100×10 kg = 1000 50×10 kg = 500 20×50 kg = 1000 Total = 2500 Divided by 24 hours = 104 mL/hr maintenance rate Using 4/2/1: 4×10 kg = 40 2×10 kg = 20 1×50 kg = 50 Total = 110 mL/hr maintenance rate

What is the common adult maintenance fluid?

D5 1/2 NS with 20 mEq KCl/L

What is the common pediatric maintenance fluid?

D5 1/4 NS with 20 mEq KCl/L (use 1/4 NS because of the decreased ability of children to concentrate urine)

Why should sugar (dextrose) be added to maintenance fluid?

To inhibit muscle breakdown

What is the best way to assess fluid status?

Urine output (unless the patient has cardiac or renal dysfunction, in which case central venous pressure or wedge pressure is often used)

What is the minimal urine output for an adult on maintenance IV?

30 mL/hr (0.5 cc/kg/hr)

What is the minimal urine output for an adult trauma patient?

50 mL/hr

How many mL are in 12 oz (beer can)?

356 mL

How many mL are in 1 oz?

30 mL

How many mL are in 1 tsp?

5 mL

What are common isotonic fluids?

NS, LR

What is a bolus?

Volume of fluid given IV rapidly (e.g., 1 L over 1 hour); used for increasing intravascular volume, and isotonic fluids should be used (i.e., NS or LR)

Why not combine bolus fluids with dextrose?

Hyperglycemia may result

What is the possible consequence of hyperglycemia in the patient with hypovolemia?	Osmotic diuresis
Why not combine bolus fluids with a significant amount of potassium?	Hyperkalemia may result (the potassium in LR is very low: 4 mEq/L)
Why should isotonic fluids be given for resuscitation (i.e., to restore intravascular volume)?	If hypotonic fluid is given, the tonicity of the intravascular space will be decreased and H_2O will freely diffuse into the interstitial and intracellular spaces; thus, use isotonic fluids to expand the intravascular space
What portion of 1 L NS will stay in the intravascular space after a laparotomy?	In 5 hours, only $\approx$200 cc (or 20%) will remain in the intravascular space!
What is the most common trauma resuscitation fluid?	LR
What is the most common postoperative IV fluid after a laparotomy?	LR or D5LR for 24 to 36 hours, followed by maintenance fluid
After a laparotomy, when should a patient's fluid be "mobilized"?	Classically, POD #3; the patient begins to "mobilize" the third-space fluid back into the intravascular space
What IVF is used to replace duodenal or pancreatic fluid loss?	LR (bicarbonate loss)

ELECTROLYTE IMBALANCES

What is a common cause of electrolyte abnormalities?	Lab error!
What is a major extracellular cation?	Na^+
What is a major intracellular cation?	K^+

HYPERKALEMIA

What is the normal range for potassium level?	3.5–5.0 mEq/L
What are the surgical causes of hyperkalemia?	Iatrogenic overdose, blood transfusion, renal failure, diuretics, acidosis, tissue destruction (injury/hemolysis)
What are the signs/ symptoms?	Decreased deep tendon reflex (DTR) or areflexia, weakness, paraesthesia, paralysis, respiratory failure
What are the ECG findings?	**Peaked T waves,** depressed ST segment, prolonged PR, wide QRS, bradycardia, ventricular fibrillation
What are the critical values?	$K^+ > 6.5$
What is the urgent treatment?	IV calcium (cardioprotective), ECG monitoring Sodium bicarbonate IV (alkalosis drives K^+ intracellularly) Glucose and insulin Albuterol Sodium polystyrene sulfonate (Kayexalate) and **furosemide** (Lasix) Dialysis
What is the nonacute treatment?	Furosemide (Lasix), sodium polystyrene sulfonate (Kayexalate)
What is the acronym for the treatment of acute symptomatic hyperkalemia?	**"CB DIAL K":** **C**alcium **B**icarbonate **D**ialysis **I**nsulin/dextrose **A**lbuterol **L**asix **K**ayexalate
What is "pseudohyper-kalemia"?	Spurious hyperkalemia as a result of falsely elevated K^+ in sample from sample hemolysis

What acid-base change lowers the serum potassium?	Alkalosis (thus, give bicarbonate for hyperkalemia)
What nebulizer treatment can help lower K+ level?	Albuterol

HYPOKALEMIA

What are the surgical causes?	Diuretics, certain antibiotics, steroids, alkalosis, diarrhea, intestinal fistulae, NG aspiration, vomiting, insulin, insufficient supplementation, amphotericin
What are the signs/symptoms?	Weakness, tetany, nausea, vomiting, **ileus,** paraesthesia
What are the ECG findings?	**Flattening of T waves, U waves,** ST segment depression, PAC, PVC, atrial fibrillation
What is a U wave?	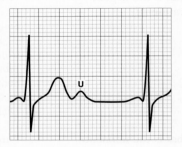
What is the rapid treatment?	KCl IV
What is the maximum amount that can be given through a peripheral IV?	10 mEq/hour
What is the maximum amount that can be given through a central line?	20 mEq/hour
What is the chronic treatment?	KCl PO
What is the most common electrolyte-mediated ileus in the surgical patient?	Hypokalemia

What electrolyte condition exacerbates digitalis toxicity?	Hypokalemia
What electrolyte deficiency can actually cause hypokalemia?	Low magnesium
What electrolyte must you replace first before replacing K$^+$?	Magnesium
Why does hypomagnesemia make replacement of K$^+$ with hypokalemia nearly impossible?	Hypomagnesemia inhibits K$^+$ reabsorption from the renal tubules

HYPERNATREMIA

What is the normal range for sodium level?	135–145 mEq/L
What are the surgical causes?	Inadequate hydration, diabetes insipidus, diuresis, vomiting, diarrhea, diaphoresis, tachypnea, iatrogenic (e.g., TPN)
What are the signs/ symptoms?	Seizures, confusion, stupor, pulmonary or peripheral edema, tremors, respiratory paralysis
What is the usual treatment supplementation slowly over days?	D5W, 1/4 NS, or 1/2 NS
How fast should you lower the sodium level in hyperna- tremia?	Guideline is <12 mEq/L per day
What is the major complica- tion of lowering the sodium level too fast?	Seizures (**not** central pontine myelinolysis)

HYPONATREMIA

What are the surgical causes of the following types:	
Hypovolemic	Diuretic excess, hypoaldosteronism, vomiting, NG suction, burns, pancreatitis, diaphoresis

Euvolemic	SIADH, CNS abnormalities, drugs
Hypervolemic	Renal failure, CHF, liver failure (cirrhosis), iatrogenic fluid overload (dilutional)
What are the signs/ symptoms?	Seizures, coma, nausea, vomiting, ileus, lethargy, confusion, weakness
What is the treatment of the following types:	
Hypovolemic	NS IV, correct underlying cause
Euvolemic	SIADH: furosemide and NS acutely, fluid restriction
Hypervolemic	Dilutional: fluid restriction and diuretics
How fast should you increase the sodium level in hyponatremia?	Guideline is <12 mEq/L per day
What may occur if you correct hyponatremia too quickly?	Central pontine myelinolysis!
What are the signs of central pontine myelinolysis?	1. Confusion 2. Spastic quadriplegia 3. Horizontal gaze paralysis
What is the most common cause of mild postoperative hyponatremia?	Fluid overload
How can the sodium level in SIADH be remembered?	**SIADH** = **S**odium **I**s **A**lways **D**own **H**ere = Hyponatremia

"PSEUDOHYPONATREMIA"

What is it?	Spurious lab value of hyponatremia as a result of hyperglycemia, hyperlipidemia, or hyperproteinemia

HYPERCALCEMIA

What are the causes?

"CHIMPANZEES":
Calcium supplementation IV
Hyperparathyroidism (1°/3°)
  hyperthyroidism
Immobility/**I**atrogenic (thiazide
  diuretics)
Mets/**M**ilk alkali syndrome
Paget's disease (bone)
Addison's disease/**A**cromegaly
Neoplasm (colon, lung, breast,
  prostate, multiple myeloma)
Zollinger-Ellison syndrome (as part of
  MEN I)
Excessive vitamin D
Excessive vitamin A
Sarcoid

**What are the signs/
symptoms?**

Hypercalcemia—"Stones, bones, abdominal groans, and psychiatric overtones"
Polydipsia, polyuria, constipation

What are the ECG findings?

Short QT interval, prolonged PR interval

**What is the acute treatment
of hypercalcemic crisis?**

Volume expansion with NS, diuresis with
furosemide (not thiazides)

**What are other options for
lowering Ca$^+$ level?**

Steroids, calcitonin, bisphosphonates
(pamidronate, etc.), mithramycin, dialysis
(last resort)

HYPOCALCEMIA

**How can the calcium level
be determined with
hypoalbuminemia?**

(4-measured albumin level) × 0.8, then
add this value to the measured calcium
level

**What are the surgical
causes?**

Short bowel syndrome, intestinal bypass,
vitamin D deficiency, sepsis, acute
pancreatitis, osteoblastic metastasis,
aminoglycosides, diuretics, renal failure,
hypomagnesemia, rhabdomyolysis

What is Chvostek's sign?

Facial muscle spasm with tapping of
facial nerve (Think: **CH**vostek = **CH**eek)

What is Trousseau's sign?	Carpal spasm after occluding blood flow in forearm with blood pressure cuff
What are the signs/ symptoms?	Chvostek's and Trousseau's signs, perioral paraesthesia (early), increased deep tendon reflexes (late), confusion, abdominal cramps, laryngospasm, stridor, seizures, tetany, psychiatric abnormalities (e.g., paranoia, depression, hallucinations)
What are the ECG findings?	Prolonged QT and ST interval (peaked T waves are also possible, as in hyperkalemia)
What is the acute treatment?	Calcium gluconate IV
What is the chronic treatment?	Calcium PO, vitamin D
What is the possible complication of infused calcium if the IV infiltrates?	**Tissue necrosis;** never administer peripherally unless absolutely necessary (calcium gluconate is less toxic than calcium chloride during an infiltration)
What is the best way to check the calcium level in the ICU?	Check ionized calcium

HYPERMAGNESEMIA

What is the normal range for magnesium level?	1.5–2.5 mEq/L
What is the surgical cause?	TPN, renal failure, IV over supplementation
What are the signs/ symptoms?	Respiratory failure, CNS depression, decreased deep tendon reflexes
What is the treatment?	Calcium gluconate IV, insulin plus glucose, dialysis (similar to treatment of hyperkalemia), furosemide (Lasix)

HYPOMAGNESEMIA

What are the surgical causes?	TPN, hypocalcemia, gastric suctioning, aminoglycosides, renal failure, diarrhea, vomiting

What are the signs/ symptoms?	Increased deep tendon reflexes, tetany, asterixis, tremor, Chvostek's sign, ventricular ectopy, vertigo, tachycardia, dysrhythmias
What is the acute treatment?	$MgSO_4$ IV
What is the chronic treatment?	Magnesium oxide PO (side effect: diarrhea)
Hypomagnesemia may make it impossible to correct what other electrolyte abnormality?	Hypokalemia (always fix hypomagnesemia with hypokalemia)

HYPERGLYCEMIA

What are the surgical causes?	Diabetes (poor control), infection, stress, TPN, drugs, lab error, drawing over IV site, somatostatinoma, glucagonoma
What are the signs/ symptoms?	Polyuria, hypovolemia, confusion/coma, polydipsia, ileus, DKA (Kussmaul breathing), abdominal pain, hyporeflexia
What is the treatment?	Insulin
What is the Weiss protocol?	Sliding scale insulin
What is the goal glucose level in the ICU?	80–110 mg/dL

HYPOGLYCEMIA

What are the surgical causes?	Excess insulin, decreased caloric intake, insulinoma, drugs, liver failure, adrenal insufficiency, gastrojejunostomy
What are the signs/ symptoms?	Sympathetic response (diaphoresis, tachycardia, palpitations), confusion, coma, headache, diplopia, neurologic deficits, seizures
What is the treatment?	Glucose (IV or PO)

HYPOPHOSPHATEMIA

What is the normal range for phosphorus level?	2.5–4.5 mg/dL
What are the signs/ symptoms?	Weakness, cardiomyopathy, neurologic dysfunction (e.g., ataxia), rhabdomyolysis, hemolysis, poor pressor response
What is a complication of severe hypophosphatemia?	Respiratory failure
What are the causes?	GI losses, inadequate supplementation, medications, sepsis, alcohol abuse, renal loss
What is the critical value?	<1.0 mg/dL
What is the treatment?	Supplement with sodium phosphate or potassium phosphate IV (depending on potassium level)

HYPERPHOSPHATEMIA

What are the signs/ symptoms?	Calcification (ectopic), heart block
What are the causes?	Renal failure, sepsis, chemotherapy, hyperthyroidism
What is the treatment?	Aluminum hydroxide (binds phosphate)

MISCELLANEOUS

This ECG pattern is consistent with which electrolyte abnormality?	Hyperkalemia: peaked T waves

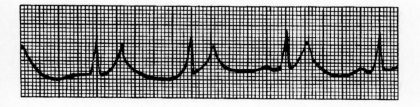

If hyperkalemia is left untreated, what can occur?

Ventricular tachycardia/fibrillation → death

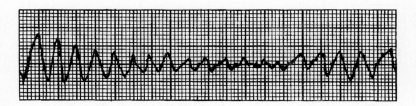

Which electrolyte is an inotrope?

Calcium

What are the major cardiac electrolytes?

Potassium (dysrhythmias), magnesium (dysrhythmias), calcium (dysrhythmias/ inotrope)

Which electrolyte must be monitored closely in patients on digitalis?

Potassium

What is the most common cause of electrolyte-mediated ileus?

Hypokalemia

What is a colloid fluid?

Protein-containing fluid (albumin)

What is the rationale for using an albumin-furosemide "sandwich"?

Albumin will pull interstitial fluid into the intravascular space and the furosemide will then help excrete the fluid as urine

An elderly patient goes into CHF (congestive heart failure) on POD #3 after a laparotomy. What is going on?

Mobilization of the "third-space" fluid into the intravascular space, resulting in fluid overload and resultant CHF (but also must rule out MI)

What fluid is used to replace NGT (gastric) aspirate?

D5 1/2 NS with 20 KCl

What electrolyte is associated with succinycholine?

Hyperkalemia

Chapter 19

Blood and Blood Products

Define the following terms:

PT

Prothrombin Time: Tests extrinsic coagulation pathway

PTT

Partial Thromboplastin Time: Tests intrinsic coagulation pathway

INR

International Normalized Ratio (reports PT results)

Packed red blood cells (PRBCs)

One unit equals ≈300 ml (±50 ml); no platelets or clotting factors; can be mixed with NS to infuse faster

Platelets

Replace platelets with units of platelets (6–10 units from single donor or random donors)

Fresh frozen plasma (FFP)

Replaces **clotting factors;** (no RBCs/WBCs/platelets)

Cryoprecipitate (cryo)

Replaces fibrinogen, von Willebrand factor, and some clotting factors

Which electrolyte is most likely to fall with the infusion of stored blood? Why?

Ionized calcium; the citrate preservative used for the storage of blood binds serum calcium

What changes occur in the storage of PRBCs?

$\downarrow Ca^+$, $\uparrow K^+$, $\downarrow$ 2,3-DPG, $\uparrow H^+$ ($\downarrow$ pH), $\downarrow$ PMNs

What are general guidelines for blood transfusion?

Acute blood loss, Hgb <10, and history of CAD/COPD **or** healthy symptomatic patient with Hgb <7

What is the rough formula for converting Hgb to Hct?

Hgb × 3 = Hct

One unit of PRBC increases Hct by how much?

≈3% to 4%

Which blood type is the "universal" donor for PRBCs?

O negative

Which blood type is the "universal" donor for FFP?

AB

What is a type and screen?

Patient's blood type is determined and the blood is screened for antibodies; a type and cross from that sample can then be ordered if needed later

What is a type and cross?

Patient's blood is sent to the blood bank and cross-matched for **specific donor units for possible blood transfusion**

Define thrombocytopenia.

Low platelet count (<100,000)

What are the common causes of thrombocytopenia in the surgical patient?

Sepsis, H_2 blockers, heparin, massive transfusion, DIC, antibiotics, spurious lab value, Swann-Ganz catheter

What can be given to help correct platelet dysfunction from uremia, aspirin, or bypass?

DDAVP (desmopressin)

What common medication causes platelets to irreversibly malfunction?

Aspirin (inhibits cyclooxygenase)

What is Plavix®?

Clopidogrel—irreversibly inhibits platelet $P2Y_{12}$ ADP receptor (blocks fibrin crosslinking of platelets)

What platelet count is associated with spontaneous bleeding?

<20,000

What should the platelet count be before surgery?

>50,000

When should "prophylactic" platelet transfusions be given?

With platelets <10,000 (old recommendation was 20,000)

What is microcytic anemia "until proven otherwise" in a man or postmenopausal woman?

Colon cancer

Why not infuse PRBCs with lactated Ringer's?

Calcium in LR may result in coagulation within the IV line (use NS)

For how long can packed RBCs be stored?

About 6 weeks (42 days)

What is the most common cause of transfusion hemolysis?

ABO incompatibility as a result of **clerical error**

What is the risk of receiving a unit of blood infected with HIV?

$\approx$1 in 1,000,000

What are the symptoms of a transfusion reaction?

Fever, chills, nausea, hypotension, lumbar pain, chest pain, abnormal bleeding

What is the treatment for transfusion hemolysis?

Stop transfusion; provide fluids; perform diuresis (Lasix) to protect kidneys; alkalinize urine (bicarbonate); give pressors as needed

What component of the blood transfusion can cause a fever?

WBCs

What is the transfusion "trigger" Hct in young healthy patients?

21%

What is the widely considered "optimal" Hct in a patient with a history of heart disease or stroke?

$\approx$30%

When should aspirin administration be discontinued preoperatively?

At 1 week because platelets live 7 to 10 days (must use judgment if patient is at risk for stroke or MI; it may be better to continue and use excellent surgical hemostasis in these patients)

What can move the oxyhemoglobin dissociation curve to the right?	Acidosis, 2,3-DPG, fever, elevated P_{CO_2} (to the right means greater ability to release the O_2 to the tissues)
What is the normal life of RBCs?	120 days
What is the normal life of platelets?	7 to 10 days
What factor is deficient in hemophilia A?	Factor VIII
How can the clotting factor for hemophilia A be remembered?	Think: "**Eight**" sounds like "**A**"
What is the preoperative treatment of hemophilia A?	Factor VIII infusion to ≥100% normal preoperative levels
What coagulation study is elevated with hemophilia A?	PTT
How do you remember which coagulation study is affected by the hemophilias?	There are two major hemophilias and two t's in PTT
What factor is deficient in hemophilia B?	Factor IX
How do you remember which factors are deficient with hemophilia A and hemophilia B?	Think alphabetically and chronologically: **A** before **B**—**8** before **9** Hemophilia **A** = factor **VIII** Hemophilia **B** = factor **IX**
How are hemophilias A and B inherited?	Sex-linked recessive
What is von Willebrand's disease?	Deficiency of von Willebrand factor (vWF) and factor VIII:C
How is von Willebrand's disease inherited?	Autosomal dominant
What is used to correct von Willebrand's disease?	DDAVP or cryoprecipitate

What coagulation is abnormal with the following disorders:	
Hemophilia A	PTT (elevated)
Hemophilia B	PTT (elevated)
von Willebrand's disease	Bleeding time
What is the effect on the coagulation system if the patient has a deficiency in protein C, protein S, or antithrombin III?	A **hyper**coagulable state
What is a "left shift" on a CBC?	Juvenile polymorphonuclear leukocytes (bands); legend has it that the old counters for all the blood cells had the lever for bands on the LEFT of the counter
What is the usual "therapeutic" PT?	With coumadin, usually shoot for an INR of 2.0–3.0
What is the acronym basis for the word WARFARIN?	**W**isconsin **A**lumni **R**esearch **F**oundation-**ARIN**
What is the most common inherited hypercoagulable state?	Factor V Leiden (Think: **LE**iden = **LE**ader)
What is Xigris®?	Activated protein C, which is used in severe sepsis

---

Chapter 20

Surgical Hemostasis

What motto is associated with surgical hemostasis?	"All bleeding stops"
What is the most immediate method to obtain hemostasis?	Pressure (finger)

What is the "Bovie"?

Electrocautery (designed by Bovie with Cushing for neurosurgery in the 1920s)

What is the CUT mode on the Bovie?

Continuous electrical current (20,000 Hz); cuts well with a decreased ability to coagulate

What is the COAG mode on the Bovie?

Intermittent electrical current (20,000 Hz); results in excellent vessel coagulation with decreased ability to cut

Where should a Bovie be applied to a clamp or pick-up to coagulate a vessel?

Anywhere on the clamp/pick-up

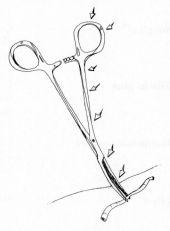

Should you ever "blindly" place a clamp in a wound to stop bleeding?

No, you may injure surrounding tissues such as nerves

Define the following terms:
   Figure-of-eight suture

Suture ligature placed **twice** in the tissue prior to being tied

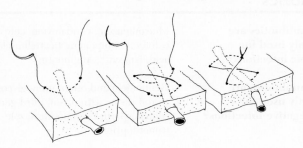

Vessel "tied in continuity"   Tie, tie, cut in between

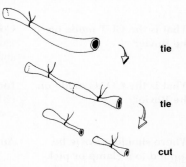

tie

tie

cut

Surgicel®   Cellulose sheets—act as a framework for clotting factors/platelets to adhere to (Think: SurgiCEL = CELlulose)

Fibrin glue   Fibrinogen and thrombin sprayed simultaneously and mixed to produce a fibrin "glue"

Harmonic scalpel   Ultrasonic scalpel that vibrates >50,000 times per second; seals vessels and cuts tissue

Clips   Metallic clips for clipping vessels

Chapter 21

Common Surgical Medications

ANTIBIOTICS

Which antibiotics are commonly used for anaerobic infections?   Metronidazole, clindamycin, cefoxitin, cefotetan, imipenem, ticarcillin-clavulanic acid, Unasyn®, Augmentin®

Which antibiotics are commonly used for gram-negative infections?   Gentamicin and other aminoglycosides, ciprofloxacin, aztreonam, third-generation cephalosporins, sulfamethoxazole-trimethoprim

Which antibiotic, if taken with alcohol, will produce a disulfiram-like reaction?

Metronidazole (Flagyl®) (disulfiram is Antabuse®)

What is the drug of choice for treating amoebic infections?

Metronidazole (Flagyl®)

Which antibiotic is associated with cholestasis?

Ceftriaxone (Rocephin®)

Which antibiotic cannot be given to children or pregnant women?

Ciprofloxacin (interferes with the growth plate)

With which common antibiotics must serum levels be determined?

Aminoglycosides and vancomycin

Is rash (only) in response to penicillins a contraindication to cephalosporins?

No, but breathing problems, urticaria, and edema in response to penicillins are contraindications to the cephalosporins

Describe the following medications:

   Augmentin®

Amoxicillin and clavulanic acid

   Unasyn®

Ampicillin and sulbactam

   Cefazolin (Ancef®)

First-generation cephalosporin; surgical prophylaxis for **skin flora**

   Cefoxitin (Mefoxin®)

Second-generation cephalosporin; used for mixed aerobic/anaerobic infections; effective against *Bacteroides fragilis* and anaerobic bacteria

   Ceftazidime (Ceftaz®)

Third-generation cephalosporin; strong activity against *Pseudomonas*

   Clindamycin

Strong activity against gram-negative **anaerobes** such as *B. fragilis*; adequate gram-positive activity

Gentamicin

Aminoglycoside used to treat **gram-negative** bacteria; nephrotoxic, ototoxic; blood peak/trough levels should be monitored

Imipenem and cilastatin (Primaxin®)

Often used as a last resort against serious, multiresistant organisms
Usually combined with cilastin, which inhibits renal excretion of imipenem
Has a very wide spectrum

Metronidazole (Flagyl®)

Used for serious **anaerobic** infections (e.g., diverticulitis); also used to treat amebiasis; patient must abstain from alcohol use during therapy

Nafcillin (Nafcil®)

Antistaphylococcal penicillin commonly used for cellulitis

Vancomycin

Used to treat methicillin-resistant *Staphylococcus aureus* (MRSA); used orally to treat *C. difficile* pseudomembranous colitis (poorly absorbed from the gut); with IV administration, peak/trough levels should be monitored

Ciprofloxacin (Cipro®)

Quinoline antibiotic with broad-spectrum activity, especially against gram-negative bacteria, including *Pseudomonas*

Aztreonam (Azactam®)

Monobactam with gram-negative spectrum

Amphotericin

IV antifungal antibiotic associated with renal toxicity, hypokalemia

Fluconazole (Diflucan®)

Antifungal agent (IV or PO) **not** associated with renal toxicity

Nystatin

PO and topical antifungal

STEROIDS

What are the side effects?	Adrenal suppression, immunosuppression, weight gain with central obesity, cushingoid facies, acne, hirsutism, purple striae, hyperglycemia, sodium retention/hypokalemia, hypertension, osteopenia, myopathy, ischemic bone necrosis (avascular necrosis of the hip), GI perforations
What are its uses?	Immunosuppression (transplant), autoimmune diseases, hormone replacement (Addison's disease), spinal cord trauma, COPD
Can steroids be stopped abruptly?	**No, steroids should never be stopped abruptly; always taper**
Which patients need stress-dose steroids before surgery?	Those who are on steroids, were on steroids in the past year, have suspected hypoadrenalism, or are about to undergo adrenalectomy
What is the "stress dose" for steroids?	**100** mg of hydrocortisone IV every 8 hours and then taper (adults)
Which vitamin helps counteract the deleterious effects of steroids on wound healing?	Vitamin A

HEPARIN

Describe the action.	Heparin binds with and activates antithrombin III
What are its uses?	Prophylaxis/treatment—DVT, pulmonary embolism, stroke, atrial fibrillation, acute arterial occlusion, cardiopulmonary bypass
What are the side effects?	Bleeding complications; can cause thrombocytopenia
What reverses the effects?	**Protamine IV (1:100, 1** mg of protamine to every **100** units of heparin)

What laboratory test should be used to follow effect?	aPTT—activated partial thromboplastin time
What is the standard lab target for therapeutic heparinization?	1.5–2.5 times control or measured antifactor X level
Who is at risk for a protamine anaphylactic reaction?	Patients with type 1 diabetes mellitus, s/p prostate surgery
What is the half-life of heparin?	≈90 minutes (1–2 hours)
How long before surgery should it be discontinued?	From 4 to 6 hours preoperatively
Does heparin dissolve clots?	No; it stops the progression of clot formation and allows the body's own fibrinolytic systems to dissolve the clot
What is LMWH?	**L**ow **M**olecular **W**eight **H**eparin
What laboratory test do you need to follow LMWH?	None, except in children, patients with obesity, and those with renal failure, which is the major advantage of LMWH (check factor X levels)

WARFARIN (COUMADIN®)

ACRONYM basis for name?	**W**isconsin **A**lumni **R**esearch **F**oundation
Describe its action.	**Inhibits vitamin K–dependent clotting factors II, VII, IX,** and **X,** (i.e., 2, 7, 9 and 10 [Think: 2 + 7 = 9 and 10]), produced in the liver
What are its uses?	Long-term anticoagulation (PO)
What are its associated risks?	Bleeding complications, teratogenic in pregnancy, skin necrosis, dermatitis
What laboratory test should be used to follow its effect?	PT (prothrombin time) as reported as INR
What is INR?	**I**nternational **N**ormalized **R**atio

What is the classic therapeutic INR?

INR of 2–3

What is the half-life of effect?

40 hours; thus, it takes about 2 days to observe a change in the PT

What reverses the action?

Cessation, vitamin K, fresh-frozen plasma (in emergencies)

How long before surgery should it be discontinued?

From 3 to 5 days preoperatively and IV heparin should be begun; heparin should be discontinued from 4 to 6 hours preoperatively and can be restarted postoperatively; Coumadin® can be restarted in a few days

How can warfarin cause skin necrosis when first started?

Initially depressed protein C and S result in a HYPERcoagulable state! Avoid by using heparin concomitantly when starting

MISCELLANEOUS AGENTS

Describe the following drugs:

Sucralfate (Carafate®)

Treats peptic ulcers by forming an acid-resistant barrier; binds to ulcer craters; needs acid to activate and thus should not be used with H_2 blockers

Cimetidine (Tagamet®)

H_2 blocker (ulcers/gastritis)

Ranitidine (Zantac®)

H_2 blocker (ulcers/gastritis)

Ondansetron (Zofran®)

Antinausea
Anti-emetic

PPI

Proton-**P**ump **I**nhibitor: Gastric acid–secretion inhibitor; works by inhibiting the K^+/H^+-ATPase (e.g., omeprazole [Prilosec®])

Promethazine (Phenergan®)

Acute antinausea agent; used postoperatively

Metoclopramide (Reglan®)	Increases gastric emptying with increase in LES pressure; **dopamine antagonist;** used in diabetic gastroparesis and to help move feeding tubes past the pylorus
Haloperidol (Haldol®)	Sedative/antipsychotic (side effects = extrapyramidal symptoms, QT prolongation)
Ondansetron (Zofran®)	Anti-emetic/serotonin receptor blocker
Albumin	5% albumin 25% albumin—draws extravascular fluid into intravascular space by oncotic pressure
Albuterol	Inhaled β_2 agonist (bronchodilator)
Octreotide	Somatostatin analog
Famotidine (Pepcid®)	H_2 blocker
Aspirin	Irreversibly inhibits platelets by irreversibly inhibiting cyclooxygenase
Furosemide (Lasix®)	Loop diuretic (watch for hypokalemia)
Dantrolene (Dantrium®)	Medication used to treat malignant hyperthermia
Misoprostol (Cytotec®)	Prostaglandin E_1 analog Gastroduodenal mucosal protection
What is an antibiotic option for colon/appendectomy coverage if the patient is allergic to penicillin?	1. IV ciprofloxacin (Cipro) AND 2. IV clindamycin or IV Flagyl
If the patient does not respond to a dose of furosemide, should the dose be repeated, increased, or decreased?	Dose should be doubled if there is no response to the initial dose

What medication is used to treat promethazine-induced dystonia?	Diphenhydramine hydrochloride IV (Benadryl®)
Which medication is classically associated with mesenteric ischemia?	Digitalis
What type of antihypertensive medication is contraindicated in patients with renal artery stenosis?	ACE inhibitors
Does acetaminophen (Tylenol®) inhibit platelets?	No
What medications are used to stop seizures?	Benzodiazepines (e.g., lorazepam [Ativan®]); phenytoin (Dilantin®)

List examples of preop antibiotics for:

Vascular prosthetic graft	Ancef® (gram-positive coverage)
Appendectomy	Cefoxitin, Unasyn® (anaerobic coverage)
Colon surgery	Cefoxitin, Unasyn® (anaerobic coverage)

NARCOTICS

What are common postoperative IV narcotics?	Morphine (most common), meperidine (Demerol®), fentanyl, Percocet®, Dilaudid®
What is Percocet®	PO narcotic pain reliever with acetaminophen and oxycodone
What is Demerol's claim to fame?	Used commonly with acute pancreatitis/ biliary pathology because classically morphine may cause sphincter of Oddi spasm/constriction
What are side effects of narcotics?	Respiratory depression, hypotension, itching, bradycardia, nausea

What is the danger of prolonged use of Demerol?	Accumulation of metabolite norme-peridine (especially with renal/hepatic dysfunction), which may result in oversedation, hallucinations, and seizures!
What medication reverses the effects of narcotic overdose?	Naloxone (Narcan®), 0.4 mg IV
Narcotic used to decrease postoperative shivering?	Demerol®

MISCELLANEOUS

What reverses the effects of benzodiazepines?	Flumazenil (Romazicon®), 0.2 mg IV
What is Toradol®?	Ketorolac = IV NSAID
What are the risks of Toradol®?	GI bleed, renal injury, platelet dysfunction
Why give patients IV Cipro if they are eating a regular diet?	No reason—500 mg of Cipro PO gives the same serum level as 400 mg Cipro IV! And PO is much cheaper!
What is clonidine "rebound"?	Abruptly stopping clonidine can cause the patient to have severe "rebound" hypertension (also seen with β-blockers)

Chapter 22   Complications

ATELECTASIS

What is it?	Collapse of the alveoli
What is the etiology?	Inadequate alveolar expansion (e.g., poor ventilation of lungs during surgery, inability to fully inspire secondary to pain), high levels of inspired oxygen

What are the signs?	Fever, decreased breath sounds with rales, tachypnea, tachycardia, and increased density on CXR
What are the risk factors?	Chronic obstructive pulmonary disease (COPD), smoking, abdominal or thoracic surgery, oversedation, poor pain control **(patient cannot breathe deeply secondary to pain on inspiration)**
What is its claim to fame?	Most common cause of fever during PODs #1 to #2
What prophylactic measures can be taken?	Preoperative smoking cessation, incentive spirometry, good pain control
What is the treatment?	Postoperative **incentive spirometry,** deep breathing, coughing, early ambulation, NT suctioning, and chest PT

POSTOPERATIVE RESPIRATORY FAILURE

What is it?	Respiratory impairment with increased respiratory rate, shortness of breath, dyspnea
What is the differential diagnosis?	Hypovolemia, pulmonary embolism, administration of supplemental O_2 to a patient with COPD, atelectasis, pneumonia, aspiration, pulmonary edema, abdominal compartment syndrome, pneumothorax, chylothorax, hemothorax, narcotic overdose, mucous plug
What is the treatment?	Supplemental O_2, chest PT; suctioning, intubation, and ventilation if necessary
What is the initial workup?	ABG, CXR, EKG, pulse oximetry, and auscultation
What are the indications for intubation and ventilation?	Cannot protect airway (unconscious), excessive work of breathing, progressive **hypoxemia** (PaO_2 <55 despite supplemental O_2), progressive **acidosis** (pH <7.3 and PCO_2 >50), RR >35

What are the possible causes of postoperative pleural effusion?	Fluid overload, pneumonia, and diaphragmatic inflammation with possible subphrenic abscess formation
What is the treatment of postoperative wheezing?	Albuterol nebulizer
Why may it be dangerous to give a patient with chronic COPD supplemental oxygen?	This patient uses relative hypoxia for respiratory drive, and supplemental O_2 may remove this drive!

PULMONARY EMBOLISM

What is a pulmonary embolism (PE)?	DVT that embolizes to the pulmonary arterial system
What is DVT?	**D**eep **V**enous **T**hrombosis—a clot forming in the pelvic or lower extremity veins
Is DVT more common in the right or left iliac vein?	Left is more common (4:1) because the aortic bifurcation crosses and possibly compresses the left iliac vein
What are the signs/symptoms of DVT?	Lower extremity pain, swelling, tenderness, Homan's sign, PE Up to 50% can be asymptomatic!
What is Homan's sign?	Calf pain with dorsiflexion of the foot seen classically with DVT, but actually found in fewer than one third of patients with DVT
What test is used to evaluate for DVT?	Duplex ultrasonography
What is Virchow's triad?	1. Stasis 2. Endothelial injury 3. Hypercoagulable state (risk factors for thrombosis)
What are the risk factors for DVT and PE?	Postoperative status, multiple trauma, paralysis, immobility, CHF, obesity, BCP/tamoxifen, cancer, advanced age, polycythemia, MI, HIT syndrome, hypercoagulable state (protein C/protein S deficiency)

What are the signs/symptoms of PE?

Shortness of breath, tachypnea, hypotension, CP, occasionally fever, loud pulmonic component of S2, hemoptysis with pulmonary infarct

What are the associated lab findings?

ABG—decreased PO_2 and PCO_2 (from hyperventilation)

Which diagnostic tests are indicated?

CT angiogram, V-Q scan (ventilation-perfusion scan), pulmonary angiogram is the gold standard

What are the associated CXR findings?

1. Westermark's sign (wedge-shaped area of decreased pulmonary vasculature resulting in hyperlucency)
2. Opacity with base at pleural edge from pulmonary infarction

What are the associated EKG findings?

>50% are abnormal; classic finding is cor pulmonale (S1Q3T3 RBBB and right-axis deviation); EKG most commonly shows flipped T waves or ST depression

What is a "saddle" embolus?

PE that "straddles" the pulmonary artery and is in the lumen of both the right and left pulmonary arteries

What is the treatment if the patient is stable?

Anticoagulation (heparin followed by long-term [3–6 months] Coumadin®) or Greenfield filter

What is a Greenfield filter?

Metallic filter placed into IVC via jugular vein to catch emboli prior to lodging in the pulmonary artery

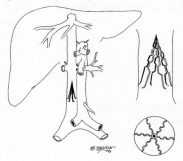

Where did Dr. Greenfield get the idea for his IVC filter?	Oil pipeline filters!
When is a Greenfield filter indicated?	If anticoagulation is contraindicated or patient has further PE on adequate anticoagulation or is high risk (e.g., pelvic and femur fractures)
What is the treatment if the patient's condition is unstable?	Consider thrombolytic therapy; consult thoracic surgeon for possible Trendelenburg operation; consider catheter suction embolectomy
What is the Trendelenburg operation?	Pulmonary artery embolectomy
What is a "retrievable" IVC filter?	IVC filter that can be removed ("retrieved")
What percentage of retrievable IVC filter are actually removed?	Only about 20%
What prophylactic measures can be taken for DVT/PE?	LMWH (Lovenox®) 40 mg SQ QD; **or** 30 mg SQ b.i.d.; subQ heparin (5000 units subQ every 8 hrs; must be started preoperatively), sequential compression device BOOTS beginning in O.R. (often used with subQ heparin), early ambulation

ASPIRATION PNEUMONIA

What is it?	Pneumonia following aspiration of vomitus
What are the risk factors?	Intubation/extubation, impaired consciousness (e.g., drug or EtOH overdose), dysphagia (esophageal disease), nonfunctioning NGT, Trendelenburg position, emergent intubation with full stomach, gastric dilatation
What are the signs/ symptoms?	Respiratory failure, CP, increased sputum production, fever, cough, mental status changes, tachycardia, cyanosis, infiltrate on CXR

What are the associated CXR findings?	Early—fluffy infiltrate or normal CXR Late—pneumonia, ARDS
Which lobes are commonly involved?	Supine—RUL Sitting/semirecumbent—RLL
Which organisms are commonly involved?	Community acquired—gram-positive/ mixed Hospital/ICU—gram-negative rods
Which diagnostic tests are indicated?	CXR, sputum, Gram stain, sputum culture, bronchoalveolar lavage
What is the treatment?	Bronchoscopy, antibiotics if pneumonia develops, intubation if respiratory failure occurs, ventilation with PEEP if ARDS develops
What is Mendelson's syndrome?	Chemical pneumonitis secondary to aspiration of stomach contents (i.e., gastric acid)
Are prophylatic antibiotics indicated for aspiration pneumonitis?	NO

GASTROINTESTINAL COMPLICATIONS

What are possible NGT complications?	Aspiration-pneumonia/atelectasis (especially if NGT is clogged) Sinusitis Minor UGI bleeding Epistaxis Pharyngeal irritation, gastric irritation

GASTRIC DILATATION

What are the risk factors?	Abdominal surgery, gastric outlet obstruction, splenectomy, narcotics
What are the signs/ symptoms?	Abdominal distension, hiccups, electrolyte abnormalities, nausea
What is the treatment?	NGT decompression

What do you do if you have a patient with high NGT output?	Check high abdominal x-ray and, if the NGT is in duodenum, pull back the NGT into the stomach

POSTOPERATIVE PANCREATITIS

What is it?	Pancreatitis resulting from manipulation of the pancreas during surgery or low blood flow during the procedure (i.e., cardiopulmonary bypass), gallstones, hypercalcemia, medications, idiopathic
What lab tests are performed?	Amylase and lipase
What is the initial treatment?	Same as that for the other causes of pancreatitis (e.g., NPO, aggressive fluid resuscitation, ± NGT PRN)

CONSTIPATION

What are the postoperative causes?	Narcotics, immobility
What is the treatment?	OBR
What is OBR?	**O**rtho **B**owel **R**outine: docusate sodium (daily), dicacodyl suppository if no bowel movement occurs, Fleet® enema if suppository is ineffective

SHORT BOWEL SYNDROME

What is it?	Malabsorption and diarrhea resulting from extensive bowel resection (≤120 cm of small bowel remaining)
What is the initial treatment?	TPN early, followed by many small meals chronically

POSTOPERATIVE SMALL BOWEL OBSTRUCTION (SBO)/ILEUS

What causes SBO?	**Adhesions** (most of which resolve spontaneously), incarcerated hernia (internal or fascial/dehiscence)

What causes ileus?   Laparotomy, hypokalemia or narcotics,
                                           intraperitoneal infection

**What are the signs of   Flatus PR, stool PR
resolving ileus/SBO?**

What is the order of recovery   **First—small intestine
of bowel function after   **Second**—stomach
abdominal surgery?**   **Third**—colon

**When can a postoperative   From 12 to 24 postoperative hours
patient be fed through a   because the small intestine recovers
J-tube?**   function first in that period

JAUNDICE

**What are the causes of the
following types of
postoperative jaundice:**
   Prehepatic   Hemolysis (prosthetic valve), resolving
                                           hematoma, transfusion reaction,
                                           postcardiopulmonary bypass, blood
                                           transfusions (decreased RBC compliance
                                           leading to cell rupture)

   Hepatic   **Drugs,** hypotension, hypoxia, sepsis,
                                           hepatitis, "sympathetic" hepatic
                                           inflammation from adjacent right lower
                                           lobe infarction of the lung or pneumonia,
                                           preexisting cirrhosis, right-sided heart
                                           failure, hepatic abscess, pylephlebitis
                                           (thrombosis of portal vein), Gilbert
                                           syndrome, Crigler-Najjar syndrome,
                                           Dubin-Johnson syndrome, fatty infiltrate
                                           from TPN

   Posthepatic   Choledocholithiasis, stricture, cholangitis,
                                           cholecystitis, biliary-duct injury,
                                           pancreatitis, sclerosing cholangitis, tumors
                                           (e.g., cholangiocarcinoma, pancreatic
                                           cancer, gallbladder cancer, metastases),
                                           biliary stasis (e.g., ceftriaxone [Rocephin®])

What blood test results would   **Decreased—Haptoglobin, Hct
support the assumption that   **Increased**—LDH, reticulocytes
hemolysis was causing   Also, fragmented RBCs on a peripheral
jaundice in a patient?**   smear

BLIND LOOP SYNDROME

What is it?	Bacterial overgrowth in the small intestine
What are the causes?	Anything that disrupts the normal flow of intestinal contents (i.e., causes stasis)
What are the surgical causes of B12 deficiency?	Blind loop syndrome, gastrectomy (decreased secretion of intrinsic factor) and excision of the terminal ileum (site of B12 absorption)

POSTVAGOTOMY DIARRHEA

What is it?	Diarrhea after a truncal vagotomy
What is the cause?	It is thought that after truncal vagotomy, a rapid transport of bile salts to the colon results in osmotic inhibition of water absorption in the colon, leading to diarrhea

DUMPING SYNDROME

What is it?	Delivery of **hyperosmotic** chyme to the small intestine causing massive fluid shifts into the bowel (normally the stomach will decrease the osmolality of the chyme prior to its emptying)
With what conditions is it associated?	Any procedure that bypasses the pylorus or compromises its function (i.e., gastroenterostomies or pyloroplasty); thus, "dumping" of chyme into small intestine
What are the signs/ symptoms?	Postprandial diaphoresis, tachycardia, abdominal pain/distention, emesis, increased flatus, dizziness, weakness
How is the diagnosis made?	History; hyperosmolar glucose load will elicit similar symptoms
What is the medical treatment?	Small, multiple, low-fat/carbohydrate meals that are high in protein content; also, **avoidance of liquids** with meals to slow gastric emptying; surgery is a last resort

What is the surgical treatment?	Conversion to Roux-en-Y ($\pm$ reversed jejunal interposition loop)
What is a reversed jejunal interposition loop?	Segment of jejunum is cut and then reversed to allow for a short segment of reversed peristalsis to slow intestinal transit

ENDOCRINE COMPLICATIONS

DIABETIC KETOACIDOSIS (DKA)

What is it?	Deficiency of body insulin, resulting in hyperglycemia, formation of ketoacids, osmotic diuresis, and metabolic acidosis
What are the signs of DKA?	Polyuria, tachypnea, dehydration, confusion, abdominal pain
What are the associated lab values?	Elevated glucose, increased anion gap, hypokalemia, urine ketones, acidosis
What is the treatment?	Insulin drip, IVF rehydration, K^+ supplementation, $\pm$ bicarbonate IV
What electrolyte must be monitored closely in DKA?	Potassium and HYPOkalemia (Remember correction of acidosis and GLC/insulin drive K^+ into cells and are treatment for HYPERkalemia!)
What must you rule out in a diabetic with DKA?	Infection (perirectal abscess is classically missed!)

ADDISONIAN CRISIS

What is it?	Acute adrenal insufficiency in the face of a stressor (i.e., surgery, trauma, infection)
How can you remember what it is?	Think: **ADD**isonian = **AD**renal **D**own
What is the cause?	Postoperatively, inadequate cortisol release usually results from steroid administration in the past year

What are the signs/ symptoms?	Tachycardia, nausea, vomiting, diarrhea, **abdominal pain,** ± fever, progressive lethargy, **hypotension, eventual hypovolemic shock**
What is its clinical claim to infamy?	Tachycardia and hypotension refractory to IVF and pressors!
Which lab values are classic?	Decreased Na^+, increased K^+ (secondary to decreased aldosterone)
How can the electrolytes with ADDisonian = ADrenal Down be remembered?	Think: **DOWN** the alphabetical electrolyte stairs

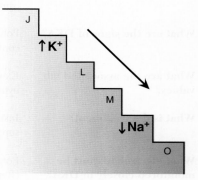

What is the treatment?	IVFs (D5 NS), hydrocortisone IV, fludrocortisone PO
What is fludrocortisone?	Mineralocorticoid replacement (aldosterone)

SIADH

What is it?	**S**yndrome of **I**nappropriate **A**nti**D**iuretic **H**ormone (ADH) secretion (think of **inappropriate increase** in ADH secretion)
What does ADH do?	ADH increases NaCl and H_2O resorption in the kidney, increasing intravascular volume (released from posterior pituitary)

| What are the causes? | **Mainly lung**/CNS: CNS trauma, oat-cell lung cancer, pancreatic cancer, duodenal cancer, pneumonia/lung abscess, increased PEEP, stroke, general anesthesia, idiopathic, postoperative, morphine |

What are the associated lab findings?

Low sodium, low chloride, low serum osmolality; increased urine osmolality

How can the serum sodium level in SIADH be remembered?

Remember, **SIADH** = **S**odium **I**s **A**lways **D**own **H**ere = hyponatremia

What is the treatment?

Treat the primary cause and restrict fluid intake

DIABETES INSIPIDUS (DI)

What is it?

Failure of ADH renal fluid conservation resulting in dilute urine in large amounts (Think: **DI** = **D**ecreased ADH)

What is the source of ADH?

POSTERIOR pituitary

What are the two major types?

1. Central (neurogenic) DI
2. Nephrogenic DI

What is the mechanism of the two types?

1. Central DI = decreased production of ADH
2. Nephrogenic DI = decreased ADH effect on kidney

What are the classic causes of central DI?

BRAIN injury, tumor, surgery, and infection

What are the classic causes of nephrogenic DI?

Amphotericin B, hypercalcemia, and chronic kidney infection

What lab values are associated with DI?

HYPERnatremia, decreased urine sodium, decreased urine osmolality, and increased serum osmolality

What is the treatment?

Fluid replacement; follow NA^+ levels and urine output; central DI warrants vasopressin; nephrogenic DI may respond to thiazide diuretics

CARDIOVASCULAR COMPLICATIONS

What are the arterial line complications?	Infection; thrombosis, which can lead to finger/hand necrosis; death/hemorrhage from catheter disconnection (remember to perform and document the **Allen test** before inserting an arterial line or obtaining a blood gas sample)
What is an Allen test?	Measures for adequate collateral blood flow to the hand via the ulnar artery:
	Patient clenches fist; clinician occludes radial and ulnar arteries; patient opens fist and clinician releases only the ulnar artery
	If the palm exhibits immediate strong blush upon release of ulnar artery, then ulnar artery can be assumed to have adequate collateral flow if the radial artery were to thrombose
What are the common causes of dyspnea following central line placement?	Pneumothorax, pericardial tamponade, carotid puncture (which can cause a hematoma that compresses the trachea), air embolism
What is the differential diagnosis of postoperative chest pain?	MI, atelectasis, pneumonia, pleurisy, esophageal reflux, PE, musculoskeletal pain, subphrenic abscess, aortic dissection, pneumo/chyle/hemothorax, gastritis
What is the differential diagnosis of postoperative atrial fibrillation?	**Fluid overload, PE, MI, pain** (excess catecholamines), atelectasis, pneumonia, digoxin toxicity, hypoxemia, thyrotoxicosis, hypercapnia, idiopathic, acidosis, electrolyte abnormalities

MYOCARDIAL INFARCTION (MI)

What is the most dangerous period for a postoperative MI following a previous MI?	Six months after an MI
What are the risk factors for postoperative MI?	History of MI, angina, Qs on EKG, S3, JVD, CHF, aortic stenosis, advanced age, extensive surgical procedure, MI within 6 months, EKG changes

How do postoperative MIs present?	**Often without chest pain** New onset **CHF,** new onset **cardiac dysrhythmia,** hypotension, chest pain, tachypnea, tachycardia, nausea/vomiting, bradycardia, neck pain, arm pain
What EKG findings are associated with cardiac ischemia/MI?	Flipped T waves, ST elevation, ST depression, dysrhythmias (e.g., new onset A fib, PVC, V tach)
Which lab tests are indicated?	Troponin I, cardiac isoenzymes (elevated CK mb fraction)
What is the treatment of postoperative MI?	Nitrates (paste or drip), as tolerated Aspirin Oxygen Pain control with IV morphine β-blocker, as tolerated Heparin (possibly; thrombolytics are contraindicated in the postoperative patient) ICU monitoring
How can the treatment of postoperative MI be remembered?	**"BEMOAN":** **BE**ta-blocker (as tolerated) **M**orphine **O**xygen **A**spirin **N**itrates
When do postoperative MIs occur?	Two thirds occur on PODs #2 to #5 (often silent and present with **dyspnea** or **dysrhythmia**)

POSTOPERATIVE CVA

What is a CVA?	**C**erebro**V**ascular **A**ccident (stroke)
What are the signs/symptoms?	Aphasia, motor/sensory deficits usually lateralizing
What is the workup?	Head CT scan; must rule out hemorrhage if anticoagulation is going to be used; carotid Doppler ultrasound study to evaluate for carotid occlusive disease

What is the treatment?	ASA, ± heparin if feasible postoperatively Thrombolytic therapy is not usually postoperative option
What is the perioperative prevention?	Avoid hypotension; continue aspirin therapy preoperatively in high-risk patients if feasible; preoperative carotid Doppler study in high-risk patients

MISCELLANEOUS

POSTOPERATIVE RENAL FAILURE

What is it?	Increase in serum creatinine and decrease in creatinine clearance; usually associated with decreased urine output
Define the following terms:	
Anuria	<50 cc urine output in 24 hours
Oliguria	Between 50 cc and 400 cc of urine output in 24 hours
What is the differential diagnosis?	
Prerenal	**Inadequate blood perfusing kidney:** inadequate fluids, hypotension, cardiac pump failure (CHF)
Renal	**Kidney parenchymal dysfunction:** acute tubular necrosis, nephrotoxic contrast or drugs
Postrenal	**Obstruction to outflow of urine from kidney:** Foley catheter obstruction/stone, ureteral/urethral injury, BPH, bladder dysfunction (e.g., medications, spinal anesthesia)
What is the workup?	Lab tests: electrolytes, BUN, Cr, urine lytes/Cr, FENa, urinalysis, renal ultrasound
What is FENa?	**F**ractional **E**xcretion of **Na**$^+$ (sodium)

What is the formula for FENa?	"YOU NEED PEE" = UNP $(U_{Na^+} \times P_{cr} / P_{Na^+} \times U_{cr}) \times 100$ (U = urine, cr = creatinine, Na^+ = sodium, P = plasma)

Define the lab results with prerenal vs renal failure:

BUN/Cr ratio	Prerenal: >20:1 Renal: <20:1
Specific gravity	Prerenal: >1.020 (as the body tries to hold on to fluid) Renal: <1.020 (kidney has decreased ability to concentrate urine)
FENa	Prerenal: <1% Renal: >2%
Urine Na$^+$ (sodium)	Prerenal: <20 Renal: >40
Urine osmolality	Prerenal: >450 Renal: <300 mOsm/kg
What are the indications for dialysis?	Fluid overload, refractory hyperkalemia, BUN >130, acidosis, uremic complication (encephalopathy, pericardial effusion)

DIC

What is it?	Activation of the coagulation cascade leading to **thrombosis** and **consumption** of clotting factors and platelets and activation of fibrinolytic system (fibrinolysis), resulting in **bleeding**
What are the causes?	Tissue necrosis, septic shock, massive large-vessel coagulation, shock, allergic reactions, massive blood transfusion reaction, cardiopulmonary bypass, cancer, obstetric complications, snake bites, trauma, burn injury, prosthetic material, liver dysfunction

What are the signs/ symptoms?	Acrocyanosis or other signs of thrombosis, then diffuse bleeding from incision sites, venipuncture sites, catheter sites, or mucous membranes
What are the associated lab findings?	Increased fibrin-degradation products, elevated PT/PTT, decreased platelets, decreased fibrinogen (level correlates well with bleeding), presence of schistocytes (fragmented RBCs), increased D-dimer
What is the treatment?	**Removal of the cause;** otherwise supportive: IVFs, O$_2$, platelets, FFP, cryoprecipitate (fibrin), Epsilon-aminocaproic acid, as needed in predominantly thrombotic cases Use of heparin is indicated in cases that are predominantly thrombotic with antithrombin III supplementation as needed

ABDOMINAL COMPARTMENT SYNDROME

What is it?	Increased intra-abdominal pressure usually seen after laparotomy or after massive IVF resuscitation (e.g., burn patients)
What are the signs/ symptoms?	Tight distended abdomen, decreased urine output, increased airway pressure, **increased intra-abdominal pressure**
How to measure intra-abdominal pressure?	Read intrabladder pressure (Foley catheter hooked up to manometry after instillation of 50–100 cc of water)
What is normal intra-abdominal pressure?	<15 mm Hg
What intra-abdominal pressure indicates need for treatment?	≥25 mm Hg, especially if signs of compromise
What is the treatment?	Release the pressure by placing drain and/or decompressive laparotomy (leaving fascia open)

What is a "Bogata Bag"?	Sheet of plastic (empty urology irrigation bag or IV bag) used to temporarily close the abdomen to allow for more intra-abdominal volume

URINARY RETENTION

What is it?	Enlarged urinary bladder resulting from medications or spinal anesthesia
How is it diagnosed?	Physical exam (palpable bladder), bladder residual volume upon placement of a Foley catheter
What is the treatment?	Foley catheter
With massive bladder distention, how much urine can be drained immediately?	Most would clamp after 1 L and then drain the rest over time to avoid a vasovagal reaction
What is the classic sign of urinary retention in an elderly patient?	Confusion

WOUND INFECTION

What are the signs/ symptoms?	Erythema, swelling, pain, heat (rubor, tumor, dolor, calor)
What is the treatment?	Open wound, leave open with wet to dry dressing changes, antibiotics if cellulitis present
What is fascial dehiscence?	Acute separation of fascia that has been sutured closed
What is the treatment?	Bring back to the O.R. emergently for reclosure of the fascia

WOUND HEMATOMA

What is it?	Collection of blood (blood clot) in operative wound
What is the treatment?	Acute: Remove with hemostasis Subacute: Observe (heat helps resorption)

WOUND SEROMA

What is it?	Postoperative collection of lymph and serum in the operative wound
What is the treatment?	Needle aspiration, repeat if necessary (prevent with closed drain)

PSEUDOMEMBRANOUS COLITIS

What are the signs/ symptoms?	**Diarrhea,** fever, hypotension/tachycardia
What is the incidence of bloody diarrhea?	10%
What *classic* antibiotic causes *C. difficile*?	Clindamycin (but almost all antibiotics can cause it)
How is it diagnosed?	*C. diff* toxin in stool, fecal WBC, flex sig (see a mucous pseudomembrane in lumen of colon = hence the name)
What is the treatment?	1. Flagyl (PO or IV) 2. PO vancomycin if refractory to Flagyl
What is the indication for emergent colectomy?	Toxic megacolon

Chapter 23

Common Causes of Ward Emergencies

What can cause hypotension?	Hypovolemia (iatrogenic, hemorrhage), sepsis, MI, cardiac dysrhythmia, hypoxia, false reading (e.g., wrong cuff/arterial line twist or clot), pneumothorax, PE, cardiac tamponade, medications (e.g., morphine)

How do you act?

ABCs, examine, recheck BP, IV access, IV bolus, labs (e.g., HCT), EKG, pulse ox/vital signs monitoring, CXR, supplemental oxygen, check medications/history, give IV antibiotics "stat" if sepsis likely, compress all bleeding sites

What are the common causes of postoperative hypertension?

Pain (from catecholamine release), anxiety, hypercapnia, hypoxia (which may also cause hypotension), preexisting condition, bladder distention

What can cause hypoxia/ shortness of breath?

Atelectasis, pneumonia, mucous plug, pneumothorax, **PE**, MI/dysrhythmia, venous blood in ABG syringe, SAT% machine malfunction/probe malposition, iatrogenic (wrong ventilator settings), severe anemia/hypovolemia, low cardiac output, CHF, ARDS, fluid overload

How do you act?

ABCs, physical exam, vital signs/pulse oximetry monitoring, supplemental oxygen, IV access, ABG, EKG, CXR

What can cause mental status change?

Hypoxia until ruled out, hypotension (e.g., cardiogenic shock), hypovolemia, iatrogenic (narcotics/benzodiazepines), drug reaction, alcohol withdrawal, drug withdrawal, seizure, ICU psychosis, CVA, sepsis, metabolic derangements, intracranial bleeding, **urinary retention in the elderly**

What are the signs of alcohol withdrawal?

Confusion, tachycardia/autonomic instability, seizure, hallucinations

What are the causes of tachycardia?

Hypovolemia/third-spacing, pain, alcohol withdrawal, anxiety/agitation, urinary retention, cardiac dysrhythmia (e.g., sinoventricular tachycardia, atrial fibrillation with rapid rate), MI, PE, β-blocker withdrawal, anastomotic leak

What are the causes of decreased urine output?

Hypovolemia, urinary retention, Foley catheter malfunction, cardiac failure, MI, acute tubular necrosis (ATN), ureteral/urethral injury, abdominal compartment syndrome, sepsis

How do you act initially in a case of decreased urine output?

Examine, vital signs, check or place Foley catheter, irrigate Foley catheter, IV fluid bolus

---

Chapter 24

Surgical Respiratory Care

What is the most common cause of fever in the first 48 hours postop?

Atelectasis

What is absorption atelectasis?

Elevated inhaled oxygen replaces the nitrogen in the alveoli resulting in collapse of the air sac (atelectasis); nitrogen keeps alveoli open by "stenting" them

What is incentive spirometry?

Patient can document tidal volume and will have an "incentive" to increase it

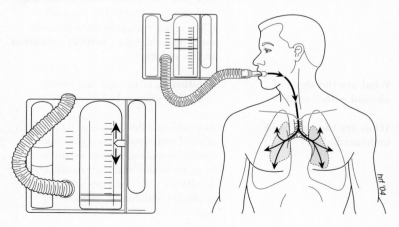

What is oxygen-induced hypoventilation?

Some patients with COPD have low oxygen as the main stimulus for the respiratory drive; if given supplemental oxygen, they will have a decreased respiratory drive and hypoventilation

Why give supplemental oxygen to a patient with a pneumothorax?

Pneumothorax is almost completely nitrogen—thus increasing the oxygen in the alveoli increases the nitrogen gradient and results in faster absorption of the pneumothorax!

What is a nonrebreather mask?

100% oxygen with a reservoir bag

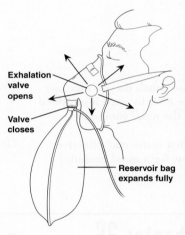

Exhalation valve opens

Valve closes

Reservoir bag expands fully

Why do nonrebreather masks have a "reservoir" bag?

Inhalation flow will exceed the delivery rate of the tubing and the bag allows for extra oxygen stores

What is the maximum oxygen FiO$_2$ delivered by a nonrebreather mask?

$\approx$80% to 90%

How do you figure out the PaO$_2$ from an O$_2$ sat?

PaO$_2$ of 40, 50, 60 roughly equals 70, 80, 90 in sats

What is an oxygen nasal cannula?

Oxygen delivered via tubing with prongs into nares

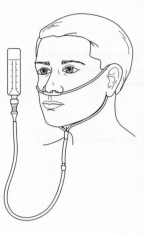

How much do you increase the FiO₂ by each liter added to the nasal cannula?

$\approx 3\%$

What is the max effective flow for a nasal cannula?

6 liters

Chapter 25

Surgical Nutrition

What is the motto of surgical nutrition?

"If the gut works, use it"

What are the normal daily dietary requirements for adults of the following:

    Protein

1 g/kg/day

    Calories

30 kcal/kg/day

By how much is basal energy expenditure (BEE) increased or decreased in the following cases:	
Severe head injury	Increased $\approx 1.7 \times$
Severe burns	Increased $\approx 2\text{--}3 \times$
What are the calorie contents of the following substances:	
Fat	9 kcal/g
Protein	4 kcal/g
Carbohydrate	4 kcal/g
What is the formula for converting nitrogen requirement/loss to protein requirement/loss?	Nitrogen $\times$ 6.25 = protein
What is RQ?	**R**espiratory **Q**uotient: ratio of CO_2 produced to O_2 consumed
What is the normal RQ?	0.8
What can be done to decrease the RQ?	More fat, less carbohydrates
What dietary change can be made to decrease CO_2 production in a patient in whom CO_2 retention is a concern?	Decrease carbohydrate calories and increase calories from **fat**
What lab tests are used to monitor nutritional status?	Blood levels of: **Prealbumin** ($t_{1/2} \approx 2\text{--}3$ days)—acute change determination Transferrin ($t_{1/2} \approx 8\text{--}9$ days) Albumin ($t_{1/2} \approx 14\text{--}20$ days)—more chronic determination Total lymphocyte count Anergy Retinol-binding protein ($t_{1/2} \approx 12$ hours)
Where is iron absorbed?	Duodenum (some in proximal jejunum)

Where is vitamin B12 absorbed?	Terminal ileum
What are the surgical causes of vitamin B12 deficiency?	Gastrectomy, excision of terminal ileum, blind loop syndrome
Where are bile salts absorbed?	Terminal ileum
Where are fat-soluble vitamins absorbed?	Terminal ileum
Which vitamins are fat soluble?	**K, A, D, E ("KADE")**

What are the signs of the following disorders:

Vitamin A deficiency	Poor wound healing
Vitamin B12/folate deficiency	Megaloblastic anemia
Vitamin C deficiency	Poor wound healing, bleeding gums
Vitamin K deficiency	↓ in the vitamin K–dependent clotting factors (II, VII, IX, and X); bleeding; elevated PT
Chromium deficiency	Diabetic state
Zinc deficiency	Poor wound healing, alopecia, dermatitis, taste disorder
Fatty acid deficiency	Dry, flaky skin; alopecia
What vitamin increases the PO absorption of iron?	PO vitamin C (ascorbic acid)
What vitamin lessens the deleterious effects of steroids on wound healing?	Vitamin A
What are the common indications for total parenteral nutrition (TPN)?	NPO >7 days Enterocutaneous fistulas Short bowel syndrome Prolonged ileus

What is TPN? **T**otal **P**arenteral **N**utrition = IV nutrition

What is in TPN? Protein
Carbohydrates
Lipids
(H_2O, electrolytes, minerals/vitamins,
$\pm$ insulin, $\pm$ H_2 blocker)

How much of each in TPN:
  Lipids 20% to 30% of calories (lipid from
soybeans, etc.)

  Protein 1.7 g/kg/day (10%–20% of calories) as
amino acids

  Carbohydrates 50% to 60% of calories as dextrose

**What are the possible
complications of TPN?** Line infection, fatty infiltration of the
liver, electrolyte/glucose problems,
pneumothorax during placement of
central line, loss of gut barrier, acalculus
cholecystitis, refeeding syndrome,
hyperosmolality

**What are the advantages of
enteral feeding?** Keeps gut barrier healthy, thought to
lessen translocation of bacteria, not
associated with complications of line
placement, associated with fewer
electrolyte/glucose problems

**What is the major nutrient
of the gut (small bowel)?** Glutamine

**What is "refeeding
syndrome"?** Decreased serum **potassium,
magnesium,** and **phosphate** after
refeeding (via TPN or enterally) a
starving patient

**What are the vitamin
K–dependent clotting factors?** 2, 7, 9, 10 (Think: 2 + 7 = 9, and then 10)

**What is an elemental tube
feed?** Very low residue tube feed in which
almost all the tube feed is absorbed

Where is calcium absorbed? Duodenum (actively)
Jejunum (passively)

What is the major nutrient of the colon?	**Butyrate** (and other short-chain fatty acids)
What must bind B12 for absorption?	Intrinsic factor from the gastric parietal cells
What sedative medication has caloric value?	Propofol delivers 1 kcal/cc in the form of lipid!
Why may all the insulin placed in a TPN bag not get to the patient?	Insulin will bind to the IV tubing
What is the best way to determine the caloric requirements of a patient on the ventilator?	Metabolic chart
How can serum bicarbonate be increased in patients on TPN?	Increase acetate (which is metabolized into bicarbonate)
What are "trophic" tube feeds?	Very low rate of tube feeds (usually 10–25 cc/hr), which are thought to keep mucosa alive and healthy
When should PO feedings be started after a laparotomy?	Classically after flatus or stool PR (usually postoperative days 3–5)
What is the best parameter to check adequacy of nutritional status?	Prealbumin

Chapter 26   Shock

What is the definition of shock?	Inadequate tissue perfusion
What are the different types (5)?	Hypovolemic Septic Cardiogenic Neurogenic Anaphylactic

What are the signs of shock?	Pale, diaphoretic, cool skin Hypotension, tachycardia, tachypnea ↓ mental status and pulse pressure Poor capillary refill Poor urine output
What are the best indicators of tissue perfusion?	Urine output, mental status
What lab tests help assess tissue perfusion?	Lactic acid (elevated with inadequate tissue perfusion), base deficit, pH from ABG (acidosis associated with inadequate tissue perfusion)

HYPOVOLEMIC SHOCK

What is the definition?	Decreased intravascular volume
What are the common causes?	Hemorrhage Burns Bowel obstruction Crush injury Pancreatitis
What are the signs?	**Early**—Orthostatic hypotension, mild tachycardia, anxiety, diaphoresis, vaso-constriction (decreased pulse pressure with increased diastolic pressure) **Late**—Changed mental status, decreased BP, marked tachycardia
What are the signs/symptoms with:	
Class I hemorrhage (<15% or 750 cc blood loss)?	Mild anxiety, normal vital signs
Class II hemorrhage (15%–30% or 750–1500 cc blood loss)?	Normal systolic BP with decreased pulse pressure, tachycardia, tachypnea, anxiety
Class III hemorrhage (30%–40% or 1500–2000 cc blood loss)?	Tachycardia (heart rate >120), tachypnea (respiratory rate >30), **decreased systolic BP,** decreased pulse pressure, confusion

Class IV hemorrhage (>40% or >2000 cc blood loss)?

Decreased systolic BP, tachycardia (heart rate >140), tachypnea (respiratory rate >35), decreased pulse pressure, confused and lethargic, no urine output

What is the treatment?

1. **Stop the bleeding**
2. **Volume:** IVF (isotonic LR) then blood products as needed

How is the effectiveness of treatment evaluated:
    Bedside indicator?

Urine output, BP, heart rate, mental status, extremity warmth, capillary refill, body temperature

    Labs?

pH, base deficit, and lactate level

What usually causes failure of resuscitation?

Persistent massive hemorrhage, requiring emergent surgical procedure

Why does decreased pulse pressure occur with early hypovolemic shock?

Pulse pressure (systolic–diastolic BP) decreases because of vasoconstriction, resulting in an elevated diastolic BP

What is the most common vital sign change associated with early hypovolemic shock?

Tachycardia

What type of patient does not mount a normal tachycardiac response to hypovolemic shock?

Patients on β-blockers, spinal shock (loss of sympathetic tone), endurance athletes

Should vasopressors be used to treat hypovolemic shock?

No

Should patients with hypovolemic shock be put into the Trendelenburg position?

No

SEPTIC SHOCK

What is the definition?	Documented infection and hypotension
What is the specific etiology?	Most common—gram-negative septicemia Less common—gram-positive septicemia, fungus
What factors increase the susceptibility to septic shock?	Any mechanism that increases susceptibility to infection (e.g., trauma, immunosuppression, corticosteroids, hematologic disease, diabetes)
What complications are major risks in septic shock?	Multiple organ failure, DIC, **death**
What are the signs/ symptoms?	Initial—vasodilation, resulting in warm skin and full pulses; normal urine output Delayed—vasoconstriction and poor urine output; mental status changes; hypotension
What percentage of blood cultures is positive in patients with bacterial septic shock?	Only about 50%!
What are the associated findings?	Fever, hyperventilation, tachycardia
What are the associated lab findings?	Early—hyperglycemia/glycosuria, respiratory alkalosis, hemoconcentration, leukopenia Late—leukocytosis, acidosis, elevated lactic acid (***Note:*** Identifying organism is important to direct treatment/antibiotics)
What is the treatment?	1. Volume (IVF) 2. Antibiotics (empiric, then by cultures) 3. Drainage of infection 4. Pressors PRN 5. Zygris® PRN

What is Zygris®?	Activated protein C, shown to decrease mortality in septic shock and multiple organ failure

CARDIOGENIC SHOCK

What is the definition?	Cardiac insufficiency; left ventricular failure (usually), resulting in inadequate tissue perfusion
What are the causes?	MI, papillary muscle dysfunction, massive cardiac contusion, cardiac tamponade, tension pneumothorax, cardiac valve failure
What are the signs/symptoms on exam?	Dyspnea Rales Pulsus alternans (increased pulse with greater filling following a weak pulse) Loud pulmonic component of S_2 Gallop rhythm
What are the associated vital signs/parameters?	Hypotension, decreased cardiac output, elevated CVP/wedge pressure, decreased urine output (low renal blood flow), tachycardia (possibly)
What are the signs on CXR?	Pulmonary edema
What is the treatment?	Based on diagnosis/mechanism: 1. CHF: diuretics and afterload reduction (e.g., ACE inhibitors), with or without pressors 2. Left ventricular failure (MI): pressors, afterload reduction
What are the last resort support mechanisms?	Intra-aortic balloon pump (IABP), ventricular assist device (VAD)

NEUROGENIC SHOCK

What is the definition?	Inadequate tissue perfusion from loss of sympathetic vasoconstrictive tone
What are the common causes?	Spinal cord injury: Complete transection of spinal cord Partial cord injury with spinal shock Spinal anesthesia

What are the signs/ symptoms?	**Hypotension** and **bradycardia**, neurologic deficit
Why are heart rate and BP decreased?	Loss of sympathetic tone (but hypovolemia [e.g., hemoperitoneum] must be ruled out)
What are the associated findings?	Neurologic deficits suggesting cord injury
What MUST be ruled out in any patient where spinal shock is suspected?	Hemorrhagic shock!
What is the treatment?	**IV fluids** (vasopressors reserved for hypotension refractory to fluid resuscitation)
What percentage of patients with hypotension and spinal neurologic deficits have hypotension of purely neurogenic origin?	About 67% (two thirds) of patients
What is spinal shock?	Complete flaccid paralysis immediately following spinal cord injury; may or may not be associated with circulatory shock
What is the lowest reflex available to the examiner?	Bulbocavernous reflex: checking for contraction of the anal sphincter upon compression of the glans penis or clitoris
What is the lowest level voluntary muscle?	External anal sphincter
What are the classic findings associated with spinal cord shock?	Hypotension Bradycardia or lack of compensatory tachycardia

MISCELLANEOUS

What is the acronym for treatment options for anaphylactic shock?	**"BASE":** **B**enadryl **A**minophylline **S**teroids **E**pinephrine

Chapter 27   **Surgical Infection**

What are the classic signs/symptoms of inflammation/infection?

Tumor (mass = swelling/edema)
Calor (heat)
Dolor (pain)
Rubor (redness = erythema)

Define:

Bacteremia

Bacteria in the blood

SIRS

Systemic Inflammatory Response Syndrome (fever, tachycardia, tachypnea, leukocytosis)

Sepsis

Documented infection and SIRS

Septic shock

Sepsis and hypotension

Cellulitis

Blanching erythema from superficial dermal/epidermal infection (usually strep more than staph)

Abscess

Collection of pus within a cavity

Superinfection

New infection arising while a patient is receiving antibiotics for the original infection at a different site (e.g., *C. difficile* colitis)

Nosocomial infection

Infection originating in the hospital

Empiric

Use of antibiotic based on previous sensitivity information or previous experience awaiting culture results in an established infection

Prophylactic

Antibiotics used to prevent an infection

What is the most common nosocomial infection?

Urinary tract infection (UTI)

What is the most common nosocomial infection causing death?

Respiratory tract infection (pneumonia)

URINARY TRACT INFECTION (UTI)

What diagnostic tests are used?	Urinalysis, culture, urine microscopy for WBC
What constitutes a POSITIVE urine analysis?	Positive nitrite (from bacteria) Positive leukocyte esterase (from WBC) >10 WBC/HPF Presence of bacteria (supportive)
What number of colony-forming units (CFU) confirms the diagnosis of UTI?	On urine culture, classically 100,000 or 10^5 CFU
What are the common organisms?	*Escherichia coli, Klebsiella, Proteus* (*Enterococcus, Staphylococcus aureus*)
What is the treatment?	Antibiotics with gram-negative spectrum (e.g., sulfamethoxazole/trimethoprim [Bactrim™], gentamicin, ciprofloxacin, aztreonam); check culture and sensitivity
What is the treatment of bladder candidiasis?	1. Remove or change Foley catheter 2. Administer systemic fluconazole or amphotericin bladder washings

CENTRAL LINE INFECTIONS

What are the signs of a central line infection?	**Unexplained hyperglycemia,** fever, mental status change, hypotension, tachycardia → **shock,** pus, and erythema at central line site
What is the most common cause of "catheter-related bloodstream infections"?	Coagulase-negative staphylococcus (33%), followed by enterococci, *Staphylococcus aureus,* gram-negative rods
When should central lines be changed?	When they are infected; there is NO advantage to changing them every 7 days in nonburn patients
What central line infusion increases the risk of infection?	Hyperal (TPN)

What is the treatment for central line infection?	1. Remove central line (send for culture) +/− IV antibiotics
	2. Place NEW central line in a different site
When should peripheral IV short angiocatheters be changed?	Every 72 to 96 hours

WOUND INFECTION (SURGICAL SITE INFECTION)

What is it?	Infection in an operative wound
When do these infections arise?	Classically, PODs #5 to #7
What are the signs/ symptoms?	**Pain** at incision site, erythema, drainage, induration, warm skin, fever
What is the treatment?	Remove skin sutures/staples, rule out fascial dehiscence, pack wound open, send wound culture, administer antibiotics
What are the most common bacteria found in postoperative wound infections?	*Staphylococcus aureus* (20%) *Escherichia coli* (10%) Enterococcus (10%) Other causes: *Staphylococcus epidermidis, Pseudomonas,* anaerobes, other gram-negative organisms, *Streptococcus*
Which bacteria cause fever and wound infection in the first 24 hours after surgery?	1. *Streptococcus*
	2. *Clostridium* (bronze-brown weeping tender wound)

CLASSIFICATION OF OPERATIVE WOUNDS

What is a "clean" wound?	Elective, nontraumatic wound without acute inflammation; usually closed primarily without the use of drains
What is the infection rate of a clean wound?	<1.5%

What is a clean-contaminated wound?

Operation on the GI or respiratory tract without unusual contamination or entry into the biliary or urinary tract

Without infection present, what is the infection rate of a clean-contaminated wound?

<3%

What is a contaminated wound?

Acute inflammation, traumatic wound, GI tract spillage, or a major break in sterile technique

What is the infection rate of a contaminated wound?

≈5%

What is a dirty wound?

Pus present, perforated viscus, or dirty traumatic wound

What is the infection rate of a dirty wound?

≈33%

What are the possible complications of wound infections?

Fistula, sinus tracts, sepsis, abscess, suppressed wound healing, superinfection (i.e., a new infection that develops during antibiotic treatment for the original infection), hernia

What factors influence the development of infections?

Foreign body (e.g., suture, drains, grafts)
Decreased blood flow (poor delivery of PMNs and antibiotics)
Strangulation of tissues with excessively tight sutures
Necrotic tissue or excessive local tissue destruction (e.g., too much Bovie)
Long operations (>2 hrs)
Hypothermia in O.R.
Hematomas or seromas
Dead space that prevents the delivery of phagocytic cells to bacterial foci
Poor approximation of tissues

What patient factors influence the development of infections?

Uremia
Hypovolemic shock
Vascular occlusive states
Advanced age
Distant area of infection

What are examples of an immunosuppressed state?	Immunosuppressant treatment Chemotherapy Systemic malignancy Trauma or burn injury Diabetes mellitus Obesity Malnutrition AIDS Uremia
Which lab tests are indicated?	CBC: leukocytosis or leukopenia (as an abscess may act as a WBC sink), blood cultures, imaging studies (e.g., CT scan to locate an abscess)
What is the treatment?	Incision and drainage—an abscess must be drained (***Note:*** fluctuation is a sign of a *subcutaneous* abscess; most abdominal abscesses are drained percutaneously) Antibiotics for deep abscesses
What are the indications for antibiotics after drainage of a subcutaneous abscess?	Diabetes mellitus, surrounding cellulitis, prosthetic heart valve, or an immunocompromised state

PERITONEAL ABSCESS

What is a peritoneal abscess?	Abscess within the peritoneal cavity
What are the causes?	Postoperative status after a laparotomy, ruptured appendix, peritonitis, any inflammatory intraperitoneal process, anastomotic leak
What are the sites of occurrence?	Pelvis, Morison's pouch, subphrenic, paracolic gutters, periappendiceal, lesser sac
What are the signs/ symptoms?	Fever (classically spiking), abdominal pain, mass
How is the diagnosis made?	Abdominal CT scan (or ultrasound)

When should an abdominal CT scan be obtained looking for a postoperative abscess?	After POD #7 (otherwise, abscess will not be "organized" and will look like a normal postoperative fluid collection)
What CT scan findings are associated with abscess?	Fluid collection with fibrous rind, **gas** in fluid collection
What is the treatment?	Percutaneous CT–guided drainage
What is an option for drainage of pelvic abscess?	Transrectal drainage (or transvaginal)
All abscesses must be drained except which type?	Amebiasis!

NECROTIZING FASCIITIS

What is it?	Bacterial infection of underlying fascia (spreads rapidly along fascial planes)
What are the causative agents?	Classically, group A *Streptococcus pyogenes,* but most often polymicrobial with anaerobes/gram-negative organisms
What are the signs/ symptoms?	Fever, pain, crepitus, cellulitis, skin discoloration, blood blisters (hemorrhagic bullae), weeping skin, increased WBCs, subcutaneous air on x-ray, septic shock
What is the treatment?	IVF, IV antibiotics and aggressive early extensive surgical débridement, cultures, tetanus prophylaxis
Is necrotizing fasciitis an emergency?	YES, patients must be taken to the O.R. immediately!

CLOSTRIDIAL MYOSITIS

What is it?	Clostridial muscle infection
What is another name for this condition?	Gas gangrene

What is the most common causative organism?	*Clostridium perfringens*
What are the signs/symptoms?	Pain, fever, shock, crepitus, foul-smelling brown fluid, subcutaneous air on x-ray
What is the treatment?	IV antibiotics, aggressive surgical débridement of involved muscle, tetanus prophylaxis

SUPPURATIVE HIDRADENITIS

What is it?	Infection/abscess formation in **apocrine** sweat glands
In what three locations does it occur?	Perineum/buttocks, inguinal area, axillae (site of apocrine glands)
What is the most common causative organism?	*Staphylococcus aureus*
What is the treatment?	Antibiotics Incision and drainage (excision of skin with glands for chronic infections)

PSEUDOMEMBRANOUS COLITIS

What is it?	Antibiotic-induced colonic overgrowth of *C. difficile,* secondary to loss of competitive nonpathogenic bacteria that comprise the normal colonic flora (***Note:*** it can be caused by any antibiotic, but especially penicillins, cephalosporins, and clindamycin)
What are the signs/symptoms?	**Diarrhea** (bloody in 10% of patients), ± fever, ± increased WBCs, ± abdominal cramps, ± abdominal distention
What causes the diarrhea?	Exotoxin released by *C. difficile*
How is the diagnosis made?	Assay stool for **exotoxin titer**; fecal leukocytes may or may not be present; on colonoscopy you may see an exudate that looks like a membrane (hence, "pseudomembranous")

What is the treatment?

PO metronidazole (Flagyl®; 93% sensitive) or PO vancomycin (97% sensitive); discontinuation of causative agent
Never give antiperistaltics

PROPHYLACTIC ANTIBIOTICS

What are the indications for prophylactic IV antibiotics?

Accidental wounds with heavy contamination and tissue damage
Accidental wounds requiring surgical therapy that has had to be delayed
Prosthetic heart valve or valve disease
Penetrating injuries of hollow intra-abdominal organs
Large bowel resections and anastomosis
Cardiovascular surgery with the use of a prosthesis/vascular procedures
Patients with open fractures (start in ER)
Traumatic wounds occurring >8 hours prior to medical attention

What must a prophylactic antibiotic cover for procedures on the large bowel/abdominal trauma/appendicitis?

Anaerobes

What commonly used antibiotics offer anaerobic coverage?

Cefoxitin (Mefoxin®), clindamycin, metronidazole (Flagyl®), cefotetan, ampicillin-sulbactam (Unasyn®), Zosyn™, Timentin®, Imipenem®

What antibiotic is used prophylactically for vascular surgery?

Ancef (if patient is significantly allergic to PCN—hives/swelling/shortness of breath—then erythromycin or clindamycin are options)

When is the appropriate time to administer prophylactic antibiotics?

Must be in adequate levels in the blood stream **prior to surgical incision!**

PAROTITIS

What is it?	Infection of the parotid gland
What is the most common causative organism?	*Staphylococcus*
What are the associated risk factors?	Age older than 65 years, malnutrition, poor oral hygiene, presence of NG tube, NPO, dehydration
What is the most common time of occurrence?	Usually 2 weeks postoperative
What are the signs?	Hot, red, tender parotid gland and increased WBCs
What is the treatment?	Antibiotics, operative drainage as necessary

MISCELLANEOUS

What is a "stitch" abscess?	Subcutaneous abscess centered around a subcutaneous stitch, which is a "foreign body"; treat with drainage and stitch removal
Which bacteria can be found in the stool (colon)?	Anaerobic—*Bacteroides fragilis* Aerobic—*Escherichia coli*
Which bacteria are found in infections from human bites?	*Streptococcus viridans, S. aureus, Peptococcus,* **Eikenella** (treat with Augmentin®)
What are the most common ICU pneumonia bacteria?	Gram-negative organisms
What is Fournier's gangrene?	Perineal infection starting classically in the scrotum in patients with diabetes; treat with triple antibiotics and wide débridement—a surgical emergency!
Does adding antibiotics to peritoneal lavage solution lower the risk of abscess formation?	No ("Dilution is the solution to pollution")

What is the classic finding associated with a *Pseudomonas* infection?

Green exudate and "fruity" smell

What are the classic antibiotics for "triple" antibiotics?

Ampicillin, gentamycin, and metronidazole (Flagyl®)

Which antibiotic is used to treat amoeba infection?

Metronidazole (Flagyl®)

Which bacteria commonly infect prosthetic material and central lines?

Staphylococcus **epidermis**

What is the antibiotic of choice for *Actinomyces*?

Penicillin G (exquisitely sensitive)

What is a furuncle?

Staphylococcal abscess that forms in a hair follicle (Think: **F**ollicle = **F**uruncle)

What is a carbuncle?

Subcutaneous staphylococcal abscess (usually an extension of a furuncle), most commonly seen in patients with diabetes (i.e., rule out diabetes)

What is a felon?

Infection of the finger pad (Think: **F**elon = **F**inger printing)

What microscopic finding is associated with *Actinomyces*?

Sulfur granules

What organism causes tetanus?

Clostridium tetani

What are the signs of tetanus?

Lockjaw, muscle spasm, laryngospasm, convulsions, respiratory failure

What are the appropriate prophylactic steps in tetanus-prone (dirty) injury in the following patients:
    Three previous immunizations?

None (tetanus toxoid only if >5 years since last toxoid)

Two previous immunizations?	Tetanus toxoid
One previous immunization?	Tetanus immunoglobulin IM and tetanus toxoid IM (at different sites!)
No previous immunizations?	Tetanus immunoglobulin IM and tetanus toxoid IM (at different sites!)
What is Fitz-Hugh-Curtis syndrome?	Right upper quadrant pain from gonococcal perihepatitis in women

Chapter 28   Fever

Define postoperative fever.	Temperature >38.5° C or 101.5° F
What are the classic W's of postoperative fever? (5)	**W**ind—atelectasis **W**ater—urinary tract infection (UTI) **W**ound—wound infection **W**alking—DVT/thrombophlebitis **W**onder drugs—drug fever
Give the classic postoperative timing for the following causes of postoperative fever:	
Atelectasis (Wind)	First 24 to 48 hours
UTI (Water)	Anytime after POD #3
Wound infection (Wound)	Usually after POD #5 (but it can be anytime!)
DVT/PE/thrombophlebitis (Walking)	PODs #7 to #10
Drug fever (Wonder drugs)	Anytime
What is the most common cause of fever on postoperative days 1 to 2?	Atelectasis

What is a "complete" fever workup?	Physical exam (look at wound, etc.), CXR, urinalysis, blood cultures, CBC
What causes fever before 24 postoperative hours?	Atelectasis, β-hemolytic streptococcal or clostridial wound infections, anastomotic leak
What causes fever from postoperative days 3 to 5?	UTI, pneumonia, IV site infection, wound infection
What is an anesthetic cause of fever INTRAoperatively?	Malignant hyperthermia—treat with **dantrolene**
What causes fever from postoperative days 5 to 10?	Wound infection, pneumonia, abscess, infected hematoma, *C. difficile* colitis, anastomotic leak **DVT, peritoneal abscess, drug fever** Pulmonary embolism, abscess, parotitis
What causes wound infection on postoperative days 1 to 2?	*Streptococcus* Clostridia (painful bronze-brown weeping wound)
What can cause fever at any time?	1. IV site infection 2. Central line infection 3. Medications

Chapter 29

Surgical Prophylaxis

What medications provide protection from postoperative GI bleeding?	H$_2$ blockers, PPI (proton-pump inhibitor)
What measures provide protection from postoperative atelectasis/pneumonia?	Incentive spirometry, coughing, **smoking cessation,** ambulation
What treatments provide protection from postoperative DVT?	Low-molecular-weight heparin (LMWH), subcutaneous low-dose unfractionated heparin, sequential compression device (SCD) for lower extremities, or both; early ambulation

What measures provide protection from wound infection?	Shower the night before surgery with chlorhexidine scrub **Never use a razor** for hair removal (electric shavers only) Ensure adequate skin prep in O.R. Do not close the skin in a contaminated case Ensure preoperative antibiotics in the bloodstream **before incision** Ensure no excess Bovie (necrotic tissue)
Why not use a razor to remove hair?	Micro cuts are a nidus for bacteria and subsequent wound infection
How long should "prophylactic antibiotics" be given?	<24 hrs
What treatment provides protection from oral/esophageal fungal infection during IV antibiotic treatment?	PO nystatin
What measures prevent ventilator-associated pneumonia (VAP)?	Head of bed >30°, handwashing, patient oral hygiene, avoidance of gastric overdistention
What is the classic preoperative "bowel prep"?	1. Bowel prep: Lower bacterial count in colon by catharsis (GoLYTELY or Fleets) 2. PO antibiotics (neomycin, erythromycin) preoperatively 3. Preoperative IV antibiotic with spectrum versus anaerobes (e.g., Cefoxitin)
Is there any evidence that a "bowel prep" decreases infections?	NO
What treatment provides protection from OPSS after splenectomy?	Immunization against *H. influenzae*, *Streptococcus*, *Meningococcus*, and penicillin when illness/fever occurs
What treatment provides protection from endocarditis with faulty heart valve or prosthetic heart valve?	Antibiotics prior to dental procedure or any surgery

What treatment provides protection from tetanus infection?	Tetanus toxoid (and tetanus immune globulin, if one or no previous toxoid with dirty wound)
What treatment provides protection from EtOH withdrawal?	Chlordiazepoxide (Librium®), also give Rally pack
What treatment provides protection from Wernicke's encephalopathy?	**Rally pack** (a.k.a. banana bag because the IV is yellow with the vitamins in it); pack includes thiamine, folate, and magnesium
What is Wernicke's encephalopathy?	Condition resulting from thiamine deficiency in patients with alcoholism, causing a **triad** of symptoms; think **"COA"**: 1. **C**onfusion 2. **O**phthalmoplegia 3. **A**taxia
What treatment decreases the risk of perioperative adrenal crisis in a patient on chronic steroids?	"Stress-dose" steroids: 100 mg hydrocortisone administered preoperatively, continued postoperatively q 8 hours, and then tapered off

Chapter 30   Surgical Radiology

CHEST

What defines a technically adequate CXR?	The film must be **"RIPE"**: **R**otation: Clavicular heads are equidistant from the thoracic spinous processes **I**nspiration: Diaphragm is at or below ribs 8–10 posteriorly and ribs 5–6 anteriorly **P**enetration: Disk spaces are visible but there is no bony detail of the spine; bronchovascular structures are seen through the heart **E**xposure: Make sure all of the lung fields are visible

How should a CXR be read?

Check the following:

    Tubes and lines: Check placement

    Patient data: Name, date, history number

    Orientation: Up/down, left-right

    Technique: AP or PA, supine or erect, decubitus

    Trachea: Midline or deviated, caliber

    Lungs: CHF, mass

    Pulmonary vessels: Artery or vein enlargement

    Mediastinum: Aortic knob, nodes

    Hila: Masses, lymphadenopathy

    Heart: Transverse diameter should be less than half the transthoracic diameter

    Pleura: Effusion, thickening, pneumothorax

    Bones: Fractures, lesions

    Soft tissues: Periphery and below the diaphragm

What CXR is better: P-A or A-P?

P-A, less magnification of the heart (heart is closer to the x-ray plate)

Classically, how much pleural fluid can the diaphragm hide on upright CXR?

It is said that the diaphragm can overshadow up to 500 cc

How can CXR confirm that the last hole on a chest tube is in the pleural cavity?

Last hole is through the radiopaque line on the chest tube; thus, look for the break in the radiopaque line to be in the rib cage

How can a loculated pleural effusion be distinguished from a free-flowing pleural effusion?

Ipsilateral decubitus CXR; if fluid is not loculated (or contained), it will layer out

How do you recognize a pneumothorax on CXR?

Air without lung markings is seen outside the white pleural line—best seen in the apices on an upright CXR

What x-ray should be obtained before feeding via a nasogastric or nasoduodenal tube?

Low CXR to ensure the tube is in the GI tract and not in the lung

What C-spine views are used to rule out bony injury?

CT scan

What is used to look for ligamentous C-spine injury?

Lateral flex and extension C-spine films, MRI

What CXR findings may provide evidence of traumatic aortic injury?

Widened mediastinum >8 cm (most common)
Apical pleural capping
Loss of aortic knob
Inferior displacement of left main bronchus; NG tube displaced to the right, tracheal deviation, hemothorax

How should a CT scan be read?

Cross section with the patient in supine position looking up from the feet

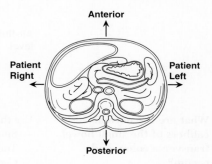

Anterior

Patient Right   **Patient Left**

Posterior

ABDOMEN

How should an abdominal x-ray (AXR) be read?

Check the following:

    Patient data: name, date, history number

    Orientation: up/down, left-right

    Technique: A-P or P-A, supine or erect, decubitus

    Air: free air under diaphragm, air-fluid levels

    Gas dilatation (3, 6, 9 rule)

    Borders: psoas shadow, preperitoneal fat stripe

    Mass: look for organomegaly, kidney shadow

    Stones/calcification: urinary, biliary, fecalith

    Stool

    Tubes

    Bones

    Foreign bodies

How can you tell the difference between a small bowel obstruction (SBO) and an ileus?

In SBO there is a transition point (cut-off sign) between the distended proximal bowel and the distal bowel of normal caliber (may be gasless), whereas the bowel in ileus is *diffusely* distended

What is the significance of an air-fluid level?

Seen in obstruction or ileus on an upright x-ray; intraluminal bowel diameter increases, allowing for separation of fluid and gas

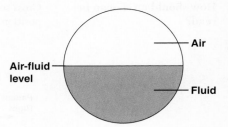

What are the normal calibers of the small bowel, transverse colon, and cecum?

Use the **"3, 6, 9 rule"**:
  Small bowel <3 cm
  Transverse colon <6 cm
  Cecum <9 cm

What is the "rule of 3s" for the small bowel?

Bowel wall should be <3 mm thick
Bowel folds should be <3 mm thick
Bowel diameter should be <3 cm wide

How can the small and large bowel be distinguished on AXR?

By the intraluminal folds: The small bowel plicae circulares are complete, whereas the plicae semilunares of the large bowel are only partially around the inner circumference of the lumen

Where does peritoneal fluid accumulate in the supine position?

Morison's pouch (hepatorenal recess), the space between the anterior surface of the right kidney and the posterior surface of the right lobe of the liver

What percentage of kidney stones are radiopaque?

≈90%

What percentage of gallstones are radiopaque?	≈10%
What percentage of patients with acute appendicitis have a radiopaque fecalith?	≈5%
What are the radiographic signs of appendicitis?	Fecalith; sentinel loops; scoliosis away from the right because of pain; mass effect (abscess); loss of psoas shadow; loss of preperitoneal fat stripe; and, very rarely, a small amount of free air, if perforated
What does KUB stand for?	**K**idneys, **U**reters, and **B**ladder—commonly used term for a plain film AXR (abdominal flat plate)
What is the "parrot's beak" or "bird's beak" sign?	Evidence of sigmoid volvulus on barium enema; evidence of achalasia on barium swallow
What is a "cut-off sign"?	Seen in obstruction, bowel distention, and distended bowel that is "cut-off" from normal bowel
What are "sentinel loops"?	Distention or air-fluid levels (or both) near a site of abdominal inflammation (e.g., seen in RLQ with appendicitis)
What is loss of the psoas shadow?	Loss of the clearly defined borders of the psoas muscle on AXR; loss signifies inflammation or ascites
What is loss of the peritoneal fat stripe (a.k.a. preperitoneal fat stripe)?	Loss of the lateral peritoneal/preperitoneal fat interface; implies inflammation
What is "thumbprinting"?	Nonspecific colonic mucosal edema resembling thumb indentations on AXR
What is pneumatosis intestinalis?	Gas within the intestinal wall (usually means **dead gut**) that can be seen in patients with congenital variant or chronic steroids

What is free air?

Air free within the peritoneal cavity (air or gas should be seen only within the bowel or stomach); results from bowel or stomach perforation

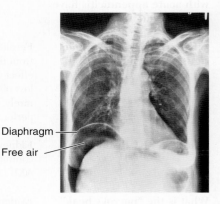

Diaphragm

Free air

What is the best position for the detection of FREE AIR (free intraperitoneal air)?

Upright CXR—air below the right diaphragm

If you cannot get an upright CXR, what is the second best plain x-ray for free air?

Left lateral decubitus, because it prevents confusion with gastric air bubble; with free air **both** sides of the bowel wall can be seen; can detect as little as 1 cc of air

How long after a laparotomy can there be free air on AXR?

Usually 7 days or less

What is Chilaiditi's sign?

Transverse colon over the liver simulating free air on x-ray

When should a postoperative abdominal/pelvic CT scan for a peritoneal abscess be performed?

POD #7 or later, to give time for the abscess to form

What is the best test to evaluate the biliary system and gallbladder?

Ultrasound (U/S)

What is the normal diameter of the common bile duct with gallbladder present?

<4 mm until age 40, then add 1 mm per decade (e.g., 7 mm at age 70)

What is the normal common bile duct diameter after removal of the gallbladder?

8 to 10 mm

What U/S findings are associated with acute cholecystitis?

Gallstones, thickened gallbladder wall (>3 mm), distended gallbladder (>4 cm A-P), impacted stone in gallbladder neck, pericholecystic fluid

What type of kidney stone is not seen on AXR?

Uric acid (Think: **U**ric acid = **U**nseen)

What medication should be given prophylactically to a patient with a true history of contrast allergy?

Methylprednisolone or dexamethasone; the patient should also receive nonionic contrast (associated with one fifth as many reactions as ionic contrast, the less expensive standard)

What is a C-C mammogram?

Cranio-**C**audal mammogram, in which the breast is compressed top to bottom

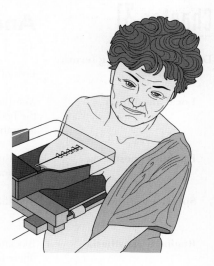

What is an MLO mammogram?

MedioLateral Oblique mammogram, in which the breast is compressed in a 45° angle from the axilla to the lower sternum

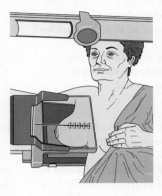

What are the best studies to evaluate for a pulmonary embolus?

Spiral thoracic CT scan, V-Q scan, pulmonary angiogram (gold standard)

Chapter 31   Anesthesia

Define the following terms:
   Anesthesia

Loss of sensation/pain

   Local anesthesia

Anesthesia of a small confined area of the body (e.g., lidocaine for an elbow laceration)

   Epidural anesthesia

Anesthetic drugs/narcotics infused into epidural space

   Spinal anesthesia

Anesthetic agents injected into the thecal sac

   Regional anesthesia

Blocking of the sensory afferent nerve fibers from a **region** of the body (e.g., radial nerve block)

General anesthesia	Triad: 1. Unconsciousness/amnesia 2. Analgesia 3. Muscle relaxation
GET or GETA	**G**eneral **E**ndo**T**racheal **A**nesthesia
Give examples of the following terms:	
Local anesthetic	Lidocaine, bupivacaine (Marcaine®)
Regional anesthetic	Lidocaine, bupivacaine (Marcaine®)
General anesthesia	Isoflurane, enflurane, sevoflurane, desflurane
Dissociative agent	Ketamine
What is cricoid pressure?	Manual pressure on cricoid cartilage occluding the esophagus and thus decreasing the chance of aspiration of gastric contents during intubation (a.k.a. Sellick's maneuver)
What is "rapid-sequence" anesthesia induction?	1. Oxygenation and short-acting induction agent 2. Muscle relaxant 3. Cricoid pressure 4. Intubation 5. Inhalation anesthetic (rapid: boom, boom, boom → to lower the risk of aspiration during intubation)
Give examples of induction agents.	Propofol, midazolam, sodium thiopental
What are contraindications of the depolarizing agent succinylcholine?	Patients with burns, neuromuscular diseases/paraplegia, eye trauma, or increased ICP
Why is succinylcholine contraindicated in these patients?	Depolarization can result in life-threatening **hyperkalemia; succinylcholine also increases intraocular pressure**
Why doesn't lidocaine work in an abscess?	Lidocaine does not work in an **acidic** environment

Why does lidocaine burn on injection and what can be done to decrease the burning sensation?

Lidocaine is acidic, which causes the burning; add sodium bicarbonate to decrease the burning sensation

Why does some lidocaine come with epinephrine?

Epinephrine vasoconstricts the small vessels, resulting in a decrease in bleeding and blood flow in the area; this prolongs retention of lidocaine and its effects

In what locations is lidocaine with epinephrine contraindicated?

Fingers, toes, penis, etc., because of the possibility of ischemic injury/necrosis resulting from vasoconstriction

What are the contraindications to nitrous oxide?

Nitrous oxide is poorly soluble in serum and thus expands into any air-filled body pockets; avoid in patients with middle ear occlusions, **pneumothorax, small bowel obstruction,** etc.

What is the feared side effect of bupivacaine (Marcaine®)?

Cardiac dysrhythmia after intravascular injection leading to fatal refractory dysrhythmia

What are the side effects of morphine?

Constipation, respiratory failure, hypotension (from histamine release), spasm of sphincter of Oddi (use Demerol® in pancreatitis and biliary surgery), decreased cough reflex

What are the side effects of meperidine?

Similar to those of morphine but causes less sphincteric spasm and can cause tachycardia and seizures

Limit to the duration of Demerol® postoperatively?

Build up of the metabolites (normeperidine)

What medication is a contraindication to Demerol®?

Monoamine oxidase inhibitor

What metabolite of Demerol® breakdown causes side effects (e.g., seizures)?

Normeperidine

What is the treatment of life-threatening respiratory depression with narcotics?	**Narcan®** IV (naloxone)
What are the side effects of epidural analgesia?	**Orthostatic hypotension,** decreased motor function, urinary retention
What is the advantage of epidural analgesia?	Analgesia without decreased cough reflex
What are the side effects of spinal anesthesia?	**Urinary retention** Hypotension (neurogenic shock)
What is the side effect of inhalational (volatile) anesthesia?	Halothane—**hypotension** (cardiac depression, decreased baroreceptor response to hypotension, and peripheral vasodilation), malignant hyperthermia

MALIGNANT HYPERTHERMIA

What is it?	Inherited predisposition to an anesthetic reaction, causing uncoupling of the excitation–contraction system in skeletal muscle, which in turn causes **malignant hyperthermia;** hypermetabolism is fatal if untreated
What is the incidence?	Very rare
What are the causative agents?	General anesthesia, succinylcholine
What are the signs/symptoms?	**Increased body temperature;** hypoxia; acidosis; tachycardia, ↑ PCO_2 (↑ end tidal CO_2)
What is the treatment?	**IV dantrolene,** body cooling, discontinuation of anesthesia

MISCELLANEOUS

What are some of the nondepolarizing muscle blockers?	Vecuronium Pancuronium

What are the antidotes to the nondepolarizing neuro-muscular blocking agents?	Edrophonium Neostigmine Pyridostigmine
How do these agents work?	They inhibit anticholinesterase
Which muscle blocker is depolarizing?	Succinylcholine
What is the duration of action of succinylcholine?	<6 minutes
What is the antidote to reverse succinylcholine?	Time; endogenous blood pseudocholines-terase (patients deficient in this enzyme may be paralyzed for hours!)
What is the maximum dose of lidocaine:	
With epinephrine?	7 mg/kg
Without epinephrine?	4 mg/kg
What is the duration of lidocaine local anesthesia?	30 to 60 minutes (up to 4 hours with epinephrine)
What are the early signs of lidocaine toxicity?	Tinnitus, perioral/tongue numbness, metallic taste, blurred vision, muscle twitches, drowsiness
What are the signs of lidocaine toxicity with large overdose (>10 mcg/mL)?	Seizures, coma, respiratory arrest Loss of consciousness Apnea
When should the Foley catheter be removed in a patient with an epidural catheter?	Several hours **after** the epidural catheter is removed (to prevent urinary retention)
What is a PCA pump?	**P**atient-**C**ontrolled **A**nalgesia; a pump delivers a set amount of pain reliever when the patient pushes a button (e.g., 1 mg of morphine every 6 minutes)

What are the advantages of a PCA pump?	Better pain control Patients actually use less pain medication with a PCA! If given a moderate dose without a basal rate, patients should not be able to overdose (They will fall asleep and not be able to push the button!)
What is a "basal rate" on the PCA?	Steady continuous infusion rate of the narcotic (e.g., 1–2 mg of morphine) continuously infused per hour; patient can supplement with additional doses as needed
What is used to reverse narcotics?	Naloxone (Narcan®)
What is used to reverse benzodiazepines?	Flumazenil
What is fentanyl?	Very potent narcotic (#1 drug of abuse by anesthesiologists)
Name an IV NSAID.	Ketorolac (has classic side effects of NSAIDs: PUD, renal insufficiency)

Chapter 32   Surgical Ulcers

Define the following terms: **Peptic ulcer**	General term for gastric/duodenal ulcer disease
Gastric ulcer	Ulcer in the stomach

Curling's ulcer

Gastric ulcer after burn injury (Think: Curling's—curling iron burn—burn)

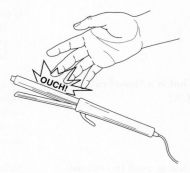

Cushing's ulcer

Peptic ulcer after neurologic insult (Think: Cushing—famous neurosurgeon)

Dieulafoy's ulcer

Pinpoint gastric mucosal defect bleeding from underlying arterial vessel malformation

Marjolin's ulcer

Squamous cell carcinoma ulceration overlying chronic osteomyelitis or burn scar

Aphthous ulcer

GI tract ulcer seen in Crohn's disease

Marginal ulcer

Mucosal ulcer seen at a site of GI tract anastomosis

Decubitus ulcer

Skin/subcutaneous ulceration from pressure necrosis, classically on the buttocks/sacrum

Venous stasis ulcer

Skin ulceration on **medial malleolus** caused by venous stasis of a lower extremity

LE arterial insufficiency ulcer

Skin ulcers usually located on the toes/feet

Chapter 33   Surgical Oncology

Define:

Surgical oncology

Surgical treatment of tumors

XRT

Radiation therapy

In situ

Not invading basement membrane

Benign

Nonmalignant tumor—does not invade or metastasize

Malignant

Tumors with anaplasia that invade and metastasize

Adjuvant RX

Treatment that aids or assists surgical treatment = Chemo or XRT

Neoadjuvant RX

Chemo, XRT, or both BEFORE surgical resection

Brachytherapy

XRT applied directly or very close to the target tissue (e.g., implantable adioactive seeds)

Metachronous tumors

Tumors occurring at different times

Synchronous tumors

Tumors occurring at the same time

What do the T, M, and N stand for in TMN staging?

T-Tumor size
M-Mets (distant)
N-Nodes

What tumor marker is associated with colon cancer?

CEA

What tumor marker is associated with hepatoma?

α-Fetoprotein

What tumor marker is associated with pancreatic carcinoma?

CA 19-9

What is paraneoplastic syndrome?	Syndrome of dysfunction not directly associated with tumor mass or mets (autoimmune or released substance)
What are the most common cancers in women?	1. Lung 2. Breast 3. Colorectal
What are the most common cancers in men?	1. Prostate 2. Lung 3. Colorectal
What is the most common cancer causing death in both men and women?	Lung!

Section II
General Surgery

Chapter 34
GI Hormones and Physiology

OVERVIEW

Define the products of the following stomach cells:	
Gastric parietal cells	HCl Intrinsic factor
Chief cells	**PEP**sinogen (Think: "a **PEP**py chief")
G cells	Gastrin, G cells are found in the antrum (Think: **G** = **G**astrin)
Mucous neck cells	Bicarbonate mucus
What is pepsin?	Proteolytic enzyme that hydrolyzes peptide bonds
What is intrinsic factor?	Protein secreted by the parietal cells that combines with vitamin B12 and enables absorption in the terminal ileum
Name three receptors on the parietal cell that stimulate HCl release.	Think: **"HAG"**: 1. **H**istamine 2. **A**cetylcholine 3. **G**astrin
What is the enterohepatic circulation?	Circulation of bile acids from the liver to the gut and back to the liver via the portal vein
Where are most of the bile acids absorbed?	Terminal ileum

How many times is the entire bile acid pool circulated during a typical meal?	Twice
What are the stimulators of gallbladder emptying?	Cholecystokinin, vagal input
What are the inhibitors of gallbladder emptying?	Somatostatin, sympathetics (it is impossible to flee and digest food at the same time), vasoactive intestinal polypeptide (VIP)

CHOLECYSTOKININ (CCK)

What is its source?	Duodenal mucosal cells
What stimulates its release?	Fat, protein, amino acids, HCl
What inhibits its release?	Trypsin and chymotrypsin
What are its actions?	Empties gallbladder Opens ampulla of Vater Slows gastric emptying Stimulates pancreatic acinar cell growth and release of exocrine products

SECRETIN

What is its source?	Duodenal cells (specifically the argyrophilic S cells)
What stimulates its release?	pH <4.5 (acid), fat in the duodenum
What inhibits its release?	High pH in the duodenum
What are its actions?	Releases pancreatic bicarbonate/enzymes/H_2O Releases bile/bicarbonate Decreases lower esophageal sphincter (LES) tone Decreases release of gastric acid

GASTRIN

What is its source?	Gastric antrum G cells

What stimulates its release?	Stomach peptides/amino acids
	Vagal input
	Calcium
What inhibits its release?	pH <3.0
	Somatostatin
What are its actions?	Release of HCl from parietal cells
	Trophic effect on mucosa of the stomach and small intestine

SOMATOSTATIN

What is its source?	Pancreatic D cells
What stimulates its release?	Food
What are its actions?	Globally inhibits GI function

MISCELLANEOUS

What is the purpose of the colon?	Reabsorption of H_2O and storage of stool
What is the main small bowel nutritional source?	Glutamine
What is the main nutritional source of the colon?	Butyrate (short-chain fatty acid)
Where is calcium absorbed?	Duodenum actively, jejunum passively
Where is iron absorbed?	Duodenum
Where is vitamin B12 absorbed?	Terminal ileum
Which hormone primarily controls gallbladder contraction?	CCK
What supplement does a patient need after removal of the terminal ileum or stomach?	Vitamin B12

Name the main constituents of bile.

Water, phospholipids (lecithins), bile acids, cholesterol, and bilirubin

What are most gallstones made of?

Cholesterol

How do opiates affect the bowel?

By stimulating sodium absorption and inhibiting secretion in the ileum as well as decreasing GI motility by incoordinated peristalsis (Therefore, place patients on stool softeners when dispensing pain medication)

Which type of muscle fibers, smooth or striated, does the esophagus contain?

Both:
    Upper third—striated muscle control of motor nerves
    Middle third—mixed
    Lower third—smooth muscle, primarily under control of vagal motor fibers

Which electrolytes does the colon actively absorb?

Na^+, Cl^-

Which electrolyte does the colon actively secrete?

HCO_3^- (plays a role in diarrhea causing the patient to have a normal anion gap acidosis)

Which electrolyte does the colon passively secrete?

K^+

What is the gastrocolic reflex?

Increased secretory and motor functions of the stomach result in increased colonic motility

What is the blood supply to the liver?

75% from the portal vein, rich in products of digestion
25% from the hepatic artery, rich in O_2 (but each provide for 50% of oxygen)

What are Peyer patches?

Nodules of lymphoid tissue with B and T lymphocytes in the small intestine that selectively sample lumenal antigens found in the terminal ileum

Chapter 35

Acute Abdomen and Referred Pain

What is an "acute abdomen"?

Acute abdominal pain so severe that the patient seeks medical attention (*Note:* Not the same as a "surgical abdomen," because most cases of acute abdominal pain do not require surgical treatment)

What are peritoneal signs?

Signs of peritoneal irritation: extreme tenderness, percussion tenderness, rebound tenderness, voluntary guarding, motion pain, **involuntary** guarding/ rigidity (late)

Define the following terms:
  Rebound tenderness

Pain upon releasing the palpating hand pushing on the abdomen

  Motion pain

Abdominal pain upon moving, pelvic rocking, moving of stretcher, or heel strike

  Voluntary guarding

Abdominal muscle contraction with palpation of the abdomen

  Involuntary guarding

Rigid abdomen as the muscles "guard" involuntarily

  Colic

Intermittent severe pain (usually because of intermittent contraction of a hollow viscus against an obstruction)

What conditions can mask abdominal pain?

Steroids, diabetes, paraplegia

What is the most common cause of acute abdominal surgery in the United States?

Acute appendicitis (7% of the population will develop it sometime during their lives)

What important questions should be asked when obtaining the history of a patient with an acute abdomen?

"Have you had this pain before?"
"On a scale from 1 to 10, how would you rank this pain?"
"Fevers/chills?"
"Duration?" (comes and goes vs. constant)
"Quality?" (sharp vs. dull)
"Does anything make the pain better or worse?"
"Migration?"
"Point of maximal pain?"
"Urinary symptoms?"
"Nausea, vomiting, or diarrhea?"
"Anorexia?"
"Constipation?"
"Last bowel movement?"
"Any change in bowel habits?"
"Any relation to eating?"
"Last menses?"
"Last meal?"
"Vaginal discharge?"
"Melena?"
"Hematochezia?"
"Hematemesis?"
"Medications?"
"Allergies?"
"Past medical history?"
"Past surgical history?"
"Family history?"
"Tobacco/EtOH/drugs?"

What should the acute abdomen physical exam include?

Inspection (e.g., surgical scars, distention)
Auscultation (e.g., bowel sounds, bruits)
Palpation (e.g., tenderness, R/O hernia, CVAT, rectal, pelvic exam, rebound, voluntary guard, motion tenderness)
Percussion (e.g., liver size, spleen size)

What is the best way to have a patient localize abdominal pain?

"Point with **one** finger to where the pain is worse"

What is the classic position of a patient with peritonitis?

Motionless (often with knees flexed)

What is the classic position of a patient with a kidney stone?

Cannot stay still, restless, writhing in pain

What is the best way to examine a scared child or histrionic adult's abdomen?

Use stethoscope to palpate abdomen

What lab tests are used to evaluate the patient with an acute abdomen?

CBC with **differential,** chem-10, amylase, type and screen, urinalysis, LFTs

What is a "left shift" on CBC differential?

Sign of inflammatory response: Immature neutrophils (bands)
Note: Many call >80% of WBCs as neutrophils a "left shift"

What lab test should every woman of childbearing age with an acute abdomen receive?

Human chorionic gonadotropin (β-hCG) to rule out pregnancy/ectopic pregnancy

Which x-rays are used to evaluate the patient with an acute abdomen?

Upright chest x-ray, upright abdominal film, supine abdominal x-ray (if patient cannot stand, left lateral decubitus abdominal film)

How is free air ruled out if the patient cannot stand?

Left lateral decubitus—free air collects over the liver and does not get confused with the gastric bubble

What diagnosis must be considered in every patient with an acute abdomen?

Appendicitis!

What are the differential diagnoses by quadrant?
  RUQ

Cholecystitis, hepatitis, PUD, perforated ulcer, pancreatitis, liver tumors, gastritis, hepatic abscess, choledocholithiasis, cholangitis, pyelonephritis, nephrolithiasis, appendicitis (**especially during pregnancy**); thoracic causes (e.g., pleurisy/pneumonia), PE, pericarditis, MI (especially inferior MI)

LUQ	PUD, perforated ulcer, gastritis, splenic injury, abscess, reflux, dissecting aortic aneurysm, thoracic causes, pyelonephritis, nephrolithiasis, hiatal hernia (strangulated paraesophageal hernia), Boerhaave's syndrome, Mallory-Weiss tear, splenic artery aneurysm, colon disease
LLQ	**Diverticulitis,** sigmoid volvulus, perforated colon, colon cancer, urinary tract infection, small bowel obstruction, inflammatory bowel disease, nephrolithiasis, pyelonephritis, fluid accumulation from aneurysm or perforation, referred hip pain, gynecologic causes, appendicitis (rare)
RLQ	**Appendicitis!** And same as LLQ; also mesenteric lymphadenitis, cecal diverticulitis, Meckel's diverticulum, intussusception
What is the differential diagnosis of epigastric pain?	PUD, gastritis, MI, pancreatitis, biliary colic, gastric volvulus, Mallory-Weiss
What is the differential diagnosis of gynecologic pain?	Ovarian cyst, ovarian torsion, PID, mittelschmerz, tubo-ovarian abscess (TOA), uterine fibroid, necrotic fibroid, pregnancy, ectopic pregnancy, endometriosis, cancer of the cervix/ uterus/ovary, endometrioma, gynecologic tumor, torsion of cyst or fallopian tube
What is the differential diagnosis of thoracic causes of abdominal pain?	MI (especially inferior), pneumonia, dissecting aorta, aortic aneurysm, empyema, esophageal rupture/tear, PTX, esophageal foreign body
What is the differential diagnosis of scrotal causes of lower abdominal pain?	Testicular torsion, epididymitis, orchitis, inguinal hernia, referred pain from nephrolithiasis or appendicitis

What are nonsurgical causes of abdominal pain?	Gastroenteritis, DKA, sickle cell crisis, rectus sheath hematoma, acute porphyria, PID, kidney stone, pyelonephritis, hepatitis, pancreatitis, pneumonia, MI, *C. difficile* colitis

What is the unique differential diagnosis for the patient with AIDS and abdominal pain?	In addition to all common abdominal conditions:
	    CMV (most **C**ommon)
	    Kaposi's sarcoma
	    Lymphoma
	    TB
	    MAI (*Mycobacterium Avium Intracellulare*)

What are the possible causes of suprapubic pain?	Cystitis, colonic pain, gynecologic causes (and, of course, appendicitis)
What causes pain limited to specific dermatomes?	Early zoster before vesicles erupt
What is referred pain?	Pain felt at a site distant from a disease process; caused by the convergence of multiple pain afferents in the posterior horn of the spinal cord
What is gastroenteritis?	Viral or bacterial infection of the GI tract, usually with vomiting and diarrhea, pain (usually **after** vomiting), nonsurgical
What is classically stated to be the "great imitator"?	Constipation
Name the classic locations of referred pain:	
Cholecystitis	Right subscapular pain (also epigastric)
Appendicitis	Early: periumbilical Rarely: testicular pain
Diaphragmatic irritation (from spleen, perforated ulcer, or abscess)	Shoulder pain (+ Kehr's sign on the left)
Pancreatitis/cancer	Back pain

Rectal disease	Pain in the small of the back
Nephrolithiasis	Testicular pain/flank pain
Rectal pain	Midline small of back pain
Small bowel	Periumbilical pain
Uterine pain	Midline small of back pain

Give the classic diagnosis for the following cases:

"Abdominal pain out of proportion to exam"	Rule out mesenteric ischemia
Hypotension and pulsatile abdominal mass	Ruptured AAA; go to the O.R.
Fever, LLQ pain, and change in bowel habits	Diverticulitis

Give the test of choice for the following conditions:

Cholelithiasis	Ultrasound (U/S)
Bile duct obstruction	U/S
Mesenteric ischemia	Mesenteric A-gram
Ruptured abdominal aortic aneurysm	NONE—emergent laparotomy
AAA	Abdominal CT scan or U/S
Abdominal abscess	Abdominal CT scan
Severe diverticulitis	Abdominal CT scan

What is the most common cause of RUQ pain?	Cholelithiasis
What is the most common cause of surgical RLQ pain?	Acute appendicitis

What is the most common cause of GI tract LLQ pain?	Diverticulitis
Classically, what endocrine problems can cause abdominal pain?	1. Addisonian crisis 2. **DKA** (**D**iabetic **K**eto**A**cidosis)

Chapter 36

Hernias

What is a hernia?	(**L. rupture**) Protrusion of a peritoneal sac through a musculoaponeurotic barrier (e.g., abdominal wall); a fascial defect
What is the incidence?	5%–10% lifetime; 50% are indirect inguinal, 25% are direct inguinal, and ≈5% are femoral
What are the precipitating factors?	Increased intra-abdominal pressure: straining at defecation or urination (rectal cancer, colon cancer, prostatic enlargement, constipation), obesity, pregnancy, ascites, valsavagenic (coughing) COPD; an abnormal congenital anatomic route (i.e., patent processus vaginalis)
Why should hernias be repaired?	To avoid complications of incarceration/ strangulation, bowel necrosis, SBO, pain
What is more dangerous: a small or large hernia defect?	Small defect is more dangerous because a tight defect is more likely to strangulate if incarcerated
Define the following descriptive terms: **Reducible**	Ability to return the displaced organ or tissue/hernia contents to their usual anatomic site
Incarcerated	Swollen or fixed within the hernia sac (incarcerated = imprisoned); may cause intestinal obstruction (i.e., an irreducible hernia)

Strangulated

Incarcerated hernia with resulting ischemia; will result in signs and symptoms of ischemia and intestinal obstruction or bowel necrosis (Think: strangulated = choked)

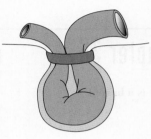

Complete

Hernia sac and its contents protrude all the way through the defect

Incomplete

Defect present without sac or contents protruding completely through it

What is reducing a hernia "en masse"?

Reducing the hernia contents and hernia sac

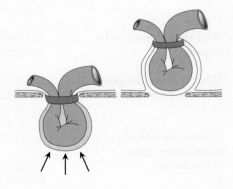

**Define the following types
of hernias:**

Sliding hernia

Hernia sac partially formed by the wall of a viscus (i.e., bladder/cecum)

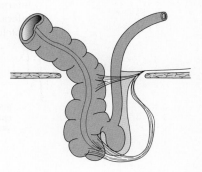

Littre's hernia

Hernia involving a Meckel's diverticulum (Think alphabetically: **L**ittre's **M**eckel's = **LM**)

Spigelian hernia

Hernia through the linea semilunaris (or spigelian fascia); also known as spontaneous lateral ventral hernia (Think: **S**pigelian = **S**emilunaris)

Internal hernia

Hernia into or involving intra-abdominal structure

Petersen's hernia

Seen after bariatric gastric bypass—internal herniation of small bowel through the mesenteric defect from the Roux limb

Obturator hernia

Hernia through obturator canal (females > males)

Lumbar hernia

Petit's hernia or Grynfeltt's hernia

Petit's hernia

(Rare) hernia through Petit's triangle (a.k.a. inferior lumbar triangle) (Think: **petit**e = small = inferior)

Grynfeltt's hernia

Hernia through Grynfeltt-Lesshaft triangle (superior lumbar triangle)

Pantaloon hernia

Hernia sac exists as **both a direct and indirect** hernia straddling the inferior epigastric vessels and protruding through the floor of the canal as well as the internal ring (two sacs separated by the inferior epigastric vessels [the pant crotch] like a pair of pantaloon pants)

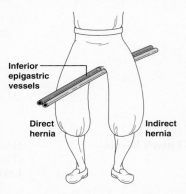

Incisional hernia

Hernia through an incisional site; most common cause is a wound infection

Ventral hernia

Incisional hernia in the ventral abdominal wall

Parastomal hernia

Hernia adjacent to an ostomy (e.g., colostomy)

Sciatic hernia

Hernia through the sciatic foramen

Richter's hernia

Incarcerated or strangulated hernia involving only **one sidewall of the bowel,** which can spontaneously reduce, resulting in gangrenous bowel and perforation within the abdomen without signs of obstruction

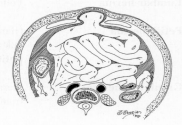

Epigastric hernia   Hernia through the linea alba above the umbilicus

Umbilical hernia   Hernia through the umbilical ring, in adults associated with ascites, pregnancy, and obesity

Intraparietal hernia   Hernia in which abdominal contents migrate between the layers of the abdominal wall

Femoral hernia   Hernia medial to femoral vessels (under inguinal ligament)

Hesselbach's hernia   Hernia under inguinal ligament **lateral** to femoral vessels

Bochdalek's hernia   Hernia through the posterior diaphragm, usually on the left (Think: Boch da lek = "back to the left" on the diaphragm)

Morgagni's hernia   Anterior parasternal diaphragmatic hernia

Properitoneal hernia   Intraparietal hernia between the peritoneum and transversalis fascia

Cooper's hernia   Hernia through the femoral canal and tracking into the scrotum or labia majus

Indirect inguinal   Inguinal hernia lateral to Hesselbach's triangle

Direct inguinal   Inguinal hernia within Hesselbach's triangle

Hiatal hernia   Hernia through esophageal hiatus

Amyand's hernia   Hernia sac containing a ruptured appendix (Think: **A**myand's = **A**ppendix)

What are the boundaries of Hesselbach's triangle?	1. Inferior epigastric vessels 2. Inguinal ligament (Poupart's) 3. Lateral border of the rectus sheath Floor consists of internal oblique and the transversus abdominis muscle
What are the layers of the abdominal wall?	Skin Subcutaneous fat Scarpa's fascia External oblique Internal oblique Transversus abdominus Transversalis fascia Preperitoneal fat Peritoneum ***Note:*** All three muscle layer aponeuroses form the anterior rectus sheath, with the posterior rectus sheath being deficient below the arcuate line
What is the differential diagnosis for a mass in a healed C-section incision?	Hernia, ENDOMETRIOMA

GROIN HERNIAS

What is the differential diagnosis of a groin mass?	Lymphadenopathy, hematoma, seroma, abscess, hydrocele, femoral artery aneurysm, EIC, undescended testicle, sarcoma, hernias, testicle torsion

DIRECT INGUINAL HERNIA

What is it?	Hernia within the floor of Hesselbach's triangle, i.e., the hernia sac does not traverse the internal ring (think **directly** through the abdominal wall)
What is the cause?	Acquired defect from mechanical breakdown over the years
What is the incidence?	≈1% of all men; frequency increases with advanced age
What nerve runs with the spermatic cord in the inguinal canal?	Ilioinguinal nerve

INDIRECT INGUINAL HERNIA

What is it?

Hernia through the internal ring of the inguinal canal, traveling down toward the external ring; it may enter the scrotum upon exiting the external ring (i.e., if complete); think of the hernia sac traveling **indirectly** through the abdominal wall from the internal ring to the external ring

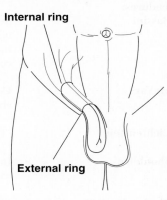

Internal ring

External ring

What is the cause?

Patent processus vaginalis (i.e., congenital)

What is the incidence?

≈5% of all men; most common hernia in both men **and** women

How is an inguinal hernia diagnosed?

Relies mainly on history and physical exam with index finger invaginated into the external ring and palpation of hernia; examine the patient standing up if diagnosis is not obvious
(**Note:** if swelling occurs below the inguinal ligament, it is possibly a femoral hernia)

What is the differential diagnosis of an inguinal hernia?

Lymphadenopathy, psoas abscess, ectopic testis, hydrocele of the cord, saphenous varix, lipoma, varicocele, testicular torsion, femoral artery aneurysm, abscess

What is the risk of strangulation?

Higher with indirect than direct inguinal hernia, but highest in femoral hernias

What is the treatment?	Emergent herniorrhaphy is indicated if strangulation is suspected or acute incarceration is present; otherwise, elective herniorrhaphy is indicated to prevent the chance of incarceration/strangulation

INGUINAL HERNIA REPAIRS

Define the following procedures:

Bassini	**Sutures** approximate reflection of inguinal ligament (Poupart's) to the transversus abdominis aponeurosis/conjoint tendon
McVay	**Cooper's** ligament sutured to transversus abdominis aponeurosis/conjoint tendon
Lichtenstein	"Tension-free repair" using mesh
Shouldice	Imbrication of the floor of the inguinal canal (a.k.a. "Canadian repair")
Plug and patch	Placing a plug of mesh in hernia defect and then overlaying a patch of mesh over inguinal floor (requires few if any sutures in mesh!)
High ligation	Ligation and transection of indirect hernia sac without repair of inguinal floor (used only in **children**)
TAPP procedure	**T**rans**A**bdominal **P**re**P**eritoneal inguinal hernia repair
TEPA procedure	**T**otally **E**xtra**P**eritoneal **A**pproach
What are the indications for laparoscopic inguinal hernia repair?	1. Bilateral inguinal hernias 2. Recurring hernia 3. Need to resume full activity as soon as possible

CLASSIC INTRAOPERATIVE INGUINAL HERNIA QUESTIONS

What is the first identifiable subcutaneous named layer?	Scarpa's fascia (thin in adults)

What is the name of the sub-cutaneous vein that is ligated?
Superficial epigastric vein

What happens if you cut the ilioinguinal nerve?
Numbness of inner thigh or lateral scrotum; usually goes away in 6 months

From what abdominal muscle layer is the cremaster muscle derived?
Internal oblique muscle

From what abdominal muscle layer is the inguinal ligament (a.k.a. Poupart's ligament) derived?
External oblique muscle aponeurosis

To what does the inguinal (Poupart's) ligament attach?
Anterior superior iliac spine to the pubic tubercle

Which nerve travels on the spermatic cord?
Ilioinguinal nerve

Why do some surgeons deliberately cut the ilioinguinal nerve?
First they obtain preoperative consent and cut so as to remove the risk of entrapment and postoperative pain

What is in the spermatic cord (6)?
1. Cremasteric muscle fibers
2. Vas deferens
3. Testicular artery
4. Testicular pampiniform venous plexus
5. ± hernia sac
6. Genital branch of the genitofemoral nerve

What is the hernia sac made of?
Peritoneum (direct) or a patent processus vaginalis (indirect)

What attaches the testicle to the scrotum?
Gubernaculum

What is the most common organ in an inguinal hernia sac in men?
Small intestine

What is the most common organ in an inguinal hernia sac in women?
Ovary/fallopian tube

What lies in the inguinal canal in the female instead of the VAS?	Round ligament
Where in the inguinal canal does the hernia sac lie in relation to the other structures?	Anteromedially
What is a "cord lipoma"?	Preperitoneal fat on the cord structures (pushed in by the hernia sac); not a real lipoma; remove surgically, if feasible
What is a small outpouching of testicular tissue off of the testicle?	Testicular appendage (a.k.a. the appendix testes); remove with electrocautery
What action should be taken if a suture is placed through the femoral artery or vein during an inguinal herniorrhaphy?	Remove the suture as soon as possible and apply pressure (i.e., do not tie the suture down!)
What nerve is found on top of the spermatic cord?	Ilioinguinal nerve
What nerve travels within the spermatic cord?	Genital branch of the genitofemoral nerve
What are the borders of Hesselbach's triangle?	1. Epigastric vessels 2. Inguinal ligament 3. Lateral border of the rectus

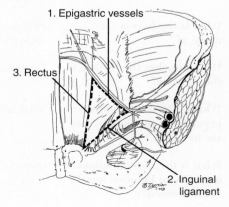

1. Epigastric vessels

3. Rectus

2. Inguinal ligament

What type of hernia goes through Hesselbach's triangle?

Direct hernia due to a weak abdominal floor

What is a "relaxing incision"?

Incision(s) in the rectus sheath to relax the conjoint tendon so that it can be approximated to the reflection of the inguinal ligament without tension

What is the conjoint tendon?

Aponeurotic attachments of the "conjoining" of the internal oblique and transversus abdominis to the pubic tubercle

Define inguinal anatomy.

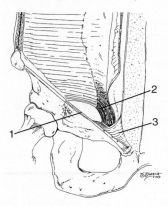

1. Inguinal ligament (Poupart's ligament)
2. Transversus aponeurosis
3. Conjoint tendon

How tight should the new internal inguinal ring be?

Should allow entrance of the tip of a Kelly clamp but not a finger (the new external inguinal ring should not be tight and should allow entrance of a finger)

What percentage of the strength of an inguinal floor repair does the external oblique aponeurosis represent?

ZERO

FEMORAL HERNIA

What is it?

Hernia traveling beneath the inguinal ligament down the femoral canal medial to the femoral vessels (Think: **FM** radio, or **F**emoral hernia = **M**edial)

What are the boundaries of the femoral canal?

1. Cooper's ligament posteriorly
2. Inguinal ligament anteriorly
3. Femoral vein laterally
4. Lacunar ligament medially

What factors are associated with femoral hernias?

Women, pregnancy, and exertion

What percentage of all hernias are femoral?

5%

What percentage of patients with a femoral hernia are female?

85%!

What are the complications?

Approximately one third incarcerate (due to narrow, unforgiving neck)

What is the most common hernia in women?

Indirect inguinal hernia

What is the repair of a femoral hernia?

McVay (Cooper's ligament repair), mesh plug repair

HERNIA REVIEW QUESTIONS

Should elective TURP or elective herniorrhaphy be performed first?

TURP

Which type of esophageal hiatal hernia is associated with GE reflux?

Sliding esophageal hiatal hernia

Classically, how can an incarcerated hernia be reduced in the ER?

1. Apply ice to incarcerated hernia
2. Sedate
3. Use the Trendelenburg position for inguinal hernias
4. Apply steady gentle manual pressure
5. Admit and observe for signs of necrotic bowel after reduction
6. Perform surgical herniorrhaphy ASAP

What is appropriate if you cannot reduce an incarcerated hernia with steady, gentle compression?

Go directly to O.R. for repair

What is the major difference in repairing a pediatric indirect inguinal hernia and an adult inguinal hernia?

In babies and children it is rarely necessary to repair the inguinal floor; repair with "high ligation" of the hernia sac

What is the Howship-Romberg sign?

Pain along the medial aspect of the proximal thigh from nerve compression caused by an obturator hernia

What is the "silk glove" sign?

Inguinal hernia sac in an infant/toddler feels like a finger of a silk glove when rolled under the examining finger

What must you do before leaving the O.R. after an inguinal hernia repair?

Pull the testicle back down to the scrotum

ESOPHAGEAL HIATAL HERNIAS

Define type I and type II hiatal hernias.

Type I = sliding
Type II = paraesophageal

SLIDING ESOPHAGEAL HIATAL HERNIA

What is it?

Both the stomach and GE junction herniate into the thorax via the esophageal hiatus; also known as type I hiatal hernia

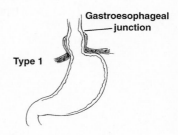

What is the incidence?	>90% of all hiatal hernias
What are the symptoms?	Most patients are asymptomatic, but the condition can cause **reflux,** dysphagia (from inflammatory edema), esophagitis, and pulmonary problems secondary to aspiration
How is it diagnosed?	UGI series, manometry, esophagogastroduodenoscopy (EGD) with biopsy for esophagitis
What are the complications?	Reflux → esophagitis → Barrett's esophagus → cancer and stricture formation; aspiration pneumonia; it can also result in UGI bleeding from esophageal ulcerations
What is the treatment?	85% of cases treated medically with antacids, H_2 blockers/PPIs, head elevation after meals, small meals, and no food prior to sleeping; 15% of cases require surgery for persistent symptoms despite adequate medical treatment
What is the surgical treatment?	Laparoscopic Nissen fundoplication (LAP NISSEN) involves wrapping the fundus around the LES and suturing it in place

PARAESOPHAGEAL HIATAL HERNIA

What is it?	Herniation of all or part of the stomach through the esophageal hiatus into the thorax without displacement of the gastroesophageal junction; also known as type II hiatal hernia

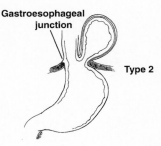

Gastroesophageal junction

Type 2

What is the incidence?	<5% of all hiatal hernias (rare)
What are the symptoms?	Derived from mechanical obstruction; dysphagia, stasis gastric ulcer, and strangulation; many cases are asymptomatic and not associated with reflux because of a relatively normal position of the GE junction
What are the complications?	Hemorrhage, incarceration, obstruction, and strangulation
What is the treatment?	Surgical, because of frequency and severity of potential complications
What is a type III hiatal hernia?	Combined type I and type II
What is a type IV hiatal hernia?	Organ (e.g., colon or spleen) +/− stomach in the chest cavity

---

Chapter 37 Laparoscopy

What is laparoscopy?	Minimally invasive surgical technique using gas to insufflate the peritoneum and instruments manipulated through ports introduced through small incisions with video camera guidance
What gas is used and why?	CO_2 because of better solubility in blood and, thus, less risk of gas embolism; noncombustible
Which operations are performed with the laparoscope?	**Frequently**—cholecystectomy; appendectomy; inguinal hernia repair; ventral hernia repair, Nissen fundoplication **Infrequently**—bowel resection, colostomy, surgery for PUD (PGV, perforation), colectomy, splenectomy, adrenalectomy

What are the contraindications?	**Absolute**—hypovolemic shock, severe cardiac decompensation **Relative**—extensive intraperitoneal adhesions, diaphragmatic hernia, COPD
What are the associated complications?	Pneumothorax, bleeding, perforating injuries, infection, intestinal injuries, solid organ injury, major vascular injury, **CO_2 embolus,** bladder injury, hernia at larger trocar sites, DVT
What are the classic findings with a CO_2 gas embolus?	Triad: 1. Hypotension 2. Decreased end tidal CO_2 (low flow to lung) 3. Mill-wheel murmur
What prophylactic measure should every patient get when they are going to have a laparoscopic procedure?	**SCD** boots—**S**equential **C**ompression **D**evice (and most add an OGT to decompress the stomach; Foley catheter is usually used for pelvic procedures)
What are the cardiovascular effects of a pneumoperitoneum?	**Increased afterload** and **decreased preload** (but the CVP and PCWP are deceivingly elevated!)
What is the effect of CO_2 insufflation on end tidal CO_2 levels?	Increased as a result of absorption of CO_2 into the bloodstream; the body compensates with increased ventilation and blows the extra CO_2 off and thus there is no acidosis
What are the advantages over laparotomy?	Shorter hospitalization, less pain and scarring, lower cost, decreased ileus
What is the Veress needle?	Needle with spring-loaded, retractable, blunt inner-protective tube that protrudes from the needle end when it enters peritoneal cavity; used for blind entrance and then insufflation of CO_2 through the Veress needle
How can it be verified that the Veress needle is in the peritoneum?	Syringe of saline; saline should flow freely without pressure through the needle "drop test"

If the Veress needle is not in the peritoneal cavity, what happens to the CO_2 flow/pressure?

Flow decreases and pressure is high

What is the Hasson technique?

No Veress needle—cut down and place trocar under **direct visualization**

What is the cause of post-laparoscopic shoulder pain?

Referred pain from CO_2 on diaphragm and diaphragm stretch

What is a laparoscopic-assisted procedure?

Laparoscopic dissection; then, part of the procedure is performed through an open incision

What is FRED®?

Fog **R**eduction **E**limination **D**evice: sponge with antifog solution used to coat the camera lens

Give some tips for "driving" the camera during laparoscopy.

1. Keep the camera centered on the action
2. Watch all trocars as they enter the peritoneal cavity (and the tissues beyond, so they can be avoided!)
3. Watch all instruments as they come through the trocars (unless directed otherwise)
4. Ask if you want to come out and clean and re-FRED the lens
5. Look outside the body at the trocars and instrument angles to reorient yourself
6. Keep the camera oriented at all times (i.e., up and down); usually the camera cord is on the bottom of the camera—orient yourself to the camera before entering the abdomen
7. You may clean the camera lens at times by lightly touching the lens to the liver or peritoneum
8. Never let the camera lens come into contact with the bowel because the camera may get very hot and you can burn a hole in the bowel or burn the drapes!

9. Put your helmet on (i.e., expect to get yelled at!)
10. Never act agitated when the surgeons are a little abrupt (e.g., "Center— center the camera!")
11. Always watch the trocars as they are removed from the abdominal wall for bleeding from the site and view the layers of the abdominal wall, looking for bleeding as you pull the camera trocar out at the end of the case

At what length must you close trocar sites?

>5 mm should be closed

How do you get the spleen out through a trocar site after a laparoscopic splenectomy?

Morcellation in a bag, then remove piecemeal

What is an IOC?

Intra**O**perative **C**holangiogram (done during a lap chole to evaluate the common bile duct anatomy and to look for any retained duct stone)

What is the safest time for laparoscopy during pregnancy?

Second trimester

Chapter 38 Trauma

What widely accepted protocol does trauma care in the United States follow?

Advanced Trauma Life Support (ATLS) precepts of the American College of Surgeons

What are the three main elements of the ATLS protocol?

1. Primary survey/resuscitation
2. Secondary survey
3. Definitive care

How and when should the patient history be obtained?	It should be obtained while completing the primary survey; often the rescue squad, witnesses, and family members must be relied upon

PRIMARY SURVEY

What are the five steps of the primary survey?	Think: **"ABCDEs"**: **A**irway (and C-spine stabilization) **B**reathing **C**irculation **D**isability **E**xposure and **E**nvironment
What principles are followed in completing the primary survey?	Life-threatening problems discovered during the primary survey are **always** addressed **before** proceeding to the next step

AIRWAY

What are the goals during assessment of the airway?	Securing the airway and protecting the spinal cord
In addition to the airway, what MUST be considered during the airway step?	Spinal immobilization
What comprises spinal immobilization?	Use of a full backboard and rigid cervical collar
In an alert patient, what is the quickest test for an adequate airway?	Ask a question: If the patient can speak, the airway is intact
What is the first maneuver used to establish an airway?	Chin lift, jaw thrust, or both; if successful, often an oral or nasal airway can be used to temporarily maintain the airway
If these methods are unsuccessful, what is the next maneuver used to establish an airway?	Endotracheal intubation

If all other methods are unsuccessful, what is the definitive airway?

Cricothyroidotomy, a.k.a. "surgical airway": Incise the cricothyroid membrane between the cricoid cartilage inferiorly and the thyroid cartilage superiorly and place an endotracheal or tracheostomy tube into the trachea

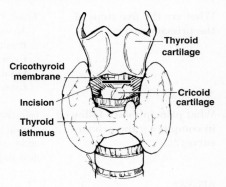

What must always be kept in mind during difficult attempts to establish an airway?

Spinal immobilization and adequate oxygenation; if at all possible, patients must be adequately ventilated with 100% oxygen using a bag and mask before any attempt to establish an airway

BREATHING

What are the goals in assessing breathing?

Securing oxygenation and ventilation
Treating life-threatening thoracic injuries

What comprises adequate assessment of breathing?

Inspection—for air movement, respiratory rate, cyanosis, tracheal shift, jugular venous distention, asymmetric chest expansion, use of accessory muscles of respiration, open chest wounds
Auscultation—for breath sounds
Percussion—for hyperresonance or dullness over either lung field
Palpation—for presence of subcutaneous emphysema, flail segments

What are the life-threatening conditions that MUST be diagnosed and treated during the breathing step?

Tension pneumothorax, open pneumothorax, massive hemothorax

Pneumothorax

What is it?

Injury to the lung, resulting in release of air into the pleural space between the normally apposed parietal and visceral pleura

How is it diagnosed?

Tension pneumothorax is a clinical diagnosis: dyspnea, jugular venous distention, tachypnea, anxiety, pleuritic chest pain, unilateral decreased or absent breath sounds, tracheal shift away from the affected side, hyperresonance on the affected side

What is the treatment of a tension pneumothorax?

Rapid thoracostomy incision or **immediate** decompression by **needle thoracostomy** in the second intercostal space midclavicular line, followed by **tube thoracostomy** placed in the anterior/midaxillary line in the fourth intercostal space (level of the nipple in men)

What is the medical term for a "sucking chest wound"?

Open pneumothorax

What is a tube thoracostomy?

"Chest tube"

How is an open pneumothorax diagnosed and treated?

Diagnosis: usually obvious, with air movement through a chest wall defect and pneumothorax on CXR
Treatment in the ER: tube thoracostomy (chest tube), occlusive dressing over chest wall defect

What does a pneumothorax look like on chest X-ray?

Loss of lung markings (Figure shows a right-sided pneumothorax; arrows point out edge of lung-air interface)

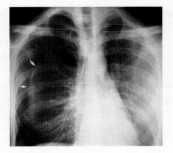

Flail Chest

What is it? Two separate fractures in three or more consecutive ribs

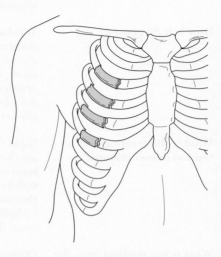

How is it diagnosed? Flail segment of chest wall that moves **paradoxically** (sucks in with inspiration and pushes out with expiration opposite the rest of the chest wall)

What is the major cause of respiratory compromise with flail chest? Underlying pulmonary contusion!

What is the treatment? **Intubation** with positive pressure ventilation and PEEP PRN (let ribs heal on their own)

Cardiac Tamponade

What is it? Bleeding into the pericardial sac, resulting in constriction of heart, decreasing inflow and resulting in decreased cardiac output (the pericardium does not stretch!)

What are the signs and symptoms? Tachycardia/shock with **Beck's triad,** pulsus paradoxus, Kussmaul's sign

Define the following:
  Beck's triad

1. Hypotension
2. Muffled heart sounds
3. JVD

  Kussmaul's sign

JVD with inspiration

How is cardiac tamponade diagnosed?

Ultrasound (echocardiogram)

What is the treatment?

Pericardial window—if blood returns then median sternotomy to rule out and treat cardiac injury

Massive Hemothorax

How is it diagnosed?

Unilaterally decreased or absent breath sounds; dullness to percussion; CXR, CT scan, chest tube output

What is the treatment?

Volume replacement
Tube thoracostomy (chest tube)
Removal of the blood (which will allow apposition of the parietal and visceral pleura, sealing the defect and slowing the bleeding)

What are indications for emergent thoracotomy for hemothorax?

Massive hemothorax =
1. >1500 cc of blood on initial placement of chest tube
2. Persistent >200 cc of bleeding via chest tube per hour × 4 hours

CIRCULATION

What are the goals in assessing circulation?

Securing adequate tissue perfusion; treatment of external bleeding

What is the initial test for adequate circulation?

Palpation of pulses: As a rough guide, if a radial pulse is palpable, then systolic pressure is at least 80 mm Hg; if a femoral or carotid pulse is palpable, then systolic pressure is at least 60 mm Hg

What comprises adequate assessment of circulation?

Heart rate, blood pressure, peripheral perfusion, urinary output, mental status, capillary refill (normal <2 seconds), exam of skin: cold, clammy = hypovolemia

Who can be hypovolemic with normal blood pressure?

Young patients; autonomic tone can maintain blood pressure until cardiovascular collapse is imminent

Which patients may not mount a tachycardic response to hypovolemic shock?

Those with concomitant spinal cord injuries
Those on β-blockers
Well-conditioned athletes

How are sites of external bleeding treated?

By direct pressure; +/− tourniquets

What is the best and preferred intravenous (IV) access in the trauma patient?

"Two large-bore IVs" (14–16 gauge), IV catheters in the upper extremities (peripheral IV access)

What are alternate sites of IV access?

Percutaneous and cutdown catheters in the lower leg saphenous; central access into femoral, jugular, subclavian veins

For a femoral vein catheter, how can the anatomy of the right groin be remembered?

Lateral to medial **"NAVEL"**:
  Nerve
  Artery
  Vein
  Empty space
  Lymphatics
Thus, the vein is medial to the femoral artery pulse (Or, think: "venous close to penis")

What is the trauma resuscitation fluid of choice?

Lactated Ringer's (LR) solution (isotonic, and the lactate helps buffer the hypovolemia-induced metabolic acidosis)

What types of decompression do trauma patients receive?

Gastric decompression with an NG tube and Foley catheter bladder decompression after **normal rectal exam**

What are the contraindications to placement of a Foley?

Signs of urethral injury:
Severe pelvic fracture in men
Blood at the urethral meatus (penile opening)
"High-riding" "ballotable" prostate (loss of urethral tethering)
Scrotal/perineal injury/ecchymosis

What test should be obtained prior to placing a Foley catheter if urethral injury is suspected?

Retrograde **U**rethro**G**ram (**RUG**): dye in penis retrograde to the bladder and x-ray looking for extravasation of dye

How is gastric decompression achieved with a maxillofacial fracture?

Not with an NG tube because the tube may perforate through the cribriform plate into the brain; place an **oral**-gastric tube (OGT), not an NG tube

DISABILITY

What are the goals in assessing disability?

Determination of neurologic injury (Think: neurologic disability)

What comprises adequate assessment of disability?

Mental status—Glasgow Coma Scale (GCS)
Pupils—a blown pupil suggests ipsilateral brain mass (blood) as herniation of the brain compresses CN III
Motor/sensory—screening exam for lateralizing extremity movement, sensory deficits

Describe the GCS scoring system.

Eye opening (E)
4—Opens spontaneously
3—Opens to voice (command)
2—Opens to painful stimulus
1—Does not open eyes

(Think: Eyes = "four eyes")

Motor response (M)
6—Obeys commands
5—Localizes painful stimulus
4—Withdraws from pain
3—Decorticate posture
2—Decerebrate posture
1—No movement

(Think: Motor = "6-cylinder motor")

Verbal response (V)
5—Appropriate and oriented
4—Confused
3—Inappropriate words
2—Incomprehensible sounds
1—No sounds

(Think: Verbal = "Jackson 5")

What is a normal human GCS?	GCS 15
What is the GCS score for a dead man?	GCS 3
What is the GCS score for a patient in a "coma"?	GCS ≤8
How does scoring differ if the patient is intubated?	Verbal evaluation is omitted and replaced with a "T"; thus, the highest score for an intubated patient is 11 T

EXPOSURE AND ENVIRONMENT

What are the goals in obtaining adequate exposure?	Complete disrobing to allow a thorough visual inspection and digital palpation of the patient during the secondary survey
What is the "environment" of the E in ABCDEs?	Keep a warm **E**nvironment (i.e., keep the patient warm; a hypothermic patient can become coagulopathic)

SECONDARY SURVEY

What principle is followed in completing the secondary survey?	Complete physical exam, including all orifices: ears, nose, mouth, vagina, rectum
Why look in the ears?	Hemotympanum is a sign of basilar skull fracture; otorrhea is a sign of basilar skull fracture
Examination of what part of the trauma patient's body is often forgotten?	Patient's back (logroll the patient and examine!)
What are typical signs of basilar skull fracture?	Raccoon eyes, Battle's sign, clear otorrhea or rhinorrhea, hemotympanum
What diagnosis in the anterior chamber must not be missed on the eye exam?	Traumatic hyphema = blood in the anterior chamber of the eye

What potentially destructive lesion must not be missed on the nasal exam?	Nasal septal hematoma: Hematoma must be evacuated; if not, it can result in pressure necrosis of the septum!
What is the best indication of a mandibular fracture?	Dental malocclusion: Tell the patient to "bite down" and ask, "Does that feel normal to you?"
What signs of thoracic trauma are often found on the neck exam?	Crepitus or subcutaneous emphysema from tracheobronchial disruption/PTX; tracheal deviation from tension pneumothorax; jugular venous distention from cardiac tamponade; carotid bruit heard with seatbelt neck injury resulting in carotid artery injury
What is the best physical exam for broken ribs or sternum?	Lateral and anterior-posterior compression of the thorax to elicit pain/instability
What physical signs are diagnostic for thoracic great vessel injury?	None: Diagnosis of great vessel injury requires a high index of suspicion based on the mechanism of injury, associated injuries, and CXR/radiographic findings (e.g., widened mediastinum)
What is the best way to diagnose or rule out aortic injury?	CT angiogram
What must be considered in every penetrating injury of the thorax at or below the level of the nipple?	Concomitant injury to the abdomen: Remember, the diaphragm extends to the level of the nipples in the male on full expiration
What is the significance of subcutaneous air?	Indicates PTX, until proven otherwise
What is the physical exam technique for examining the thoracic and lumbar spine?	Logrolling the patient to allow complete visualization of the back and palpation of the spine to elicit pain over fractures, step off (spine deformity)
What conditions must exist to pronounce an abdominal physical exam negative?	Alert patient without any evidence of head/spinal cord injury or drug/EtOH intoxication (even then, the abdominal exam is not 100% accurate)

What physical signs may indicate intra-abdominal injury?

Tenderness; guarding; peritoneal signs; progressive distention (always use a gastric tube for decompression of air); seatbelt sign

What is the seatbelt sign?

Ecchymosis on lower abdomen from wearing a seatbelt ($\approx$10% of patients with this sign have a small bowel perforation!)

What must be documented from the rectal exam?

Sphincter tone (as an indication of spinal cord function); presence of blood (as an indication of colon or rectal injury); prostate position (as an indication of urethral injury)

What is the best physical exam technique to test for pelvic fractures?

Lateral compression of the iliac crests and greater trochanters and anterior-posterior compression of the symphysis pubis to elicit pain/instability

What is the "halo" sign?

Cerebrospinal fluid from nose/ear will form a clear "halo" around the blood on a cloth

What physical signs indicate possible urethral injury, thus contraindicating placement of a Foley catheter?

High-riding ballotable prostate on rectal exam; presence of blood at the meatus; scrotal or perineal ecchymosis

What must be documented from the extremity exam?

Any fractures or joint injuries; any open wounds; motor and sensory exam, particularly distal to any fractures; distal pulses; peripheral perfusion

What complication after prolonged ischemia to the lower extremity must be treated immediately?

Compartment syndrome

What is the treatment for this condition?

Fasciotomy (four compartments below the knee)

What injuries must be suspected in a trauma patient with a progressive decline in mental status?

Epidural hematoma, subdural hematoma, brain swelling with rising intracranial pressure

But **hypoxia/hypotension must be ruled out!**

TRAUMA STUDIES

What are the classic blunt trauma ER x-rays?	1. AP (anterior-to-posterior) chest film 2. AP pelvis film
What are the common trauma labs?	Blood for complete blood count, chemistries, amylase, liver function tests, lactic acid, coagulation studies, and **type and crossmatch;** urine for urinalysis
Will the hematocrit be low after an acute massive hemorrhage?	No (no time to equilibrate)
How can a C-spine be evaluated?	1. Clinically by physical exam 2. Radiographically
What patients can have their C-spines cleared by a physical exam?	No neck pain on palpation with full range of motion (FROM) with no neurologic injury (GCS 15), no EtOH/drugs, no distracting injury, no pain meds
How do you rule out a C-spine bony fracture?	With a CT scan of the C-spine
What do you do if no bony C-spine fracture is apparent on CT scan and you cannot obtain an MRI in a COMATOSE patient?	This is controversial; the easiest answer is to leave the patient in a cervical collar
Which x-rays are used for evaluation of cervical spine LIGAMENTOUS injury?	MRI, lateral flexion and extension C-spine films
What findings on chest film are suggestive of thoracic aortic injury?	**Widened mediastinum (most common finding),** apical pleural capping, loss of aortic contour/KNOB/AP window, depression of left main stem bronchus, nasogastric tube/tracheal deviation, pleural fluid, elevation of right mainstem bronchus, clinical suspicion, high-speed mechanism

What study is used to rule out thoracic aortic injury?	Spiral CT scan of mediastinum looking for mediastinal hematoma with CTA Thoracic arch aortogram (gold standard)
What is the most common site of thoracic aortic traumatic tear?	Just distal to the take-off of the left subclavian artery
What studies are available to evaluate for intra-abdominal injury?	FAST, CT scan, DPL
What is a FAST exam?	Ultrasound: **F**ocused **A**ssessment with **S**onography for **T**rauma = **FAST**
What does the FAST exam look for?	Blood in the peritoneal cavity looking at Morison's pouch, bladder, spleen, and pericardial sac
What does DPL stand for?	**D**iagnostic **P**eritoneal **L**avage
What diagnostic test is the test of choice for evaluation of the unstable patient with blunt abdominal trauma?	FAST
What is the indication for abdominal CT scan in blunt trauma?	Normal vital signs with abdominal pain/tenderness/mechanism
What is the indication for DPL or FAST in blunt trauma?	Unstable vital signs (hypotension)
How is a DPL performed?	Place a catheter below the umbilicus (in patients without a pelvic fracture) into the peritoneal cavity Aspirate for blood and if <10 cc are aspirated, infuse 1 L of saline or LR Drain the fluid (by gravity) and analyze
What is a "grossly positive" DPL?	≥10 cc blood aspirated

Where should the DPL catheter be placed in a patient with a pelvic fracture?

Above the umbilicus

Common error: If you go below the umbilicus, you may get into a pelvic hematoma tracking between the fascia layers and thus obtain a false-positive DPL

What constitutes a positive peritoneal tap?

Prior to starting a peritoneal lavage, the DPL catheter should be aspirated; if >10 mL of blood or any enteric contents are aspirated, then this constitutes a positive tap and requires laparotomy

What are the indicators of a positive peritoneal lavage in blunt trauma?

Classic:
  Inability to read newsprint through lavaged fluid
  RBC ≥100,000/mm^3
  WBC ≥500/mm^3 (***Note:*** mm^3, not mm^2)
  Lavage fluid (LR/NS) drained from chest tube, Foley, NG tube

Less common:
  Bile present
  Bacteria present
  Feces present
  Vegetable matter present
  Elevated amylase level

What must be in place before a DPL is performed?

NG tube and Foley catheter (to remove the stomach and bladder from the line of fire!)

What injuries does CT scan miss?

Small bowel injuries and diaphragm injuries

What injuries does DPL miss?

Retroperitoneal injuries

What study is used to evaluate the urethra in cases of possible disruption due to blunt trauma?

Retrograde urethrogram (RUG)

What are the most emergent orthopaedic injuries?

1. Hip dislocation—must be reduced immediately
2. Exsanguinating pelvic fracture (binder or external fixator)

What findings would require a celiotomy in a blunt trauma victim?

Peritoneal signs, free air on CXR/CT scan, unstable patient with positive FAST exam or positive DPL results

What is the treatment of a gunshot wound to the belly?

Exploratory laparotomy

What is the evaluation of a stab wound to the belly?

If there are peritoneal signs, heavy bleeding, shock, perform exploratory laparotomy; otherwise, many surgeons either observe the asymptomatic stab wound patient closely, use local wound exploration to rule out fascial penetration, or use DPL

PENETRATING NECK INJURIES

What depth of neck injury must be further evaluated?

Penetrating injury through the platysma

Define the anatomy of the neck by trauma zones:
    Zone III

Angle of the mandible and up

    Zone II

Angle of the mandible to the cricoid cartilage

    Zone I

Below the cricoid cartilage

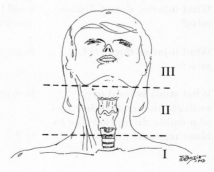

How do most surgeons treat penetrating neck injuries (those that penetrate the platysma) by neck zone:

Zone III — Selective exploration

Zone II — Surgical exploration vs. selective exploration

Zone I — Selective exploration

What is selective exploration? — Selective exploration is based on diagnostic studies that include A-gram or CT A-gram, bronchoscopy, esophagoscopy

What are the indications for surgical exploration in all penetrating neck wounds (Zones I, II, III)? — "**Hard** signs" of significant neck damage: **shock,** exsanguinating hemorrhage, expanding hematoma, pulsatile hematoma, neurologic injury, subQ emphysema

How can you remember the order of the neck trauma zones and Le Forte fractures? — In the direction of carotid blood flow

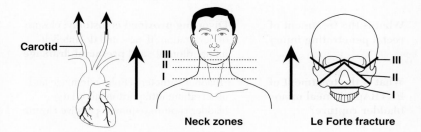

Carotid

Neck zones

Le Forte fracture

MISCELLANEOUS TRAUMA FACTS

What is the "3-for-1" rule? — Trauma patient in hypovolemic shock acutely requires 3 L of crystalloid (LR) for every 1 L of blood loss

What is the minimal urine output for an adult trauma patient? — 50 mL/hr

How much blood can be lost into the thigh with a closed femur fracture?

Up to 1.5 L of blood

Can an adult lose enough blood in the "closed" skull from a brain injury to cause hypovolemic shock?

Absolutely not! But infants can lose enough blood from a brain injury to cause shock

Can a patient be hypotensive after an isolated head injury?

Yes, but rule out hemorrhagic shock!

What is the brief ATLS history?

"AMPLE" history:
  Allergies
  Medications
  PMH
  Last meal (when)
  Events (of injury, etc.)

In what population is a surgical cricothyroidotomy not recommended?

Any patient younger than 12 years; instead perform needle cricothyroidotomy

What are the signs of a laryngeal fracture?

Subcutaneous emphysema in neck
Altered voice
Palpable laryngeal fracture

What is the treatment of rectal penetrating injury?

Diverting proximal colostomy; closure of perforation (if easy, and definitely if intraperitoneal); and **presacral drainage**

What is the treatment of EXTRAperitoneal minor bladder rupture?

"Bladder catheter" (Foley) drainage and observation; intraperitoneal or large bladder rupture requires operative closure

What intra-abdominal injury is associated with seatbelt use?

Small bowel injuries (L2 fracture, pancreatic injury)

What is the treatment of a pelvic fracture?

+/− pelvic binder until the external fixator is placed; IVF/blood; +/− A-gram to embolize bleeding pelvic vessels

Bleeding from pelvic fractures is most commonly caused by arterial or venous bleeding?

Venous ($\approx 85\%$)

If a patient has a laceration through an eyebrow, should you shave the eyebrow prior to suturing it closed?	No—20% of the time, the eyebrow will not grow back if shaved!
What is the treatment of extensive irreparable biliary, duodenal, and pancreatic head injury?	Trauma Whipple
What is the most common intra-abdominal organ injured with penetrating trauma?	Small bowel
How high up do the diaphragms go?	To the nipples (intercostal space #4); thus, intra-abdominal injury with penetrating injury below the nipples must be ruled out
Classic trauma question: "If you have only one vial of blood from a trauma victim to send to the lab, what test should be ordered?"	Type and cross (for blood transfusion)
What is the treatment of penetrating injury to the colon?	If the patient is in shock, resection and colostomy If the patient is stable, the trend is primary anastomosis/repair
What is the treatment of small bowel injury?	Primary closure or resection and primary anastomosis
What is the treatment of minor pancreatic injury?	Drainage (e.g., JP drains)
What is the most commonly injured abdominal organ with blunt trauma?	Liver (in recent studies)
What is the treatment for significant duodenal injury?	Pyloric exclusion: 1. Close duodenal injury 2. Staple off pylorus 3. Gastrojejunostomy

What is the treatment for massive tail of pancreas injury?

Distal pancreatectomy (usually perform splenectomy also)

What is "damage control" surgery?

Stop major hemorrhage and GI soilage
Pack and get out of the O.R. ASAP to bring the patient to the ICU to warm, correct coags, and resuscitate
Return patient to O.R. when stable, warm, and not acidotic

What is the "lethal triad"?

"ACH":
1. **A**cidosis
2. **C**oagulopathy
3. **H**ypothermia

(Think: **ACH**e = **A**cidosis, **C**oagulopathy, **H**ypothermia)

What comprises the workup/ treatment of a stable parasternal chest gunshot/ stab wound?

1. CXR
2. FAST, chest tube, +/− O.R. for sub-xiphoid window; if blood returns, then sternotomy to assess for cardiac injury

What is the diagnosis with NGT in chest on CXR?

Ruptured diaphragm with stomach in pleural cavity (go to ex lap)

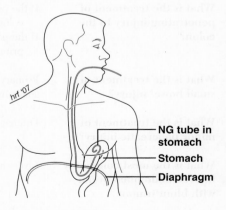

What films are typically obtained to evaluate extremity fractures?

Complete views of the involved extremity, including the joints above and below the fracture

Outline basic workup for a victim of severe blunt trauma
In ER: Airway, physical exam. IV X 2, labs, type and cross,
OGT/NGT, Foley, chest tube PRN
X-rays: CXR, pelvic, femur
(if femur fracture is suspected)

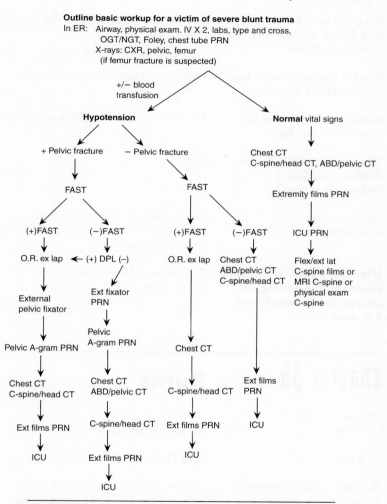

[Note: AP = anteroposterior; Ext = extremity; OGT = orogastric tube;
FAST = Focused Assessment Sonogram for Trauma; lat = lateral; C = cervical.]

What finding on ABD/pelvic CT scan requires ex lap in the blunt trauma patient with normal vital signs?

Free air; also strongly consider in the patient with no solid organ injury but lots of free fluid = both to rule out hollow viscus injury

Can you rely on a negative FAST in the unstable patient with a pelvic fracture?

No—perform DPL (above umbilicus)

What lab tests are used to look for intra-abdominal injury in children?	Liver function tests (LFTs) = ↑AST and/or ↑ALT
What is the only real indication for MAST trousers?	Prehospitalization, pelvic fracture
What is the treatment for human and dog bites?	Leave wound open, irrigation, antibiotics
What percentage of pelvic fracture bleeding is exclusively venous?	85%
What is sympathetic ophthalmia?	Blindness in one eye that results in subsequent blindness in the contralateral eye (autoimmune)
What can present after blunt trauma with neurological deficits and a normal brain CT scan?	**D**iffuse **A**xonal **I**njury (**DAI**), carotid artery injury

Chapter 39   Burns

Define:	
TBSA	**T**otal **B**ody **S**urface **A**rea
STSG	**S**plit **T**hickness **S**kin **G**raft
Are acid or alkali chemical burns more serious?	In general, **ALKALI** burns are more serious because the body cannot buffer the alkali, thus allowing them to burn for much longer
Why are electrical burns so dangerous?	Most of the destruction from electrical burns is internal because the route of least electrical resistance follows nerves, blood vessels, and fascia; injury is usually worse than external burns at entrance and exit sites would indicate; **cardiac dysrhythmias,** myoglobinuria, acidosis, and renal failure are common

How is myoglobinuria treated?	To avoid renal injury, think **"HAM"**:
	    Hydration with IV fluids
	    Alkalization of urine with IV
	        bicarbonate
	    Mannitol diuresis

Define level of burn injury: **First-degree burns**	Epidermis only
Second-degree burns	Epidermis and varying levels of dermis
Third-degree burns	A.k.a. "full thickness"; all layers of the skin including the entire dermis (Think: "getting the third degree")
Fourth-degree burns	Burn injury into bone or muscle
How do first-degree burns present?	Painful, dry, red areas that do not form blisters (think of sunburn)
How do second-degree burns present?	Painful, hypersensitive, swollen, mottled areas with **blisters** and open weeping surfaces
How do third-degree burns present?	Painless, insensate, swollen, dry, mottled white, and charred areas; often described as dried leather
What is the major clinical difference between second- and third-degree burns?	Third-degree burns are painless, and second-degree burns are painful
By which measure is burn severity determined?	Depth of burn and TBSA affected by second- and third-degree burns TBSA is calculated by the "rule of nines" in adults and by a modified rule in children to account for the disproportionate size of the head and trunk

What is the "rule of nines"?

In an adult, the total body surface area that is burned can be estimated by the following:

    Each upper limb = 9%
    Each lower limb = 18%
    Anterior and posterior trunk = 18% each
    Head and neck = 9%
    Perineum and genitalia = 1%

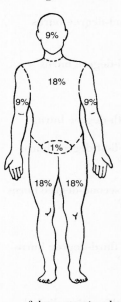

What is the "rule of the palm"?

Surface area of the patient's palm is ≈1% of the TBSA used for estimating size of small burns

What is the burn center referral criteria for the following?
    Second-degree burns

>20% TBSA

    Third-degree burns

>5% TBSA
Second degree >10% TBSA in children and the elderly
Any burns involving the face, hands, feet, or perineum
Any burns with inhalation injury
Any burns with associated trauma
Any electrical burns

What is the treatment of first-degree burns?

Keep clean, ± Neosporin®, pain meds

What is the treatment of second-degree burns?

Remove blisters; apply antibiotic ointment (usually Silvadene®) and dressing; pain meds

Most second-degree burns do not require skin grafting (epidermis grows from hair follicles and from margins)

What are some newer options for treating a second-degree burn?

1. Biobrane® (silicone artificial epidermis—temporary)
2. Silverlon® (silver ion dressings)

What is the treatment of third-degree burns?

Early excision of eschar (within first week postburn) and STSG

How can you decrease bleeding during excision?

Tourniquets as possible, topical epinephrine, topical thrombin

What is an autograft STSG?

STSG from the patient's own skin

What is an allograft STSG?

STSG from a cadaver (temporary coverage)

What thickness is the STSG?

10/1000 to 15/1000 of an inch (down to the dermal layer)

What prophylaxis should the burn patient get in the ER?

Tetanus

What is used to evaluate the eyes after a third-degree burn?

Fluorescein

What principles guide the initial assessment and resuscitation of the burn patient?

ABCDEs, then urine output; check for eschar and compartment syndromes

What are the signs of smoke inhalation?

Smoke and soot in sputum/mouth/nose, nasal/facial hair burns, carboxyhemoglobin, throat/mouth erythema, history of loss of consciousness/explosion/fire in small enclosed area, dyspnea, low O_2 saturation, confusion, headache, coma

What diagnostic imaging is used for smoke inhalation?

Bronchoscopy

What lab value assesses smoke inhalation?

Carboxyhemoglobin level (a carboxy-hemoglobin level of >60% is associated with a 50% mortality); treat with 100% O_2 and time

How should the airway be managed in the burn patient with an inhalational injury?

With a low threshold for **intubation;** oropharyngeal swelling may occlude the airway so that intubation is impossible; 100% oxygen should be administered immediately and continued until signifi-cant carboxyhemoglobin is ruled out

What is "burn shock"?

Burn shock describes the loss of fluid from the intravascular space as a result of burn injury, which causes "leaking capillaries" that require crystalloid infusion

What is the "Parkland formula"?

V = TBSA Burn (%) × Weight (kg) × 4
Formula widely used to estimate the volume (V) of crystalloid necessary for the initial resuscitation of the burn patient; half of the calculated volume is given in the **first 8 hours,** the rest in the next 16 hours

What burns qualify for the Parkland formula?

≥20% TBSA second- and third-degree burns only

What is the Brooke formula for burn resuscitation?

Replace 2 cc for the 4 cc in the Parkland formula

How is the crystalloid given?

Through two large-bore peripheral venous catheters

Can you place an IV or central line through burned skin?

YES

What is the adult urine output goal?

30–50 cc (titrate IVF)

Why is glucose-containing IVF contraindicated in burn patients in the first 24 hours postburn?

Patient's serum glucose will be elevated on its own because of the stress response

What fluid is used after the first 24 hours postburn?

Colloid; use D5W **and** 5% albumin at 0.5 cc/kg/% burn surface area

Why should D5W IV be administered after 24 hours postburn?

Because of the massive sodium load in the first 24 hrs of LR infusion and because of the massive evaporation of H_2O from the burn injury, the patient will need free water; after 24 hours, the capillaries begin to work and then the patient can usually benefit from **albumin** and D5W

What is the minimal urine output for burn patients?

Adults 30 cc; children 1–2 cc/kg/hr

How is volume status monitored in the burn patient?

Urine output, blood pressure, heart rate, peripheral perfusion, and mental status; Foley catheter is mandatory and may be supplemented by central venous pressure and pulmonary capillary wedge pressure monitoring

Why do most severely burned patients require nasogastric decompression?

Patients with greater than 20% TBSA burns usually develop a paralytic ileus → vomiting → aspiration risk → pneumonia

What stress prophylaxis must be given to the burn patient?

H_2 blocker to prevent burn stress ulcer (Curling's ulcer)

What are the signs of burn wound infection?

Increased WBC with left shift, **discoloration of burn eschar** (most common sign), green pigment, necrotic skin lesion in unburned skin, edema, ecchymosis tissue below eschar, second-degree burns that turn into third-degree burns, hypotension

Is fever a good sign of infection in burn patients?

NO

What are the common organisms found in burn wound infections?

Staphylococcus aureus, Pseudomonas, Streptococcus, Candida albicans

How is a burn wound infection diagnosed?

Send burned tissue in question to the laboratory for quantitative burn wound bacterial count; if the count is $>10^5$/gram, infection is present and IV antibiotics should be administered

How are minor burns dressed?

Gentle cleaning with nonionic detergent and débridement of loose skin and broken blisters; the burn is dressed with a topical antibacterial (e.g., neomycin) and covered with a sterile dressing

How are major burns dressed?

Cleansing and application of topical antibacterial agent

Why are systemic IV antibiotics contraindicated in fresh burns?

Bacteria live in the eschar, which is avascular (the systemic antibiotic will not be delivered to the eschar); thus, apply topical antimicrobial agents

Note some advantages and disadvantages of the following topical antibiotic agents:

Silver sulfadiazine (Silvadene®)

Painless, but little eschar penetration, misses *Pseudomonas*, and has idiosyncratic **neutropenia**; sulfa allergy is contraindication

Mafenide acetate (Sulfamylon®)

Penetrates eschars, broad spectrum (but misses *Staphylococcus*), causes pain on application; triggers allergic reaction in 7% of patients; may cause **acid-base imbalances** (Think: **M**afenide **AC**etate = **M**etabolic **AC**idosis); agent of choice in already-contaminated burn wounds

Polysporin®

Polymyxin B sulfate; painless, clear, used for facial burns; does not have a wide antimicrobial spectrum

Are prophylactic systemic antibiotics administered to burn patients?

No—prophylactic antibiotics have not been shown to reduce the incidence of sepsis, but rather have been shown to select for resistant organisms; IV antibiotics are reserved for established wound infections, pneumonia, urinary tract infections, etc.

Are prophylactic antibiotics administered for inhalational injury?

No

Circumferential, full-thickness burns to the extremities are at risk for what complication?

Distal neurovascular impairment

How is it treated?

Escharotomy: full-thickness longitudinal incision through the eschar with scalpel or electrocautery

What is the major infection complication (other than wound infection) in burn patients?

Pneumonia, central line infection (change central lines prophylactically every 3 to 4 days)

Is tetanus prophylaxis required in the burn patient?

Yes, it is mandatory in all patients except those actively immunized within the past 12 months (with incomplete immunization: toxoid × 3)

From which burn wound is water evaporation highest?

Third degree

Can infection convert a partial-thickness injury into a full-thickness injury?

Yes!

How is carbon monoxide inhalation overdose treated?

100% O_2 ($\pm$ hyperbaric O_2)

Which electrolyte must be closely followed acutely after a burn?

Na^+ (sodium)

When should central lines be changed in the burn patient?	Most burn centers change them every 3 to 4 days
What is the name of the gastric/duodenal ulcer associated with burn injury?	Curling's ulcer (Think: **CURLING** iron burn = **CURLING**'s burn ulcer)
How are STSGs nourished in the first 24 hours?	IMBIBITION (fed from wound bed exudate)

Chapter 40   Upper GI Bleeding

What is it?	Bleeding into the lumen of the proximal GI tract, proximal to the ligament of Treitz
What are the signs/ symptoms?	Hematemesis, melena, syncope, shock, fatigue, coffee-ground emesis, hematochezia, epigastric discomfort, epigastric tenderness, signs of hypovolemia, guaiac-positive stools
Why is it possible to have hematochezia?	Blood is a cathartic and hematochezia usually indicates a vigorous rate of bleeding from the UGI source
Are stools melenic or melanotic?	Melenic (melanotic is incorrect)
How much blood do you need to have melena?	>50 cc of blood
What are the risk factors?	Alcohol, cigarettes, liver disease, burn/ trauma, aspirin/NSAIDs, vomiting, sepsis, steroids, previous UGI bleeding, history of peptic ulcer disease (PUD), esophageal varices, portal hypertension, splenic vein thrombosis, abdominal aortic aneurysm repair (aortoenteric fistula), burn injury, trauma

What is the most common cause of significant UGI bleeding?

PUD—duodenal and gastric ulcers (50%)

What is the *common* differential diagnosis of UGI bleeding?

1. **Acute gastritis**
2. **Duodenal ulcer**
3. Esophageal varices
4. Gastric ulcer
5. Esophageal
6. Mallory-Weiss tear

What is the *uncommon* differential diagnosis of UGI bleeding?

Gastric cancer, hemobilia, duodenal diverticula, gastric volvulus, Boerhaave's syndrome, aortoenteric fistula, paraesophageal hiatal hernia, epistaxis, NGT irritation, Dieulafoy's ulcer, angiodysplasia

Which diagnostic tests are useful?

History, NGT aspirate, abdominal x-ray, endoscopy (EGD)

What is the diagnostic test of choice with UGI bleeding?

EGD (>95% diagnosis rate)

What are the treatment options with the endoscope during an EGD?

Coagulation, injection of epinephrine (for vasoconstriction), injection of sclerosing agents (varices), variceal ligation (banding)

Which lab tests should be performed?

Chem-7, bilirubin, LFTs, CBC, **type & cross,** PT/PTT, amylase

Why is BUN elevated?

Because of absorption of blood by the GI tract

What is the initial treatment?

1. **IVFs** (16 G or larger peripheral IVS $\times$ 2), **Foley** catheter (monitor fluid status)
2. **NGT** suction (determine rate and amount of blood)
3. Water lavage (use warm H_2O—will remove clots)
4. **EGD:** endoscopy (determine etiology/location of bleeding and possible treatment—coagulate bleeders)

Why irrigate in an upper GI bleed?

To remove the blood clot so you can see the mucosa

What test may help identify the site of MASSIVE UGI bleeding when EGD fails to diagnose cause and blood continues per NGT?

Selective mesenteric angiography

What are the indications for surgical intervention in UGI bleeding?

Refractory or recurrent bleeding and site known, >3 u PRBCS to stabilize or >6 u PRBCs overall

What percentage of patients require surgery?

$\approx$10%

What percentage of patients spontaneously stop bleeding?

$\approx$80% to 85%

What is the mortality of acute UGI bleeding?

Overall 10%, 60–80 years of age 15%, older than 80 years of age 25%

What are the risk factors for death following UGI bleed?

Age older than 60 years
Shock
>5 units of PRBC transfusion
Concomitant health problems

PEPTIC ULCER DISEASE (PUD)

What is it?

Gastric and duodenal ulcers

What is the incidence in the United States?

$\approx$10% of the population will suffer from PUD during their lifetime!

What are the possible consequences of PUD?

Pain, hemorrhage, perforation, obstruction

What percentage of patients with PUD develops bleeding from the ulcer?

$\approx$20%

Which bacteria are associated with PUD?

Helicobacter pylori

What is the treatment?	Treat *H. pylori* with MOC or ACO 2-week antibiotic regimens: **MOC: M**etronidazole, **O**meprazole, **C**larithromycin (Think: **MOC**k) or **ACO: A**mpicillin, **C**larithromycin, **O**meprazole
What is the name of the sign with RLQ pain/peritonitis as a result of succus collecting from a perforated peptic ulcer?	Valentino's sign

DUODENAL ULCERS

In which age group are these ulcers most common?	40–65 years of age (younger than patients with gastric ulcer)
What is the ratio of male to female patients?	Men > women (3:1)
What is the most common location?	Most are within 2 cm of the pylorus in the duodenal bulb
What is the classic pain response to food intake?	Food classically relieves duodenal ulcer pain (Think: **D**uodenum = **D**ecreased with food)
What is the cause?	Increased production of gastric acid
What syndrome must you always think of with a duodenal ulcer?	Zollinger-Ellison syndrome
What are the associated risk factors?	Male gender, smoking, aspirin and other NSAIDs, uremia, Z-E syndrome, *H. pylori,* trauma, burn injury
What are the symptoms?	Epigastric pain—burning or aching, usually several hours after a meal (food, milk, or antacids initially relieve pain) Bleeding Back pain Nausea, vomiting, and anorexia ↓ appetite

What are the signs?

Tenderness in epigastric area (possibly), guaiac-positive stool, melena, hematochezia, hematemesis

What is the differential diagnosis?

Acute abdomen, pancreatitis, cholecystitis, **all causes of UGI bleeding,** Z-E syndrome, gastritis, MI, gastric ulcer, reflux

How is the diagnosis made?

History, PE, EGD, UGI series **(if patient is not actively bleeding)**

When is surgery indicated with a bleeding duodenal ulcer?

Most surgeons use: >6 u PRBC transfusions, >3 u PRBCs needed to stabilize, or significant rebleed

What EGD finding is associated with rebleeding?

Visible vessel in the ulcer crater, recent clot, active oozing

What is the medical treatment?

PPIs (proton pump inhibitors) or H_2 receptor antagonists—heal ulcers in 4 to 6 weeks in most cases
Treatment for *H. pylori*

When is surgery indicated?

The acronym **"I HOP":**
Intractability

Hemorrhage (massive or relentless)
Obstruction (gastric outlet obstruction)
Perforation

How is a bleeding duodenal ulcer surgically corrected?

Opening of the duodenum through the pylorus
Oversewing of the bleeding vessel

What artery is involved with bleeding duodenal ulcers?

Gastroduodenal artery

What are the common surgical options for the following conditions:
Truncal vagotomy?

Pyloroplasty

Duodenal perforation?

Graham patch (poor candidates, shock, prolonged perforation)

Truncal vagotomy and pyloroplasty incorporating ulcer

Graham patch and highly selective vagotomy

Truncal vagotomy and antrectomy (higher mortality rate, but lowest recurrence rate)

Duodenal obstruction resulting from duodenal ulcer scarring (gastric outlet obstruction)?

Truncal vagotomy, antrectomy, and gastroduodenostomy (BI or BII)

Truncal vagotomy and drainage procedure (gastrojejunostomy)

Duodenal ulcer intractability?

PGV (highly selective vagotomy)

Vagotomy and pyloroplasty

Vagotomy and antrectomy BI or BII (especially if there is a coexistent pyloric/prepyloric ulcer) but associated with a higher mortality

Which ulcer operation has the highest ulcer recurrence rate and the lowest dumping syndrome rate?

PGV (proximal gastric vagotomy)

Which ulcer operation has the lowest ulcer recurrence rate and the highest dumping syndrome rate?

Vagotomy and antrectomy

Why must you perform a drainage procedure (pyloroplasty, antrectomy) after a truncal vagotomy?

Pylorus will not open after a truncal vagotomy

Which duodenal ulcer operation has the lowest mortality rate?

PGV (1/200 mortality), truncal vagotomy and pyloroplasty (1–2/200), vagotomy and antrectomy (1%–2% mortality)

Thus, PGV is the operation of choice for intractable duodenal ulcers with the cost of increased risk of ulcer recurrence

What is a "kissing" ulcer?	Two ulcers, each on opposite sides of the lumen so that they can "kiss"
Why may a duodenal rupture be initially painless?	Fluid can be sterile, with a nonirritating pH of 7.0 initially
Why may a perforated duodenal ulcer present as lower quadrant abdominal pain?	Fluid from stomach/bile drains down paracolic gutters to lower quadrants and causes localized irritation

GASTRIC ULCERS

In which age group are these ulcers most common?	40–70 years old (older than the duodenal ulcer population) Rare in patients younger than 40 years
How does the incidence in men compare with that of women?	Men > women
Which is more common overall: gastric or duodenal ulcers?	Duodenal ulcers are more than twice as common as gastric ulcers (Think: **D**uodenal = **D**ouble rate)
What is the classic pain response to food?	Food classically increases gastric ulcer pain
What is the cause?	**Decreased cytoprotection** or gastric protection (i.e., decreased bicarbonate/ mucous production)
Is gastric acid production high or low?	Gastric acid production is normal or low!
Which gastric ulcers are associated with increased gastric acid?	Prepyloric Pyloric Coexist with duodenal ulcers
What are the associated risk factors?	Smoking, alcohol, burns, trauma, CNS tumor/trauma, NSAIDs, steroids, shock, severe illness, male gender, advanced age
What are the symptoms?	Epigastric pain +/− Vomiting, anorexia, and nausea

How is the diagnosis made?

History, PE, EGD with multiple biopsy (looking for gastric cancer)

What is the most common location?

≈70% are on the lesser curvature; 5% are on the greater curvature

When and why should biopsy be performed?

With all gastric ulcers, to rule out gastric cancer

If the ulcer does not heal in 6 weeks after medical treatment, **rebiopsy** (always biopsy in O.R. also) must be performed

What is the medical treatment?

Similar to that of duodenal ulcer—PPIs or H$_2$ blockers, *Helicobacter pylori* treatment

When do patients with gastric ulcers need to have an EGD?

1. For diagnosis with biopsies
2. 6 weeks postdiagnosis to confirm healing and rule out gastric cancer!

What are the indications for surgery?

The acronym **"I CHOP":**
    Intractability

    Cancer (rule out)
    Hemorrhage (massive or relentless)
    Obstruction (gastric outlet obstruction)
    Perforation
(**Note:** Surgery is indicated if gastric cancer cannot be ruled out)

What is the common operation for hemorrhage, obstruction, and perforation?

Distal gastrectomy with excision of the ulcer **without** vagotomy unless there is duodenal disease (i.e., BI or BII)

What are the options for concomitant duodenal and gastric ulcers?

Resect (BI, BII) and **truncal vagotomy**

What is a common option for surgical treatment of a pyloric gastric ulcer?

Truncal vagotomy and antrectomy (i.e., BI or BII)

What is a common option for a poor operative candidate with a perforated gastric ulcer?

Graham patch

What must be performed in every operation for gastric ulcers?	Biopsy looking for gastric cancer
Define the following terms:	
Cushing's ulcer	PUD/gastritis associated with neurologic trauma or tumor (Think: Dr. **C**ushing = Neuro**S**urgeon = **CNS**)
Curling's ulcer	PUD/gastritis associated with major burn injury (Think: curling iron burn)
Marginal ulcer	Ulcer at the margin of a GI anastomosis
Dieulafoy's ulcer	Pinpoint gastric mucosal defect bleeding from an underlying vascular malformation

PERFORATED PEPTIC ULCER

What are the symptoms?	**Acute** onset of upper abdominal pain
What causes pain in the lower quadrants?	Passage of perforated fluid along colic gutters
What are the signs?	Decreased bowel sounds, tympanic sound over the liver (air), peritoneal signs, tender abdomen
What are the signs of posterior duodenal erosion/ perforation?	Bleeding from gastroduodenal artery (and possibly acute pancreatitis)
What sign indicates anterior duodenal perforation?	Free air (anterior perforation is more common than posterior)
What is the differential diagnosis?	Acute pancreatitis, acute cholecystitis, perforated acute appendicitis, colonic diverticulitis, MI, any perforated viscus
Which diagnostic tests are indicated?	X-ray: free air under diaphragm or in lesser sac in an upright CXR (if upright CXR is not possible, then left lateral decubitus can be performed because air can be seen over the liver and not confused with the gastric bubble)

What are the associated lab findings?	Leukocytosis, high amylase serum (secondary to absorption into the blood stream from the peritoneum)
What is the initial treatment?	NPO: NGT ($\downarrow$ contamination of the peritoneal cavity) IVF/Foley catheter Antibiotics/PPIs Surgery
What is a Graham patch?	Piece of omentum incorporated into the suture closure of perforation
What are the surgical options for treatment of a duodenal perforation?	Graham patch (open or laparoscopic) Truncal vagotomy and pyloroplasty incorporating ulcer Graham patch and highly selective vagotomy
What are the surgical options for perforated gastric ulcer?	Antrectomy incorporating perforated ulcer, Graham patch or wedge resection in unstable/poor operative candidates
What is the significance of hemorrhage and perforation with duodenal ulcer?	May indicate two ulcers (kissing); posterior is bleeding and anterior is perforated with free air
What type of perforated ulcer may present just like acute pancreatitis?	Posterior perforated duodenal ulcer into the pancreas (i.e., epigastric pain radiating to the back; high serum amylase)
What is the classic difference between duodenal and gastric ulcer symptoms as related to food ingestion?	Duodenal = decreased pain Gastric = increased pain (Think: **D**uodenal = **D**ecreased pain)

TYPES OF SURGERIES

Define the following terms:

Graham patch For treatment of duodenal perforation in poor operative candidates/unstable patients

Place viable omentum over perforation and tack into place with sutures

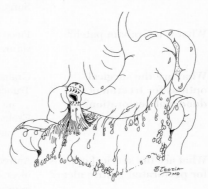

Truncal vagotomy Resection of a 1- to 2-cm segment of each vagal **trunk** as it enters the abdomen on the distal esophagus, decreasing gastric acid secretion

What other procedure must be performed along with a truncal vagotomy? "Drainage procedure" (pyloroplasty, antrectomy, or gastrojejunostomy), because vagal fibers provide relaxation of the pylorus, and, if you cut them, the pylorus will not open

Define the following terms:

Vagotomy and pyloroplasty Pyloroplasty performed with vagotomy to compensate for decreased gastric emptying

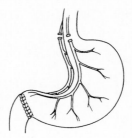

Vagotomy and antrectomy

Remove antrum and pylorus in addition to vagotomy; reconstruct as a Billroth I or II

What is the goal of duodenal ulcer surgery?

Decrease gastric acid secretion (and fix IHOP)

What is the advantage of proximal gastric vagotomy (highly selective vagotomy)?

No drainage procedure is needed; vagal fibers to the pylorus are preserved; rate of dumping syndrome is low

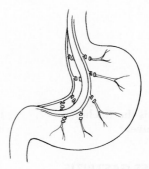

What is a Billroth I (BI)?

Truncal vagotomy, antrectomy, and gastroduodenostomy (Think: B**I** = **ONE** limb off of the stomach remnant)

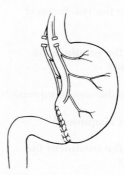

What are the contraindications for a Billroth I?

Gastric cancer or suspicion of gastric cancer

What is a Billroth II (BII)?   Truncal vagotomy, antrectomy, and gastrojejunostomy (Think: B**II** = **TWO** limbs off of the stomach remnant)

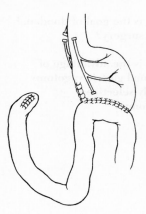

What is the Kocher maneuver?   Dissect the left lateral peritoneal attachments to the duodenum to allow visualization of posterior duodenum

STRESS GASTRITIS

What is it?   **Superficial** mucosal erosions in the stressed patient

What are the risk factors?   Sepsis, intubation, trauma, shock, burn, brain injury

What is the prophylactic treatment? H_2 blockers, PPIs, antacids, sucralfate

What are the signs/symptoms?   NGT blood (usually), painless (usually)

How is it diagnosed?   EGD, if bleeding is significant

What is the treatment for gastritis?   LAVAGE out blood clots, give a maximum dose of PPI in a 24-hour IV drip

MALLORY-WEISS SYNDROME

What is it?   Post-retching, postemesis longitudinal tear (submucosa and mucosa) of the stomach near the GE junction; approximately three fourths are in the stomach

For what percentage of all upper GI bleeds does this syndrome account?	≈10%
What are the causes of a tear?	Increased gastric pressure, often aggravated by hiatal hernia
What are the risk factors?	Retching, alcoholism (50%), >50% of patients have hiatal hernia
What are the symptoms?	Epigastric pain, thoracic substernal pain, emesis, hematemesis
What percentage of patients will have hematemesis?	85%
How is the diagnosis made?	EGD
What is the "classic" history?	Alcoholic patient after binge drinking—first, vomit food and gastric contents, followed by forceful retching and bloody vomitus
What is the treatment?	Room temperature water lavage (90% of patients stop bleeding), electrocautery, arterial embolization, or surgery for refractory bleeding
When is surgery indicated?	When medical/endoscopic treatment fails (>6 u PRBCs infused)
Can the Sengstaken-Blakemore tamponade balloon be used for treatment of Mallory-Weiss tear bleeding?	No, it makes bleeding worse Use the balloon only for bleeding from esophageal varices

ESOPHAGEAL VARICEAL BLEEDING

What is it?	Bleeding from formation of esophageal varices from back up of portal pressure via the coronary vein to the submucosal esophageal venous plexuses secondary to portal hypertension from liver cirrhosis

What is the "rule of two thirds" of esophageal variceal hemorrhage?

Two thirds of patients with portal hypertension develop esophageal varices

Two thirds of patients with esophageal varices bleed

What are the signs/ symptoms?

Liver disease, portal hypertension, hematemesis, caput medusa, ascites

How is the diagnosis made?

EGD (very important because only 50% of UGI bleeding in patients with known esophageal varices are bleeding from the varices; the other 50% have bleeding from ulcers, etc.)

What is the acute medical treatment?

Lower portal pressure with somatostatin and vasopressin

In the patient with CAD, what must you give in addition to the vasopressin?

Nitroglycerin—to prevent coronary artery vasoconstriction that may result in an MI

What are the treatment options?

Sclerotherapy or band ligation via endoscope, TIPS, liver transplant

What is the Sengstaken-Blakemore balloon?

Tamponades with an esophageal balloon and a gastric balloon

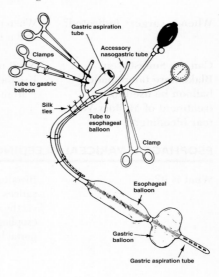

Gastric aspiration tube

Clamps

Accessory nasogastric tube

Tube to gastric balloon

Silk ties

Tube to esophageal balloon

Clamp

Esophageal balloon

Gastric balloon

Gastric aspiration tube

What is the problem with shunts?	Decreased portal pressure, but increased encephalopathy

BOERHAAVE'S SYNDROME

What is it?	Postemetic esophageal rupture
Who was Dr. Boerhaave?	Dutch physician who first described the syndrome in the Dutch Grand Admiral Van Wassenaer in 1724
Why is the esophagus susceptible to perforation and more likely to break down an anastomosis?	No serosa
What is the most common location?	Posterolateral aspect of the esophagus (on the left), 3 to 5 cm above the GE junction
What is the cause of rupture?	Increased intraluminal pressure, usually caused by violent retching and vomiting
What is the associated risk factor?	Esophageal reflux disease (50%)
What are the symptoms?	Pain postemesis (may radiate to the back, dysphagia)
What are the signs?	Left pneumothorax, Hamman's sign, left pleural effusion, subcutaneous/mediastinal emphysema, fever, tachypnea, tachycardia, signs of infection by 24 hours, neck crepitus, widened mediastinum on CXR
What is Mackler's triad?	1. Emesis 2. Lower chest pain 3. Cervical emphysema (subQ air)
What is Hamman's sign?	"Mediastinal crunch or clicking" produced by the heart beating against air-filled tissues
How is the diagnosis made?	History, physical examination, CXR, esophagram with water-soluble contrast

What is the treatment?	Surgery within 24 hours to **drain** the mediastinum and surgically close the perforation and placement of pleural patch; broad-spectrum antibiotics
What is the mortality rate if less than 24 hours until surgery for perforated esophagus?	≈15%
What is the mortality rate if more than 24 hours until surgery for perforated esophagus?	≈33%
Overall, what is the most common cause of esophageal perforation?	Iatrogenic (most commonly cervical esophagus)

Chapter 41   Stomach

ANATOMY

Identify the parts of the stomach:

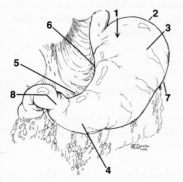

1. Cardia
2. Fundus
3. Body
4. Antrum
5. Incisura angularis
6. Lesser curvature
7. Greater curvature
8. Pylorus

Identify the blood supply to the stomach:

1. Left gastric artery
2. Right gastric artery
3. Right gastroepiploic artery
4. Left gastroepiploic artery
5. Short gastrics (from spleen)

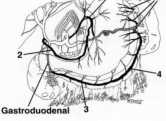

Gastroduodenal 3

What space lies behind the stomach?

Lesser sac; the pancreas lies behind the stomach

What is the opening into the lesser sac?

Foramen of Winslow

What are the folds of gastric mucosa called?

Rugae

GASTRIC PHYSIOLOGY

Define the products of the following stomach cells:

    Gastric parietal cells

HCl
Intrinsic factor

    Chief cells

PEPsinogen (Think: "a **PEP**py chief")

    Mucous neck cells

Bicarbonate
Mucus

    G cells

Gastrin (Think: **G** cells = **G**astrin)

Where are G cells located?

Antrum

What is pepsin?

Proteolytic enzyme that hydrolyzes peptide bonds

What is intrinsic factor?

Protein secreted by the parietal cells that combines with vitamin B12 and allows for absorption in the terminal ileum

GASTROESOPHAGEAL REFLUX DISEASE (GERD)

What is it?	Excessive reflux of gastric contents into the esophagus, "heartburn"
What is pyrosis?	Medical term for heartburn
What are the causes?	Decreased lower esophageal sphincter (LES) tone (>50% of cases) Decreased esophageal motility to clear refluxed fluid Gastric outlet obstruction Hiatal hernia in ≈50% of patients
What are the signs/symptoms?	Heartburn, regurgitation, respiratory problems/pneumonia from aspiration of refluxed gastric contents; substernal pain
What disease must be ruled out when the symptoms of GERD are present?	Coronary artery disease
What tests are included in the workup?	EGD UGI contrast study with esophagogram 24-hour acid analysis (pH probe in esophagus) Manometry, EKG, CXR
What is the medical treatment?	Small meals PPIs (proton-pump inhibitors) or H_2 blockers Elevation of head at night and no meals prior to sleeping
What are the indications for surgery?	Intractability (failure of medical treatment) Respiratory problems as a result of reflux and aspiration of gastric contents (e.g., pneumonia) Severe esophageal injury (e.g., ulcers, hemorrhage, stricture, ± Barrett's esophagus)
What is Barrett's esophagus?	Columnar metaplasia from the normal squamous epithelium as a result of chronic irritation from reflux

What is the major concern with Barrett's esophagus?

Developing cancer

What type of cancer develops in Barrett's esophagus?

Adenocarcinoma

What percentage of patients with GERD develops Barrett's esophagus?

10%

What percentage of patients with Barrett's esophagus will develop adenocarcinoma?

7% lifetime (5%–10%)

What is the treatment of Barrett's esophagus with dysplasia?

Nonsurgical: endoscopic mucosal resection and photodynamic therapy; other options include radiofrequency ablation, cryoablation (these methods are also often used for mucosal adenocarcinoma)

Define the following surgical options for severe GERD:
　　Lap Nissen

360° fundoplication—2 cm long (laparoscopically)

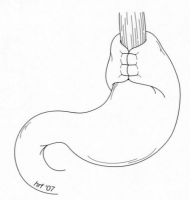

Belsey mark IV

240° to 270° fundoplication performed through a **thoracic** approach

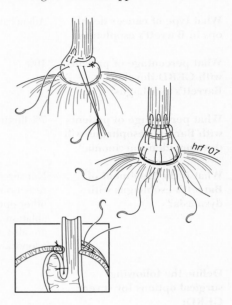

Hill

Arcuate ligament repair (close large esophageal hiatus) and gastropexy to diaphragm (suture stomach to diaphragm)

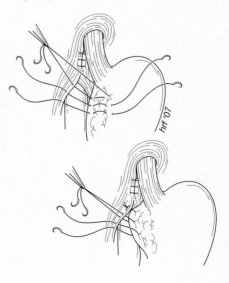

Toupet

Incomplete (around 200°) posterior wrap (laparoscopic) often used with severe decreased esophageal motility

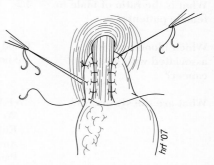

How does the Nissen wrap work?

Thought to work by improving the lower esophageal sphincter:
1. Increasing LES tone
2. Elongating LES ≈3 cm
3. Returning LES into abdominal cavity

In what percentage of patients does Lap Nissen work?

85% (70%–95%)

What are the postoperative complications of Lap Nissen?

1. Gas-bloat syndrome
2. Stricture
3. Dysphagia
4. Spleen injury requiring splenectomy
5. Esophageal perforation
6. Pneumothorax

What is gas-bloat syndrome?

Inability to burp or vomit

GASTRIC CANCER

What is the incidence?

Low in United States (10/100,000); high in Japan (78/100,000)

What are the associated risk factors?

Diet—smoked meats, high nitrates, low fruits and vegetables, alcohol, tobacco
Environment—raised in high-risk area, poor socioeconomic status, atrophic gastritis, male gender, blood type A, previous partial gastrectomy, pernicious anemia, polyps, *Helicobacter pylori*

What is the average age at the time of discovery?	>60 years
What is the ratio of male to female patients?	3:2
Which blood type is associated with gastric cancer?	Blood type A (there is an "**A**" in gastric but no "O" or "B" = g**A**stric = type "**A**")
What are the symptoms?	"**WEAPON**": **W**eight loss **E**mesis **A**norexia **P**ain/epigastric discomfort **O**bstruction **N**ausea
What are the most common early symptoms?	Mild epigastric discomfort and indigestion
What is the most common symptom?	Weight loss
What are the signs?	Anemia, melena, heme occult, epigastric mass (in advanced disease), hepatomegaly, coffee-ground emesis, Blumer's shelf, Virchow's node, enlarged ovaries, axillary adenopathy
What does the patient with gastric cancer have if he or she has proximal colon distension?	Colonic obstruction by direct invasion (rare)
What is the symptom of proximal gastric cancer?	Dysphagia (gastroesophageal junction/cardia)
What is a Blumer's shelf?	Solid peritoneal deposit anterior to the rectum, forming a "shelf," palpated on **rectal examination**
What is a Virchow's node?	Metastatic gastric cancer to the nodes in the left supraclavicular fossa

What is Sister Mary Joseph's sign?

Periumbilical lymph node gastric cancer metastases; presents as periumbilical mass

What is a Krukenberg's tumor?

Gastric cancer (or other adenocarcinoma) that has metastasized to the ovary

What is "Irish's" node?

Left axillary adenopathy from gastric cancer metastasis

What is a surveillance laboratory finding?

CEA elevated in 30% of cases (if +, useful for postoperative surveillance)

What is the initial workup?

EGD with biopsy, endoscopic U/S to evaluate the level of invasion, CT of abdomen/pelvis for metastasis, CXR, labs

What is the histology?

Adenocarcinoma

What is the differential diagnosis for gastric tumors?

Adenocarcinoma, leiomyoma, leiomyosarcoma, lymphoma, carcinoid, ectopic pancreatic tissue, gastrinoma, benign gastric ulcer, polyp

What are the two histologic types?

1. Intestinal (glands)
2. Diffuse (no glands)

What is the morphology?

Ulcerative (75%)
Polypoid (10%)
Scirrhous (10%)
Superficial (5%)

Are gastric cancers more common on the lesser or greater curvatures?

Lesser ("less is more")

What is more common, proximal or distal gastric cancer?

Proximal

Which morphologic type is named after a "leather bottle"?

Linitis plastica—the entire stomach is involved and looks thickened (10% of cancers)

How do gastric adenocarcinomas metastasize?

Hematogenously and lymphatically

Which patients with gastric cancer are NONoperative?

1. Distant metastasis (e.g., liver metastasis)
2. Peritoneal implants

What is the role of laparoscopy?

To rule out peritoneal implants and to evaluate for liver metastasis

What is the genetic alteration seen in >50% of patients with gastric cancer?

P53

How can you remember P53 for gastric cancer?

Gastric **C**ancer = **GC** = P53; or, think: "GCP . . . 53"—it sings!

What is the treatment?

Surgical resection with wide (>5 cm checked by frozen section) margins and lymph node dissection

What operation is performed for tumor in the:
    Antrum?

Distal subtotal gastrectomy

    Midbody?

Total gastrectomy

    Proximal?

Total gastrectomy

What is a subtotal gastrectomy?

Subtotal gastrectomy = 75% of stomach removed

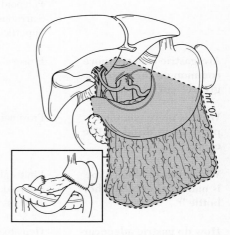

What is a total gastrectomy? Stomach is removed and a Roux-en-Y limb is sewn to the esophagus

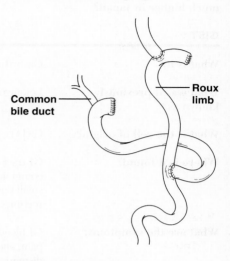

What type of anastomosis? Billroth II or Roux-en-Y (never use a Billroth I)

When should splenectomy be performed? When the tumor directly invades the spleen/splenic hilum or with splenic hilar adenopathy

Define "extended lymph node dissection." Usually D1 and D2:
  D1 are perigastric LNs
  D2 include: splenic artery LNs, hepatic artery LNs, anterior mesocolon LNs, anterior pancreas LNs, crural LNs

What percentage of patients are inoperable at presentation? ≈10% to 15%

What is the adjuvant treatment? Stages II and III: postoperative chemotherapy and radiation

What is the 5-year survival rate for gastric cancer? 25% of patients are alive 5 years after diagnosis in the United States (in Japan, 50% are alive at 5 years)

Why is it thought that the postoperative survival is so much higher in Japan?	Aggressive screening and capturing early cancers

GIST

What is it?	**G**astro**I**ntestinal **S**tromal **T**umor
What was it previously known as?	Leiomyosarcoma
What is the cell of origin?	CAJAL, interstitial cells of Cajal
Where is it found?	GI tract—"esophagus to rectum"—most commonly found in **stomach** (60%), small bowel (30%), duodenum (5%), rectum (3%), colon (2%), esophagus (1%)
What are the symptoms?	GI bleed, occult GI bleed, abdominal pain, abdominal mass, nausea, distention
How is it diagnosed?	CT scan, EGD, colonoscopy
How are distant metastases diagnosed?	PET scan
What is the tumor marker?	C-KIT (CD117 antigen)
What is the prognosis?	Local spread, distant metastases Poor long-term prognosis: size >5cm, mitotic rate >5 per 50 HPF (high power field)
What is the treatment?	Resect with negative margins, +/− chemotherapy
Is there a need for lymph node dissection?	NO
What is the chemotherapy for metastatic or advanced disease?	Imatinib—tyrosine kinase inhibitor

MALTOMA

What is it?	**M**ucosal-**A**ssociated **L**ymphoproliferative Tissue
What is the most common site?	Stomach (70%)
What is the causative agent?	*H. pylori*
What is the medical treatment?	Nonsurgical—treat for *H. pylori* with triple therapy and chemotherapy/XRT in refractory cases

GASTRIC VOLVULUS

What is it?	Twisting of the stomach
What are the symptoms?	Borchardt's triad:

1. Distention of epigastrium
2. Cannot pass an NGT
3. Emesis followed by inability to vomit

What is the treatment?	Exploratory laparotomy to untwist, and gastropexy

---

Chapter 42   Bariatric Surgery

What is it?	Weight reduction surgery for the morbidly obese
Define morbid obesity.	1. BMI >40 (basically, >100 pounds above ideal body weight) or

2. BMI >35 with a medical problem related to morbid obesity

What is the BMI?	**B**ody **M**ass **I**ndex
What is the formula for BMI?	Body weight in kg divided by height in meters squared

What is a formula for a rough estimate of BMI without using metric measures?

$$\frac{Wt\ (pounds) \times 703}{(Ht\ in\ inches)^2}$$

What medical conditions are associated with morbid obesity?

Sleep apnea, coronary artery disease, pulmonary disease, diabetes mellitus, venous stasis ulcers, arthritis, infections, sex-hormone abnormalities, HTN, breast cancer, colon cancer

What are the current options for surgery?

Gastric bypass (malabsorptive)
Vertical-banded gastroplasty

Define gastric bypass.

Stapling off of small gastric pouch (restrictive)
Roux-en-Y limb to gastric pouch (bypass)

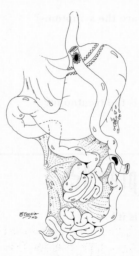

How does gastric bypass work?

1. Creates a small gastric reservoir
2. Causes dumping symptoms when a patient eats too much food or high-calorie foods; the food is "dumped" into the Roux-en-Y limb
3. Bypass of small bowel by Roux-en-Y limb

Which operation works best overall?

Gastric bypass (mean weight loss 50% of excess weight)

What are the possible postoperative complications after weight reduction surgery?

Gallstones (if gallbladder in situ), anastomotic leak, marginal ulcer, stenosis of pouch/anastomosis, malnutrition, incisional hernia, spleen injury, iron deficiency, B12 deficiency

What is the most common sign of an anastomotic leak after a gastric bypass?

Tachycardia

What is the incidence of anastomotic leak?

≈3% (1%–5%)

What is the mortality rate of an anastomotic leak?

≈10%

What is a lap-band?

Laparoscopically placed **band** around stomach with a subcutaneous port to adjust constriction; results in smaller gastric reservoir

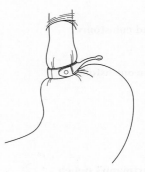

What is a Petersen's hernia?

Seen after bariatric gastric bypass— internal herniation of small bowel through the mesenteric defect from the Roux-en-Y limb

Chapter 43   Ostomies

Define the following terms:

Ostomy

Operation that connects the GI tract to abdominal wall skin or the lumen of another hollow organ; a man-made fistula

Stoma

Opening of the ostomy (Gr. "mouth")

Gastrostomy

G-tube through the abdominal wall to the stomach for drainage or feeding

Jejunostomy

J-tube through the abdominal wall to the jejunum for feeding

Kock pouch

"Continent ileostomy"
Pouch is made of several ileal loops
Patient must access the pouch with a
    tube intermittently

Colostomy

Connection of colon mucosa to the abdominal wall skin for stool drainage

End colostomy

Proximal end of colon brought to the skin for stool drainage

Mucous fistula

Distal end of transected colon brought to the skin for decompression; the mucosa produces mucus, an ostomy is a fistula, and, hence, the term **mucous fistula** (proximal colon brought up as a colostomy or, if the proximal colon is removed, an ileostomy)

Hartmann's pouch

Distal end of transected colon stapled and dropped back into the peritoneal cavity, resulting in a blind pouch; mucus is decompressed through the anus (proximal colon is brought up as an end colostomy or, if proximal colon is removed, an end ileostomy)

Double-barrel colostomy

End colostomy and a mucous fistula (i.e., two barrels brought up to the skin)

Loop colostomy

Loop of large bowel is brought up to the abdominal wall skin and a plastic rod is placed underneath the loop; the colon is then opened and sewn to the abdominal wall skin as a colostomy

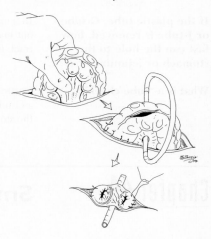

Ileal conduit

Loops of stapled-off ileum made into a pouch, anastomosed to the ureters, and then brought to the abdominal wall skin to allow drainage of urine in patients who undergo removal of the bladder (cystectomy)

Brooke ileostomy

Ileostomy folded over itself to provide clearance from skin

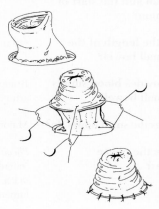

Why doesn't an ileostomy or colostomy close?	**E**pithelialization (mucosa to skin) from the acronym **FRIEND** (see page 305)
Why doesn't a gastrostomy close?	**F**oreign body (the plastic tube) from the acronym **FRIEND**
If the plastic tube, G-tube, or J-tube is removed, how fast can the hole to the stomach or jejunum close?	In a matter of hours! (Thus, if it comes out inadvertently from a well-established tract, it must be replaced immediately)
What is a "tube check"?	Gastrografin contrast study to confirm that a G-tube or J-tube is within the lumen of the stomach or jejunum, respectively

Chapter 44   Small Intestine

SMALL BOWEL

ANATOMY

What comprises the small bowel?	Duodenum, jejunum, and ileum
How long is the duodenum?	≈12 inches—thus the name: duodenum!
What marks the end of the duodenum and the start of the jejunum?	Ligament of Treitz
What is the length of the entire small bowel?	≈6 meters (20 feet)
What provides blood supply to the small bowel?	Branches of the superior mesenteric artery
What does the small bowel do?	Major site of digestion and absorption
What are the plicae circulares?	*Plicae* means "folds," *circulares* means "circular"; thus, circular folds of mucosa (a.k.a. valvulae conniventes) in small bowel lumen

What are the major structural differences between the jejunum and the ileum?	Jejunum—long vasa rectae, large plicae circulares, thicker wall
	Ileum—shorter vasa rectae, smaller plicae circulares, thinner wall
	(Think: **I**leum = **I**nferior vasa rectae, **I**nferior plicae circulares, and **I**nferior wall thickness in comparison to the jejunum)

What does the terminal ileum absorb? B12, fatty acids, bile salts

SMALL BOWEL OBSTRUCTION

What is small bowel obstruction (SBO)? Mechanical obstruction to the passage of intraluminal contents

What are the signs/ symptoms? Abdominal discomfort, cramping, nausea, abdominal distention, emesis, high-pitched bowel sounds

What lab tests are performed with SBO? Electrolytes, CBC, type and screen, urinalysis

What are classic electrolyte/ acid-base findings with proximal obstruction? Hypovolemic, hypochloremic, hypokalemia, alkalosis

What must be ruled out on physical exam in patients with SBO? Incarcerated hernia (also look for surgical scars)

What major AXR findings are associated with SBO? Distended loops of small bowel air-fluid levels on upright film

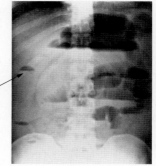

Air-fluid level

Define complete SBO.   Complete obstruction of the lumen; usually paucity or no colon gas

What is the danger of complete SBO?   Closed loop strangulation of the bowel leading to bowel necrosis

Define partial SBO.   Incomplete SBO; some colon gas

What is initial management of all patients with SBO?   NPO, NGT, IVF, Foley

What tests can differentiate partial from complete bowel obstruction?   CT with oral contrast, small bowel follow-through

What are the ABCs of SBO?   Causes of SBO:
1. **A**dhesions
2. **B**ulge (hernias)
3. **C**ancer and tumors

What are other causes of SBO?   The acronym **"GIVES BAD CRAMPS"**:
Gallstone ileus
Intussusception
Volvulus
External compression
SMA syndrome

Bezoars, **B**owel wall hematoma
Abscesses
Diverticulitis

Crohn's disease
Radiation enteritis
Annular pancreas
Meckel's diverticulum
Peritoneal adhesions
Stricture

What is superior mesenteric artery (SMA) syndrome?   Seen with weight loss—SMA compresses duodenum, causing obstruction

What is the treatment of complete SBO?   Laparotomy and lysis of adhesions

What is LOA?   **L**ysis **O**f **A**dhesions

What is the treatment of incomplete SBO?

Initially, conservative treatment with close observation plus NGT decompression

Intraoperatively, how can the level of obstruction be determined in patients with SBO?

Transition from dilated bowel proximal to the decompressed bowel distal to the obstruction

What is the most common indication for abdominal surgery in patients with Crohn's disease?

SBO

Can a patient have complete SBO and bowel movements and flatus?

Yes; the bowel distal to the obstruction can clear out gas and stool

After a small bowel resection, why should the mesenteric defect always be closed?

To prevent an internal hernia

What may cause SBO if patient is on coumadin?

Bowel wall hematoma

What is the #1 cause of SBO in adults (industrialized nations)?

Postoperative adhesions

What is the #1 cause of SBO around the world?

Hernias

What is the #1 cause of SBO in children?

Hernias

What are the signs of strangulated bowel with SBO?

Fever, severe/continuous pain, hematemesis, **shock,** gas in the bowel wall or portal vein, abdominal free air, **peritoneal signs, acidosis** (increased lactic acid)

What are the clinical parameters that will lower the threshold to operate on a partial SBO?

Increasing **WBC**
Fever
Tachycardia/tachypnea
Abdominal pain

What is an absolute indication for operation with partial SBO?

Peritoneal signs, free air on AXR

What classic saying is associated with complete SBO?

"Never let the sun set or rise on complete SBO"

What condition commonly mimics SBO?

Paralytic ileus (AXR reveals gas distention throughout, including the colon)

What is the differential diagnosis of paralytic (nonobstructive) ileus?

Postoperative ileus after abdominal surgery (normally resolves in 3–5 days)
Electrolyte abnormalities (hypokalemia is most common)
Medications (anticholinergic, narcotics)
Inflammatory intra-abdominal process
Sepsis/shock
Spine injury/spinal cord injury
Retroperitoneal hemorrhage

What tumor classically causes SBO due to "mesenteric fibrosis"?

Carcinoid tumor

SMALL BOWEL TUMORS

What is the differential diagnosis of benign tumors of the small intestine?

Leiomyoma, lipoma, lymphangioma, fibroma, adenomas, hemangiomas

What are the signs and symptoms of small bowel tumors?

Abdominal pain, weight loss, obstruction (SBO), and perforation

What is the most common benign small bowel tumor?

Leiomyoma

What is the most common malignant small bowel tumor?

Adenocarcinoma

What is the differential diagnosis of malignant tumors of the small intestine?

1. Adenocarcinoma (50%)
2. Carcinoid (25%)
3. Lymphoma (20%)
4. Sarcomas (<5%)

What is the workup of a small bowel tumor?	UGI with small bowel follow-through, enteroclysis, CT scan, enteroscopy
What is the treatment for malignant small bowel tumor?	Resection and removal of mesenteric draining lymph nodes
What malignancy is classically associated with metastasis to small bowel?	Melanoma

MECKEL'S DIVERTICULUM

What is it?	Remnant of the omphalomesenteric duct/vitelline duct, which connects the yolk sac with the primitive midgut in the embryo

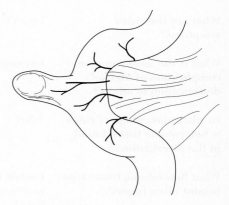

What is its claim to fame?	Most common small bowel congenital abnormality
What is the usual location?	Within ≈2 feet of the ileocecal valve on the **antimesenteric** border of the bowel
What is the major differential diagnosis?	Appendicitis
Is it a true diverticulum?	**Yes;** all layers of the intestine are found in the wall
What is the incidence?	≈2% of the population at autopsy

What is the gender ratio?

Twice as common in **men**

What is the average age at onset of symptoms?

Most frequently in the first **2 years of life,** but can occur at any age

What are the possible complications?

Intestinal hemorrhage (painless)— 50%; accounts for half of all lower GI bleeding in patients younger than 2 years

Bleeding results from ectopic gastric mucosa secreting acid → ulcer → bleeding

Intestinal obstruction—25%; most common complication in adults; includes volvulus and intussusception

Inflammation (± perforations)—20%

What are the signs/ symptoms?

Lower GI bleeding, abdominal pain, SBO

What is the most common complication of Meckel's diverticulum in adults?

Intestinal obstruction

In what percentage of cases is heterotopic tissue found in the diverticulum?

>50%

What heterotopic tissue type is most often found?

Gastric mucosa (60%), but duodenal, pancreatic, and colonic mucosa are also found

What is the "rule of 2s"?

2% of patients are **symptomatic**
Found ≈**2** feet from the ileocecal valve
Found in **2**% of the population
Most symptoms occur before age **2** years
Ectopic tissue found in 1 of **2** patients
Most diverticula are ≈**2** inches long
2 to 1 male:female ratio

What is the role of incidental Meckel's diverticulectomy (surgical removal upon finding asymptomatic diverticulum)?

Most experts would remove in children (very controversial in adults)

What is a Meckel's scan?

Scan for ectopic gastric mucosa in Meckel's diverticulum; uses **technetium pertechnetate** IV, which is preferentially taken up by gastric mucosa

What is the treatment of a Meckel's diverticulum that is causing bleeding and obstruction?

Surgical resection, with small bowel resection as the actual ulcer is usually on the mesenteric wall opposite the diverticulum!

What is the name of the hernia associated with incarcerated Meckel's diverticulum?

Littre's hernia (Think alphabetically: Littre's, then Meckel's)

In patients with guaiac-positive stools and a negative upper- and lower-GI workup, what must be ruled out?

Small bowel tumor; evaluate with enteroclysis (small bowel contrast study)

What is the most common cause of small bowel bleeding?

Small bowel angiodysplasia

Chapter 45

Appendix

What vessel provides blood supply to the appendix?

Appendiceal artery—branch of the ileocolic artery

Name the mesentery of the appendix.

Mesoappendix (contains the appendiceal artery)

How can the appendix be located if the cecum has been identified?

Follow the taenia coli down to the appendix; The taeniae converge on the appendix

APPENDICITIS

What is it?	Inflammation of the appendix caused by **obstruction** of the appendiceal lumen, producing a closed loop with resultant inflammation that can lead to necrosis and perforation
What are the causes?	**Lymphoid hyperplasia, fecalith** (a.k.a. appendicolith) Rare—parasite, foreign body, tumor (e.g., carcinoid)
What is the lifetime incidence of acute appendicitis in the United States?	≈7%!
What is the most common cause of emergent abdominal surgery in the United States?	Acute appendicitis
How does appendicitis classically present?	Classic chronologic order: 1. Periumbilical pain (intermittent and crampy) 2. Nausea/vomiting 3. Anorexia 4. Pain migrates to RLQ (constant and intense pain), usually in <24 hours
Why does periumbilical pain occur?	Referred pain
Why does RLQ pain occur?	Peritoneal irritation
What are the signs/symptoms?	Signs of peritoneal irritation may be present: guarding, muscle spasm, rebound tenderness, obturator and psoas signs, low-grade fever (high grade if perforation occurs), RLQ hyperesthesia
Define the following terms: Obturator sign	Pain upon internal rotation of the leg with the hip and knee flexed; seen in patients with pelvic appendicitis

Psoas sign   Pain elicited by extending the hip with
                              the knee in full extension or by flexing
                              the hip against resistance; seen classically
                              c̄ retrocecal appendicitis

Rovsing's sign   Palpation or rebound pressure of the
                              LLQ results in pain in the RLQ; seen in
                              appendicitis

Valentino's sign   RLQ pain/peritonitis from succus
                              draining down to the RLQ from a
                              perforated gastric or duodenal ulcer

McBurney's point   Point one third from the anterior
                              superior iliac spine to the umbilicus
                              (often the point of maximal tenderness)

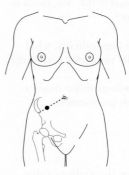

**What is the differential
diagnosis for:**

Everyone?   Meckel's diverticulum, Crohn's
                              disease, perforated ulcer, pancreatitis,
                              mesenteric lymphadenitis, constipation,
                              gastroenteritis, intussusception, volvulus,
                              tumors, UTI (e.g., cystitis), pyelonephritis,
                              torsed epiploicae, cholecystitis, cecal
                              tumor, diverticulitis (floppy sigmoid)

Females?   Ovarian cyst, ovarian torsion, tuboovarian
                              abscess, mittelschmerz, pelvic inflamma-
                              tory disease (PID), ectopic pregnancy,
                              ruptured pregnancy

What lab tests should be performed?

CBC: increased WBC ($>$10,000 per mm^3 in $>$90% of cases), most often with a "left shift"

Urinalysis: to evaluate for pyelonephritis or renal calculus

Can you have an abnormal urinalysis with appendicitis?

Yes; mild hematuria and pyuria are common in appendicitis with pelvic inflammation, resulting in inflammation of the ureter

Does a positive urinalysis rule out appendicitis?

No; ureteral inflammation resulting from the periappendiceal inflammation can cause abnormal urinalysis

What additional tests can be performed if the diagnosis is not clear?

Spiral CT, U/S (may see a large, noncompressible appendix or fecalith), AXR

In acute appendicitis, what classically precedes vomiting?

Pain (in gastroenteritis, the pain classically follows vomiting)

What radiographic studies are often performed?

CXR: to rule out RML or RLL pneumonia, free air

AXR: abdominal films are usually nonspecific, but calcified fecalith present in about 5% of cases

What are the radiographic signs of appendicitis on AXR?

Fecalith, sentinel loops, **scoliosis** away from the right because of pain, mass effect (abscess), loss of psoas shadow, loss of preperitoneal fat stripe, and (very rarely) a small amount of free air if perforated

With acute appendicitis, in what percentage of cases will a radiopaque fecalith be on AXR?

Only $\approx$5% of the time!

What are the CT findings with acute appendicitis?

Periappendiceal fat stranding, appendiceal diameter $>$6 mm, periappendiceal fluid, fecalith

What are the preoperative medications/preparation?

1. Rehydration with **IV fluids** (LR)
2. Preoperative **antibiotics** with anaerobic coverage (appendix is considered part of the colon)

What is a lap appy?

Laparoscopic appendectomy; used in most cases in women (can see adnexa) or if patient has a need to quickly return to physical activity, or is obese

What is the treatment for *non*perforated acute appendicitis?

Nonperforated—prompt appendectomy (prevents perforation), 24 hours of antibiotics, discharge home usually on POD #1

What is the treatment for *perforated* acute appendicitis?

Perforated—IV fluid resuscitation and prompt appendectomy; all pus is drained with postoperative antibiotics continued for 3 to 7 days; wound is left open in most cases of perforation after closing the fascia (heals by secondary intention or delayed primary closure)

How is an appendiceal abscess that is diagnosed preoperatively treated?

Usually by **percutaneous** drainage of the abscess, antibiotic administration, and elective appendectomy ≈6 weeks later (a.k.a. interval appendectomy)

If a normal appendix is found upon exploration, should you take out the normal appendix?

Yes

How long after removal of a NONRUPTURED appendix should antibiotics continue postoperatively?

For 24 hours

Which antibiotic is used for NONPERFORATED appendicitis?

Anaerobic coverage: Cefoxitin®, Cefotetan®, Unasyn®, Cipro®, and Flagyl®

What antibiotic is used for a PERFORATED appendix?

Broad-spectrum antibiotics (e.g., Amp/ Cipro®/Clinda or a penicillin such as Zosyn®)

How long do you give antibiotics for perforated appendicitis?

Until the patient has a normal WBC count and is afebrile, ambulating, and eating a regular diet (usually 3–7 days)

What is the risk of perforation?

≈25% by 24 hours from onset of symptoms, ≈50% by 36 hours, and ≈75% by 48 hours

What is the most common general surgical abdominal emergency in pregnancy?

Appendicitis (about 1/1750; **appendix may be in the RUQ because of the enlarged uterus**)

What are the possible complications of appendicitis?

Pelvic abscess, liver abscess, free perforation, portal pylethrombophlebitis (very rare)

What percentage of the population has a retrocecal, retroperitoneal appendix?

≈15%

What percentage of negative appendectomies is acceptable?

Up to 20%; taking out some normal appendixes is better than missing a case of acute appendicitis that eventually ruptures

Who is at risk of dying from acute appendicitis?

Very old and very young patients

What bacteria are associated with "mesenteric adenitis" that can closely mimic acute appendicitis?

Yersinia enterolytica

What is an "incidental appendectomy"?

Removal of normal appendix during abdominal operation for different procedure

What are complications of an appendectomy?

SBO, enterocutaneous fistula, wound infection, infertility with perforation in women, increased incidence of right inguinal hernia, stump abscess

What is the most common postoperative complication?

Wound infection

CLASSIC INTRAOPERATIVE QUESTIONS

What is the difference between a McBurney's incision and a Rocky-Davis incision?	McBurney's is angled down (follows ext oblique fibers), and Rocky-Davis is straight across (transverse)
What are the layers of the abdominal wall during a McBurney incision?	1. Skin 2. Subcutaneous fat 3. Scarpa's fascia 4. External oblique 5. Internal oblique 6. Transversus muscle 7. Transversalis fascia 8. Preperitoneal fat 9. Peritoneum
What are the steps in laparoscopic appendectomy (lap appy)?	1. Identify the appendix 2. Staple the mesoappendix (or coagulate) 3. Staple and transect the appendix at the base (or use Endoloop® and cut between) 4. Remove the appendix from the abdomen 5. Irrigate and aspirate until clear
Do you routinely get peritoneal cultures for acute appendicitis (nonperforated)?	No
How can you find the appendix after identifying the cecum?	Follow the taeniae down to where they converge on the appendix
Which way should your finger sweep trying to find the appendix?	Lateral to medial along the lateral peritoneum—this way you will not tear the mesoappendix that lies medially!
How do you get to a retrocecal and retroperitoneal appendix?	Divide the lateral peritoneal attachments of the cecum
Why use electrocautery on the exposed mucosa on the appendiceal stump?	To kill the mucosal cells so they do not form a mucocele

If you find Crohn's disease in the terminal ileum, will you remove the appendix?	Yes, if the cecal/appendiceal base is not involved
If the appendix is normal what do you inspect intraoperatively?	Terminal ileum: Meckel's diverticulum, Crohn's disease, intussusception Gynecologic: Cysts, torsion, etc. Groin: hernia, rectus sheath hematoma, adenopathy (adenitis)
Who first described the classic history and treatment for acute appendicitis?	Reginald Fitz
Who performed the first appendectomy?	Harry Hancock in 1848 (McBurney popularized the procedure in 1880s)
Who performed the first lap appy?	Dr. Semm (GYN) in 1983

APPENDICEAL TUMORS

What is the most common appendiceal tumor?	Carcinoid tumor
What is the treatment of appendiceal carcinoid less than 1.5 cm?	Appendectomy (if not through the bowel wall)
What is the treatment of appendiceal carcinoid larger than 1.5 cm?	Right hemicolectomy
What percentage of appendiceal carcinoids are malignant?	<5%
What is the differential diagnosis of appendiceal tumor?	Carcinoid, adenocarcinoma, malignant mucoid adenocarcinoma
What type of appendiceal tumor can cause the dreaded pseudomyxoma peritonei if the appendix ruptures?	Malignant mucoid adenocarcinoma

What is "mittelschmerz"?	Pelvic pain caused by ovulation
Should one remove the normal appendix with Crohn's disease found intraoperatively?	Yes, unless the base of the appendix is involved with Crohn's disease, the normal appendix should be removed to avoid diagnostic confusion with appendicitis in the future

Chapter 46

Carcinoid Tumors

What is a carcinoid tumor?	Tumor arising from neuroendocrine cells (APUDomas), a.k.a. **Kulchitsky cells;** basically, a tumor that secretes **serotonin**
Why is it called "carcinoid"?	Suffix "-oid" means "resembling"; thus, carcinoid resembles a carcinoma but is clinically and histologically less aggressive than most GI carcinomas
How can you remember that Kulchitsky cells are found in carcinoid tumors?	Think: **"COOL CAR"** or **KUL**chitsky **CAR**cinoid
What is the incidence?	Between 0.2% and 1.0% and about 25% of all small bowel tumors
What are the common sites of occurrence?	"AIR": 1. **A**ppendix (most common) 2. **I**leum 3. **R**ectum 4. Bronchus Other sites: jejunum, stomach, duodenum, colon, ovary, testicle, pancreas, thymus
What are the signs/ symptoms?	Depends on location; most cases are asymptomatic; also SBO, abdominal pain, bleeding, weight loss, diaphoresis, **pellagra skin changes,** intussusception, carcinoid syndrome, wheezing
Why SBO with carcinoid?	Classically = severe mesenteric fibrosis

What are the pellagra-like symptoms?	Think "3-D": 1. **D**ermatitis 2. **D**iarrhea 3. **D**ementia
What causes pellagra in carcinoid patients?	Decreased **niacin** production
What is carcinoid syndrome?	Syndrome of symptoms caused by release of substances from a carcinoid tumor
What are the symptoms of carcinoid syndrome?	Remember the acronym "**B FDR**": **B**ronchospasm **F**lushing (skin) **D**iarrhea **R**ight-sided heart failure (from valve failure)
What is a complete memory aid for carcinoid?	Think: **B FDR** = **CAR**cinoid, or "**Be FDR** in a **cool CAR**" (COOL = **KUL**chitsky cells)

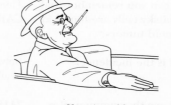

Why does right-sided heart failure develop but not left-sided heart failure?	Lungs act as a filter (just like the liver); thus, the left heart doesn't see all the vasoactive compounds
What is the incidence of carcinoid SYNDROME in patients who have a carcinoid TUMOR?	≈10%
What released substances cause carcinoid syndrome?	**Serotonin** and vasoactive peptides
What is the medical treatment for carcinoid syndrome?	Octreotide IV
What is the medical treatment of diarrhea alone?	Odansetron (Zofran®)—serotonin **antagonist**

How does the liver prevent carcinoid syndrome?

By degradation of serotonin and the other vasoactive peptides when the **tumor drains into the portal vein**

Why does carcinoid syndrome occur in some tumors and not in others?

Occurs when **venous drainage from the tumor gains access to the systemic circulation** by avoiding hepatic degradation of the vasoactive substances

What tumors can produce carcinoid syndrome?

Liver metastases
Retroperitoneal disease draining into
    paravertebral veins
Primary tumor outside the GI tract,
    portal venous drainage (e.g., ovary,
    testicular, bronchus), or both

What does the liver break down serotonin into?

5-hydroxyindoleacetic acid **(5-HIAA)**

What percentage of patients with a carcinoid have an elevated urine 5-HIAA level?

50%

What are the associated diagnostic lab findings?

Elevated urine 5-HIAA as well as elevated urine and blood **serotonin** levels

How do you remember 5-HIAA for carcinoid?

Think of a **5-HIGH CAR** pile up = **5-HIAA CAR**cinoid

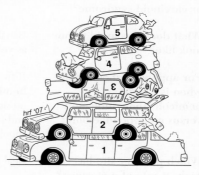

What stimulation test can often elevate serotonin levels and cause symptoms of carcinoid syndrome?

Pentagastrin stimulation

How do you localize a GI carcinoid?

Barium enema, upper GI series with small bowel follow-through, colonoscopy, enteroscopy, enteroclysis, EGD, radiology tests

What are the special radiologic (scintigraphy) localization tests?

^{131}I-MIBG (131 metaiodobenzylguanidine)
^{111}In-octreotide
PET scan utilizing ^{11}C-labeled HTP

What is the surgical treatment?

Excision of the primary tumor and single or feasible metastasis in the liver (liver transplant is an option with unresectable liver metastasis); chemotherapy for advanced disease

What is the medical treatment?

Medical therapy for palliation of the carcinoid syndrome (serotonin antagonists, somatostatin analogue [**octreotide**])

How effective is octreotide?

It relieves diarrhea and flushing in more than 85% of cases and may shrink tumor in 10% to 20% of cases

What is a common antiserotonin drug?

Cyproheptadine

What is the overall prognosis?

Two thirds of patients are alive at 5 years

What is the prognosis of patients with liver metastasis or carcinoid syndrome?

50% are alive at 3 years

What does carcinoid tumor look like?

Usually intramural bowel mass; appears as **yellowish** tumor upon incision

For appendiceal carcinoid, when is a right hemicolectomy indicated versus an appendectomy?

If the tumor is >1.5 cm, right **hemicolectomy** is indicated; if there are no signs of serosal or cecal involvement and tumor is <1.5 cm, appendectomy should be performed

Which primary site has the highest rate of metastasis?

Ileal primary tumor

Can a carcinoid tumor be confirmed malignant by looking at the histology?

No, metastasis must be present to diagnose malignancy

What is the correlation between tumor size and malignancy potential?

Vast majority of tumors <2 cm are benign; in tumors >2 cm, malignancy potential is significant

What treatments might you use for the patient with unresectable liver metastasis that is refractory to medical treatment?

Chemoembolization or radiofrequency ablation

What are the overall survival rates for carcinoid tumors at 5 years? 10 years?

5 years = 70%; 10 years = 50%

What are the side effects of colorectal carcinoid?

Most common side effect is rectal bleeding +/− vague abdominal pain/discomfort

---

Chapter 47 — Fistulas

What is a fistula?

Abnormal **communication** between two hollow organs or a hollow organ and the skin (i.e., two epithelial cell layers)

What are the predisposing factors and conditions that maintain patency of a fistula?

The acronym **"HIS FRIEND"**:
High output fistula (>500 cc/day)
Intestinal destruction (>50% of circumference)
Short segment fistula <2.5 cm

Foreign body (e.g., G-tube)
Radiation
Infection
Epithelization (e.g., colostomy)
Neoplasm
Distal obstruction

SPECIFIC TYPES OF FISTULAS

ENTEROCUTANEOUS

What is it?

Fistula from GI tract to skin
(entero—cutaneous = **bowel to skin**)

What are the causes?	Anastomotic leak, trauma/injury to the bowel/colon, Crohn's disease, abscess, diverticulitis, inflammation/infection, inadvertent suture through bowel
What is the workup?	1. CT scan to rule out abscess/inflammatory process 2. Fistulagram
What are the possible complications?	High-output fistulas, malnutrition, skin breakdown
What is the treatment?	NPO; TPN; drain abscesses, rule out and correct underlying causes; may feed distally (or if fistula is distal, feed elemental diet proximally); half will close spontaneously, but the other half require operation and resection of the involved bowel segment
Which enterocutaneous fistula closes faster: short or long?	Long fistula (may be counterintuitive—but true)

COLONIC FISTULAS

What are they?	Include colovesical, colocutaneous, colovaginal, and coloenteric fistulas
What are the most common causes?	**Diverticulitis** (most common cause), cancer, IBD, foreign body, and irradiation
What is the most common type?	**Colovesical fistula,** which often presents with recurrent urinary tract infections; other signs include pneumaturia, dysuria, and fecaluria
How is the diagnosis made?	Via BE and cystoscopy
What is the treatment?	Surgery: segmental colon resection and primary anastomosis; repair/resection of the involved organ
What is a cholecystenteric fistula?	Connection between gallbladder and duodenum or other loop of small bowel due to large gallstone erosion, often resulting in SBO as the gallstone lodges in the ileocecal valve (gallstone ileus)

What are the common causes of a gastrocolic fistula?	Penetrating ulcers, **gastric** or **colonic cancer,** and Crohn's disease
What are the possible complications of gastrocolic fistulas?	Malnutrition and severe **enteritis** due to reflux of colonic contents into the stomach and small bowel with subsequent bacterial overgrowth

PANCREATIC ENTERIC FISTULA

What is it?	Decompression of a **pseudocyst** or **abscess** into an adjacent organ (a **rare** complication); usually done surgically or endoscopically to treat a pancreatic pseudocyst

EXTERNAL PANCREATIC FISTULA

What is it?	Pancreaticocutaneous fistula; drainage of pancreatic exocrine secretions through to abdominal skin (usually through drain tract/wound)
What is the treatment?	NPO, TPN, skin protection, **octreotide**
What is a "refractory" pancreatic fistula?	Pancreaticocutaneous fistula that does not resolve with conservative medical management (the minority of cases)
What is the diagnostic test for "refractory" pancreatic fistulas?	ERCP to define site of fistula tract (i.e., tail versus head of pancreas)
How is refractory tail of a pancreas fistula treated?	Resection of the tail of the pancreas and the fistula
How is refractory head of a pancreas fistula treated?	Pancreaticojejunostomy

BLADDER FISTULAS

What are the specific types?	**Vesicoenteric** (50% due to sigmoid diverticulitis); signs include pneumaturia, fecaluria **Vesicovaginal** (most are secondary to gynecologic procedures); signs include urinary leak through vagina

Chapter 48

Colon and Rectum

ANATOMY

Identify the arterial blood supply to the colon:

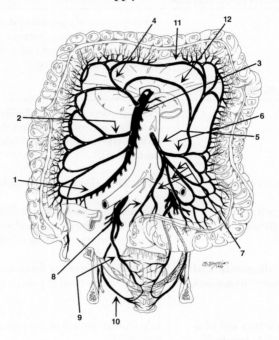

1. Ileocolic artery
2. Right colic artery
3. Superior mesenteric artery (SMA)
4. Middle colic artery
5. Inferior mesenteric artery (IMA)
6. Left colic artery
7. Sigmoidal artery
8. Superior hemorrhoidal artery (superior rectal)
9. Middle hemorrhoidal artery
10. Inferior hemorrhoidal artery
11. Marginal artery of Drummond
12. Meandering artery of Gonzalez

What are the white lines of Toldt?	Lateral peritoneal reflections of the ascending and descending colon
What parts of the GI tract do not have a serosa?	Esophagus, middle and distal **rectum**
What are the major anatomic differences between the colon and the small bowel?	Colon has taeniae coli, haustra, and appendices epiploicae (fat appendages), whereas the small intestine is smooth
What is the blood supply to the rectum:	
Proximal?	Superior hemorrhoidal (or superior rectal) from the IMA
Middle?	Middle hemorrhoidal (or middle rectal) from the hypogastric (internal iliac)
Distal?	Inferior hemorrhoidal (or inferior rectal) from the pudendal artery (a branch of the hypogastric artery)
What is the venous drainage of the rectum:	
Proximal?	Via the IMV to the splenic vein, then **to the portal vein**
Middle?	Via the iliac vein to the **IVC**
Distal?	Via the iliac vein to the **IVC**

COLORECTAL CARCINOMA

What is it?	Adenocarcinoma of the colon or rectum
What is the incidence?	Most common GI cancer Second most common cancer in the United States Incidence increases with age starting at 40 and peaks at 70 to 80 years
How common is it as a cause of cancer deaths?	Second most common cause of cancer deaths

What is the lifetime risk of colorectal cancer? 6%

What is the male to female ratio? ≈1:1

What are the risk factors? **Dietary:** Low-fiber, high-fat diets correlate with increased rates
Genetic: Family history is important when taking history
FAP, Lynch's syndrome
IBD: Ulcerative colitis > Crohn's disease, age, previous colon cancer

What is Lynch's syndrome? **HNPCC** = **H**ereditary **N**on**P**olyposis **C**olon **C**ancer—autosomal-dominant inheritance of high risk for development of colon cancer

What are current ACS recommendations for polyp/colorectal screening in asymptomatic patients without family (first-degree) history of colorectal cancer? Starting at age 50, at least one of the following test regimens is recommended:
Colonoscopy q 10 yrs
Double contrast barium enema (DCBE) q 5 yrs
Flex sigmoidoscopy q 5 yrs
CT colonography q 5 yrs

What are the current recommendations for colorectal cancer screening if there is a history of colorectal cancer in a first-degree relative less than 60 years old? Colonoscopy at age 40, or 10 years before the age at diagnosis of the youngest first-degree relative, and every 5 years thereafter

What percentage of adults will have a guaiac-positive stool test? ≈2%

What percentage of patients with a guaiac-positive stool test will have colon cancer? ≈10%

What signs/symptoms are associated with the following conditions:

Right-sided lesions?

Right side of bowel has a large luminal diameter, so a tumor may attain a large size before causing problems

Microcytic anemia, occult/melena more than hematochezia PR, postprandial discomfort, fatigue

Left-sided lesions?

Left side of bowel has smaller lumen and semisolid contents

Change in bowel habits (small-caliber stools), colicky pain, signs of obstruction, abdominal mass, heme(+) or gross red blood

Nausea, vomiting, constipation

From which site is melena more common?

Right-sided colon cancer

From which site is hematochezia more common?

Left-sided colon cancer

What is the incidence of rectal cancer?

Comprises 20% to 30% of all colorectal cancer

What are the signs/ symptoms of rectal cancer?

Most common symptom is hematochezia (passage of red blood ± stool) or mucus; also tenesmus, feeling of incomplete evacuation of stool (because of the mass), and rectal mass

What is the differential diagnosis of a colon tumor/ mass?

Adenocarcinoma, carcinoid tumor, lipoma, liposarcoma, leiomyoma, leiomyosarcoma, lymphoma, diverticular disease, ulcerative colitis, Crohn's disease, polyps

Which diagnostic tests are helpful?

History and physical exam (***Note:* ≈10% of cancers are palpable on rectal exam**), heme occult, CBC, barium enema, colonoscopy

What disease does microcytic anemia signify until proven otherwise in a man or postmenopausal woman?

Colon cancer

What tests help find metastases?

CXR (lung metastases), LFTs (liver metastases), abdominal CT (liver metastases), other tests based on history and physical exam (e.g., head CT for left arm weakness looking for brain metastasis)

What is the preoperative workup for colorectal cancer?

History, physical exam, LFTs, CEA, CBC, Chem 10, PT/PTT, type and cross 2 u PRBCs, CXR, U/A, abdominopelvic CT

What are the means by which the cancer spreads?

Direct extension: circumferentially and then through bowel wall to later invade other abdominoperineal organs
Hematogenous: portal circulation to liver; lumbar/vertebral veins to lungs
Lymphogenous: regional lymph nodes
Transperitoneal
Intraluminal

Is CEA useful?

Not for screening but for baseline and recurrence surveillance (but offers no proven survival benefit)

What unique diagnostic test is helpful in patients with rectal cancer?

Endorectal ultrasound (probe is placed transanally and depth of invasion and nodes are evaluated)

How are tumors staged?

TMN staging system

Give the TNM stages:
 Stage I

Invades submucosa or muscularis propria (T1–2 N0 M0)

 Stage II

Invades through muscularis propria or surrounding structures but with negative nodes (T3–4, N0, M0)

Stage III	**Positive nodes,** no distant metastasis (any T, N1–3, M0)
Stage IV	Positive **distant metastasis** (any T, any N, M1)

**What is the approximate
5-year survival by stage:**

Stage I?	**90%**
Stage II?	**70%**
Stage III?	**50%**
Stage IV?	**10%**

What percentage of patients with colorectal cancer have liver metastases on diagnosis?	≈20%

Define the preoperative "bowel prep."	Preoperative preparation for colon/rectal resection: 1. Golytely colonic lavage or Fleets Phospho-Soda until clear effluent per rectum 2. PO antibiotics (1 gm neomycin and 1 gm erythromycin × 3 doses) ***Note:*** Patient should also receive preoperative and 24-hr IV antibiotics
What are the common preoperative IV antibiotics?	Cefoxitin, Unasyn®
If the patient is allergic (hives, swelling), what antibiotics should be prescribed?	IV Cipro® and Flagyl®
What are the treatment options?	Resection: wide surgical resection of lesion and its regional lymphatic drainage

What decides low anterior resection (LAR) versus abdominal perineal resection (APR)?

Distance from the anal verge, pelvis size

What do all rectal cancer operations include?

Total mesorectal excision—remove the rectal mesentery, including the lymph nodes (LNs)

What is the lowest LAR possible?

Coloanal anastomosis (anastomosis normal colon directly to anus)

What do some surgeons do with any anastomosis less than 5 cm from the anus?

Temporary ileostomy to "protect" the anastomosis

What surgical margins are needed for colon cancer?

Traditionally >5 cm; margins must be at least 2 cm

What is the minimal surgical margin for rectal cancer?

2 cm

How many lymph nodes should be resected with a colon cancer mass?

12 LNs minimum = for staging, and may improve prognosis

What is the adjuvant treatment of stage III colon cancer?

5-FU and leucovorin (or levamisole) chemotherapy (if there is nodal metastasis postoperatively)

What is the adjuvant treatment for T3–T4 rectal cancer?

Preoperative radiation therapy and 5-FU chemotherapy as a "radiosensitizer"

What is the most common site of distant (hematogenous) metastasis from colorectal cancer?

Liver

What is the treatment of liver metastases from colorectal cancer?

Resect with ≥1-cm margins and administer chemotherapy if feasible

What is the surveillance regimen?

Physical exam, stool guaiac, CBC, CEA, LFTs (every 3 months for 3 years, then every 6 months for 2 years), CXR every 6 months for 2 years and then yearly, colonoscopy at years 1 and 3 postoperatively, CT scans directed by exam

Why is follow-up so important the first 3 postoperative years?

≈90% of colorectal recurrences are within 3 years of surgery

What are the most common causes of colonic obstruction in the adult population?

Colon cancer, diverticular disease, colonic volvulus

What is the 5-year survival rate after liver resection with clean margins for colon cancer liver metastasis?

≈33% (28%–50%)

What is the 5-year survival rate after diagnosis of unresectable colon cancer liver metastasis?

0%

COLONIC AND RECTAL POLYPS

What are they?

Tissue growth into bowel lumen, usually consisting of mucosa, submucosa, or both

How are they anatomically classified?

Sessile (flat)
Pedunculated (on a stalk)

What are the histologic classifications of the following types:
    Inflammatory (pseudopolyp)?

As in Crohn's disease or ulcerative colitis

    Hamartomatous?

Normal tissue in abnormal configuration

    Hyperplastic?

Benign—normal cells—no malignant potential

Neoplastic?	Proliferation of undifferentiated cells; premalignant or malignant cells
What are the subtypes of neoplastic polyps?	Tubular adenomas (usually pedunculated) Tubulovillous adenomas Villous adenomas (usually sessile and look like broccoli heads)
What determines malignant potential of an adenomatous polyp?	Size Histologic type Atypia of cells
What is the most common type of adenomatous polyp?	Tubular 85%
What is the correlation between size and malignancy?	Polyps larger than 2 cm have a high risk of carcinoma (33%–55%)
What about histology and cancer potential of an adenomatous polyp?	Villous > tubovillous > tubular (Think: **VILL**ous = **VILL**ain)
What is the approximate percentage of carcinomas found in the following polyps overall:	
Tubular adenoma?	5%
Tubulovillous adenoma?	20%
Villous adenoma?	40%
Where are most polyps found?	Rectosigmoid (30%)
What are the signs/ symptoms?	Bleeding (red or dark blood), change in bowel habits, mucus per rectum, electrolyte loss, totally asymptomatic
What are the diagnostic tests?	Best = colonoscopy Less sensitive for small polyps = barium enema and sigmoidoscopy

What is the treatment?	Endoscopic resection (snared) if polyps; large sessile villous adenomas should be removed with bowel resection and lymph node resection

POLYPOSIS SYNDROMES

FAMILIAL POLYPOSIS

What is another name for this condition?	Familial adenomatous polyposis (FAP)
What are the characteristics?	Hundreds of adenomatous polyps within the rectum and colon that begin developing at puberty; all undiagnosed; untreated patients develop cancer by ages 40 to 50
What is the inheritance pattern?	Autosomal dominant (i.e., 50% of offspring)
What is the genetic defect?	APC (adenomatous polyposis coli) gene
What is the treatment?	Total proctocolectomy and ileostomy Total colectomy and rectal mucosal removal (mucosal proctectomy) and ileoanal anastomosis

GARDNER'S SYNDROME

What are the characteristics?	Neoplastic polyps of the **small bowel** and **colon;** cancer by age 40 in 100% of undiagnosed patients, as in FAP
What are the other associated findings?	**Desmoid** tumors (in abdominal wall or cavity), **osteomas** of skull (seen on x-ray), **sebaceous** cysts, adrenal and thyroid tumors, retroperitoneal fibrosis, duodenal and periampullary tumors
How can the findings associated with Gardner's syndrome be remembered?	Think of a gardener planting **"SOD":** **S**ebaceous cysts **O**steomas **D**esmoid tumors

What is a desmoid tumor?	Tumor of the musculoaponeurotic sheath, usually of the abdominal wall; benign, but grows locally; treated by wide resection
What medications may slow the growth of a desmoid tumor?	Tamoxifen, sulindac, steroids
What is the inheritance pattern?	Varying degree of penetrance from an autosomal-dominant gene
What is the treatment of colon polyps in patients with Gardner's syndrome?	Total proctocolectomy and ileostomy Total colectomy and rectal mucosal removal (mucosal proctectomy) and ileoanal anastomosis

PEUTZ-JEGHERS' SYNDROME

What are the characteristics?	Hamartomas throughout the GI tract (jejunum/ileum > colon > stomach)
What is the associated cancer risk from polyps?	Increased
What is the associated cancer risk for women with Peutz-Jeghers?	Ovarian cancer (granulosa cell tumor is most common)
What is the inheritance pattern?	Autosomal dominant
What are the other signs?	Melanotic pigmentation (black/brown) of buccal mucosa (mouth), lips, digits, palms, feet (soles) (Think: **P**eutz = **P**igmented)
What is the treatment?	Removal of polyps, if symptomatic (i.e., bleeding, intussusception, or obstruction) or large (>1.5 cm)
What are juvenile polyps?	Benign hamartomas in the small bowel and colon; not premalignant; also known as "retention polyps"

What is Cronkhite-Canada syndrome?	Diffuse GI hamartoma polyps (i.e., no cancer potential) associated with malabsorption/weight loss, diarrhea, and **loss of electrolytes/protein;** signs include alopecia, nail atrophy, skin pigmentation
What is Turcot's syndrome?	Colon polyps with malignant **CNS tumors** (glioblastoma multiforme)

DIVERTICULAR DISEASE OF THE COLON

DIVERTICULOSIS

What is diverticulosis?	Condition in which diverticula can be found within the colon, especially the sigmoid; diverticula are actually **false diverticula** in that only mucosa and submucosa herniate through the bowel musculature; true diverticula involve all layers of the bowel wall and are rare in the colon

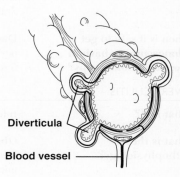

Diverticula

Blood vessel

Describe the pathophysiology.	**Weakness** in the bowel wall develops at points where nutrient **blood vessels** enter between antimesenteric and mesenteric taeniae; increased intraluminal pressures then cause herniation through these areas
What is the incidence?	≈50% to 60% in the United States by age 60, with only 10% to 20% becoming symptomatic
What is the most common site?	95% of people with diverticulosis have **sigmoid** colon involvement

Who is at risk?	People with **low-fiber diets,** chronic constipation, and a positive family history; incidence increases with age
What are the symptoms/ complications?	**Bleeding:** may be massive Diverticulitis, asymptomatic (80% of cases)
What is the diagnostic approach: **Bleeding?**	Without signs of inflammation: colonoscopy
Pain and signs of inflammation?	Abdominal/pelvic CT scan
What is the treatment of diverticulosis?	High-fiber diet is recommended
What are the indications for operation with diverticulosis?	Complications of diverticulitis (e.g., fistula, obstruction, stricture); recurrent episodes; hemorrhage; suspected carcinoma; prolonged symptoms; abscess not drainable by percutaneous approach
When is it safe to get a colonoscopy or barium enema/sigmoidoscopy?	Due to risk of perforation, this is performed 6 weeks after inflammation resolves to rule out colon cancer

DIVERTICULITIS

What is it?	Infection or perforation of a diverticulum
What is the pathophysiology?	**Obstruction** of diverticulum by a fecalith leading to inflammation and microperforation
What are the signs/ symptoms?	LLQ pain (cramping or steady), change in bowel habits **(diarrhea),** fever, chills, anorexia, LLQ mass, nausea/vomiting, dysuria
What are the associated lab findings?	Increased WBCs
What are the associated radiographic findings?	On x-ray: ileus, partially obstructed colon, air-fluid levels, free air if perforated On abdominal/pelvic CT scan: swollen, edematous bowel wall; particularly helpful in diagnosing an abscess

What are the associated barium enema findings?	Barium enema should be avoided in acute cases
Is colonoscopy safe in an acute setting?	No, there is increased risk of perforation
What are the possible complications?	Abscess, diffuse peritonitis, fistula, obstruction, perforation, stricture
What is the most common fistula with diverticulitis?	Colovesical fistula (to bladder)
What is the best test for diverticulitis?	CT scan
What is the initial therapy?	IV fluids, NPO, broad-spectrum antibiotics with anaerobic coverage, NG suction (as needed for emesis/ileus)
When is surgery warranted?	Obstruction, fistula, free perforation, abscess not amenable to percutaneous drainage, sepsis, deterioration with initial conservative treatment
What is the lifelong risk of recurrence after:	
First episode?	33%
Second episode?	50%
What are the indications for elective resection?	Two episodes of diverticulitis; should be considered after the **first** episode in a young, diabetic, or immunosuppressed patient
What surgery is usually performed ELECTIVELY for recurrent bouts?	One-stage operation: resection of involved segment and primary anastomosis (with preoperative bowel prep)
What type of surgery is usually performed for an acute case of diverticulitis with a complication (e.g., perforation, obstruction)?	**Hartmann's procedure:** resection of involved segment with an end colostomy and stapled rectal stump (will need subsequent reanastomosis of colon usually after 2–3 postoperative months)

What is the treatment of diverticular abscess?

Percutaneous drainage; if abscess is not amenable to percutaneous drainage, then surgical approach for drainage is necessary

How common is massive lower GI bleeding with diverticulitis?

Very **rare**! Massive lower GI bleeding is seen with divertic**ulosis,** not diverticulitis

What are the most common causes of massive lower GI bleeding in adults?

Diverticulosis (especially right sided), vascular ectasia

What must you rule out in any patient with diverticulitis/diverticulosis?

Colon cancer

COLONIC VOLVULUS

What is it?

Twisting of colon on itself about its mesentery, resulting in obstruction and, if complete, vascular compromise with potential necrosis, perforation, or both

What is the most common type of colonic volvulus?

Sigmoid volvulus (makes sense because the sigmoid is a redundant/"floppy" structure!)

SIGMOID VOLVULUS

What is it?

Volvulus or "twist" in the sigmoid colon

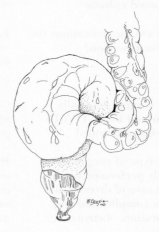

What is the incidence? ≈75% of colonic volvulus cases (Think: **S**igmoid = **S**uperior)

What are the etiologic factors? High-residue diet resulting in bulky stools and tortuous, elongated colon; chronic constipation; laxative abuse; pregnancy; seen most commonly in bedridden elderly or institutionalized patients, many of whom have history of prior abdominal surgery or distal colonic obstruction

What are the signs/ symptoms? Acute abdominal pain, progressive abdominal distention, anorexia, obstipation, cramps, nausea/vomiting

What findings are evident on abdominal plain film? Distended loop of sigmoid colon, often in the classic "bent inner tube" or "omega" sign with the loop aiming toward the RUQ

What are the signs of necrotic bowel in colonic volvulus? Free air, pneumatosis (air in bowel wall)

How is the diagnosis made? Sigmoidoscopy or radiographic exam with gastrografin enema

Under what conditions is gastrografin enema useful? If sigmoidoscopy and plain films fail to confirm the diagnosis; **"bird's beak"** is pathognomonic seen on enema contrast study as the contrast comes to a sharp end

What are the signs of strangulation? Discolored or hemorrhagic mucosa on sigmoidoscopy, bloody fluid in the rectum, frank ulceration or necrosis at the point of the twist, peritoneal signs, fever, hypotension, ↑ WBCs

What is the initial treatment? **Nonoperative:** If there is no strangulation, sigmoidoscopic reduction is successful in ≈85% of cases; enema study will occasionally reduce (5%)

What is the percentage of recurrence after nonoperative reduction of a sigmoid volvulus? ≈40%!

What are the indications for surgery?

Emergently if strangulation is suspected or nonoperative reduction unsuccessful (Hartmann's procedure); most patients should undergo resection during same hospitalization of redundant sigmoid after successful nonoperative reduction because of high recurrence rate (40%)

CECAL VOLVULUS

What is it?

Twisting of the cecum upon itself and the mesentery

What is a cecal "bascule" volvulus?

Instead of the more common axial twist, the cecum folds upward (lies on the ascending colon)

What is the incidence?

≈25% of colonic volvulus (i.e., much less common than sigmoid volvulus)

What is the etiology?

Idiopathic, poor fixation of the right colon, many patients have history of abdominal surgery

What are the signs/symptoms?

Acute onset of abdominal or colicky pain beginning in the RLQ and progressing to a constant pain, vomiting, obstipation, abdominal distention, and SBO; many patients will have had previous similar episodes

How is the diagnosis made?

Abdominal plain film; dilated, ovoid colon with large air/fluid level in the RLQ often forming the classic **"coffee bean"** sign with the apex aiming toward the epigastrium or LUQ (must rule out gastric dilation with NG aspiration)

What diagnostic studies should be performed?

Water-soluble contrast study (gastrografin), if diagnosis cannot be made by AXR

What is the treatment?

Emergent surgery, right colectomy with primary anastomosis or ileostomy and mucous fistula (primary anastomosis may be performed in stable patients)

What are the major differences in the EMERGENT management of cecal volvulus versus sigmoid?

Patients with cecal volvulus require **surgical** reduction, whereas the vast majority of patients with sigmoid volvulus undergo initial **endoscopic** reduction of the twist

Chapter 49   **Anus**

ANATOMY

Identify the following:

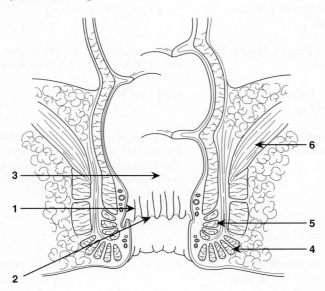

1. Anal columns
2. Dentate line
3. Rectum
4. External sphincter
5. Internal sphincter
6. Levator ani muscle

ANAL CANCER

What is the most common carcinoma of the anus?	Squamous cell carcinoma (80%) (Think: **ASS** = **A**nal **S**quamous **S**uperior)
What cell types are found in carcinomas of the anus?	1. Squamous cell carcinoma (80%) 2. Cloacogenic (transitional cell) 3. Adenocarcinoma/melanoma/ mucoepidermal
What is the incidence of anal carcinoma?	Rare (1% of colon cancers incidence)
What is anal Bowen's disease?	Squamous cell carcinoma in situ (Think: **B.S.** = **B**owen **S**quamous)
How is Bowen's disease treated?	With local wide excision
What is Paget's disease of the anus?	Adenocarcinoma in situ of the anus (Think: **P.A.** = **P**aget's **A**denocarcinoma)
How is Paget's disease treated?	With local wide excision
What are the risk factors for anal cancer?	Human papilloma virus, condyloma, herpes, HIV, chronic inflammation (fistulae/Crohn's disease) immunosuppression, homosexuality in males, cervical/ vaginal cancer, STDs, smoking
What is the most common symptom of anal carcinoma?	Anal bleeding
What are the other signs/symptoms of anal carcinoma?	Pain, mass, mucus per rectum, pruritus
What percentage of patients with anal cancer is asymptomatic?	$\approx 25\%$
To what locations do anal canal cancers metastasize?	Lymph nodes, liver, bone, lung

What is the lymphatic drainage below the dentate line?

Below to inguinal lymph nodes (above to pelvic chains)

Are most patients with anal cancer diagnosed early or late?

Late (diagnosis is often missed)

What is the workup of a patient with suspected anal carcinoma?

History
Physical exam: digital rectal exam, proctoscopic exam, and colonoscopy
Biopsy of mass
Abdominal/pelvic CT scan, transanal U/S
CXR
LFTs

Define:

Margin cancer

Anal verge out 5 cm onto the perianal skin

Canal cancer

Proximal to anal verge up to the border of the internal sphincter

How is an anal canal epidermal carcinoma treated?

NIGRO protocol:
1. Chemotherapy (5-FU and mitomycin C)
2. Radiation
3. Postradiation therapy scar biopsy (6–8 weeks post XRT)

What percentage of patients have a "complete" response with the NIGRO protocol?

90%

What is the 5-year survival with the NIGRO protocol?

85%

What is the treatment for local recurrence of anal cancer after the NIGRO protocol?

May repeat chemotherapy/XRT or salvage APR

How is a small (<5 cm) anal margin cancer treated?

Surgical excision with 1-cm margins

How is a large (>5 cm) anal margin cancer treated?

Chemoradiation

What is the treatment of anal melanoma?

Wide excision or APR (especially if tumor is large) +/− XRT, chemotherapy, postoperatively

What is the 5-year survival rate with anal melanoma?

<10%

How many patients with anal melanoma have an amelanotic anal tumor?

Approximately one third, thus making diagnosis difficult without pathology

What is the prognosis of anal melanoma?

<5% 5-year survival rate

FISTULA IN ANO

What is it?

Anal fistula, from rectum to perianal skin

What are the causes?

Usually anal crypt/gland infection (usually perianal abscess)

What are the signs/ symptoms?

Perianal drainage, perirectal abscess, recurrent perirectal abscess, "diaper rash," itching

What disease should be considered with fistula in ano?

Crohn's disease

How is the diagnosis made?

Exam, proctoscope

What is Goodsall's rule?

Fistulas originating **anterior** to a transverse line through the anus will course **straight** ahead and exit anteriorly, whereas those exiting **posteriorly** have a **curved** tract

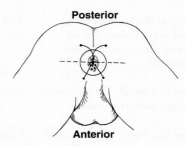

Posterior

Anterior

How can Goodsall's rule be remembered?

Think of a dog with a **straight** nose (anterior) and **curved** tail (posterior)

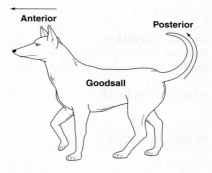

What is the management of anorectal fistulas?

1. Define the anatomy
2. Marsupialization of fistula tract (i.e., fillet tract open)
3. Wound care: routine Sitz baths and dressing changes
4. Seton placement if fistula is through the sphincter muscle

What is a seton?

Thick suture placed through fistula tract to allow slow transection of sphincter muscle; scar tissue formed will hold the sphincter muscle in place and allow for continence after transection

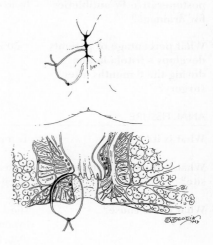

What percentage of patients with a perirectal abscess develop a fistula in ano after drainage?	≈50%
How do you find the internal rectal opening of an anorectal fistula in the O.R.?	Inject H_2O_2 (or methylene blue) in external opening—then look for bubbles (or blue dye) coming out of internal opening!
What is a sitz bath?	Sitting in a warm bath (usually done after bowel movement and TID

PERIRECTAL ABSCESS

What is it?	Abscess formation around the anus/rectum
What are the signs/ symptoms?	Rectal pain, drainage of pus, fever, perianal mass
How is the diagnosis made?	Physical/digital exam reveals perianal/ rectal submucosal mass/fluctuance
What is the cause?	Crypt abscess in dentate line with spread
What is the treatment?	As with all abscesses (except simple liver amebic abscess) **drainage,** sitz bath, anal hygiene, stool softeners
What is the indication for postoperative IV antibiotics for drainage?	Cellulitis, immunosuppression, diabetes, heart valve abnormality
What percentage of patients develops a fistula in ano during the 6 months after surgery?	≈50%

ANAL FISSURE

What is it?	Tear or fissure in the anal epithelium
What is the most common site?	Posterior midline (comparatively low blood flow)
What is the cause?	Hard stool passage (constipation), hyperactive sphincter, disease process (e.g., Crohn's disease)

What are the signs/symptoms?

Pain in the anus, painful (can be excruciating) bowel movement, rectal bleeding, blood on toilet tissue after bowel movement, sentinel tag, tear in the anal skin, extremely painful rectal exam, sentinel pile, hypertrophic papilla

What is a sentinel pile?

Thickened mucosa/skin at the distal end of an anal fissure that is often confused with a small hemorrhoid

What is the anal fissure triad for a chronic fissure?

1. Fissure
2. Sentinel pile
3. Hypertrophied anal papilla

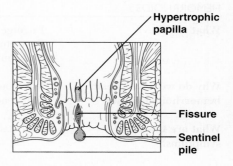

What is the conservative treatment?

Sitz baths, stool softeners, high fiber diet, excellent anal hygiene, topical nifedipine, Botox®

What disease processes must be considered with a chronic anal fissure?

Crohn's disease, anal cancer, sexually transmitted disease, ulcerative colitis, AIDS

What are the indications for surgery?

Chronic fissure refractory to conservative treatment

What is one surgical option?

Lateral internal sphincterotomy (LIS)—cut the internal sphincter to release it from spasm

What is the "rule of 90%" for anal fissures?

90% occur posteriorly
90% heal with medical treatment alone
90% of patients who undergo an LIS heal successfully

PERIANAL WARTS

What are they?	Warts around the anus/perineum
What is the cause?	Condyloma acuminatum (human papilloma virus)
What is the major risk?	Squamous cell carcinoma
What is the treatment if warts are small?	Topical podophyllin, imiquimod (Aldara®)
What is the treatment if warts are large?	Surgical resection or laser ablation

HEMORRHOIDS

What are they?	Engorgement of the venous plexuses of the rectum, anus, or both; with protrusion of the mucosa, anal margin, or both
Why do we have "healthy" hemorrhoidal tissue?	It is thought to be involved with fluid/air continence
What are the signs/ symptoms?	Anal mass/prolapse, bleeding, itching, pain
Which type, internal or external, is painful?	External, below the dentate line
If a patient has excruciating anal pain and history of hemorrhoids, what is the likely diagnosis?	Thrombosed external hemorrhoid (treat by excision)
What are the causes of hemorrhoids?	Constipation/straining, portal hypertension, pregnancy
What is an internal hemorrhoid?	Hemorrhoid above the (proximal) dentate line
What is an external hemorrhoid?	Hemorrhoid below the dentate line
What are the three "hemorrhoid quadrants"?	1. Left lateral 2. Right posterior 3. Right anterior

Classification by Degrees

**Define the following terms
for internal hemorrhoids:**

    First-degree hemorrhoid   Hemorrhoid that does not prolapse

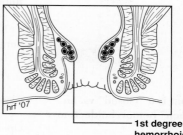

1st degree
hemorrhoid

**Second-degree
hemorrhoid**   Prolapses with defecation, but returns on
its own

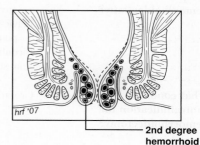

2nd degree
hemorrhoid

Third-degree hemorrhoid   Prolapses with defecation or any type of
Valsalva maneuver and requires active
manual reduction (eat fiber!)

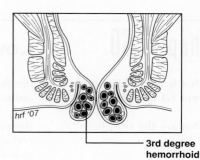

3rd degree
hemorrhoid

Fourth-degree hemorrhoid

Prolapsed hemorrhoid that cannot be reduced

What is the treatment?

High-fiber diet, anal hygiene, topical steroids, sitz baths
Rubber band ligation (in most cases anesthetic is not necessary for internal hemorrhoids)
Surgical resection for large refractory hemorrhoids, infrared coagulation, harmonic scalpel

What is a "closed" vs. an "open" hemorrhoidectomy?

Closed (Ferguson) "closes" the mucosa with sutures after hemorrhoid tissue removal
Open (Milligan-Morgan) leaves mucosa "open"

What are the dreaded complications of hemorrhoidectomy?

Exsanguination (bleeding may pool proximally in lumen of colon without any signs of external bleeding)
Pelvic infection (may be extensive and potentially fatal)
Incontinence (injury to sphincter complex)
Anal stricture

What condition is a contraindication for hemorrhoidectomy?

Crohn's disease

Classically, what must be ruled out with lower GI bleeding believed to be caused by hemorrhoids?

Colon cancer (colonoscopy)

Chapter 50

Lower GI Bleeding

What is the definition of lower GI bleeding?

Bleeding distal to the ligament of Treitz; vast majority occurs in the colon

What are the symptoms?

Hematochezia (bright red blood per rectum [BRBPR]), with or without abdominal pain, melena, anorexia, fatigue, syncope, shortness of breath, shock

What are the signs?   BRBPR, positive hemoccult, abdominal
                                        tenderness, hypovolemic shock, orthostasis

What are the causes?   Diverticulosis (usually **right**-sided in
                                        severe hemorrhage), vascular ectasia,
                                        colon cancer, hemorrhoids, trauma,
                                        hereditary hemorrhagic telangiectasia,
                                        intussusception, volvulus, ischemic colitis,
                                        IBD (especially ulcerative colitis),
                                        anticoagulation, rectal cancer, Meckel's
                                        diverticulum (with ectopic gastric
                                        mucosa), stercoral ulcer (ulcer from hard
                                        stool), infectious colitis, aortoenteric
                                        fistula, chemotherapy, irradiation injury,
                                        infarcted bowel, strangulated hernia, anal
                                        fissure

**What medicines should be   Coumadin®, aspirin, Plavix®
looked for causally with a
lower GI bleed?**

What are the most common   1. **Diverticulosis
causes of massive lower GI   2. Vascular ectasia
bleeding?**

**What lab tests should be   CBC, Chem-7, PT/PTT, type and cross
performed?**

What is the initial treatment?   IVFs: lactated Ringer's; packed red blood
                                        cells as needed, IV × 2, Foley catheter to
                                        follow urine output, d/c aspirin, NGT

**What diagnostic tests should   History, physical exam, NGT aspiration
be performed for all lower   (to rule out UGI bleeding; bile or blood
GI bleeds?**   must be seen; otherwise, perform EGD),
                                        anoscopy/proctoscopic exam

What must be ruled out in   **Upper GI bleeding! Remember, NGT
patients with lower GI   aspiration is not 100% accurate (even if
bleeding?**   you get bile without blood)

**How can you have a UGI   Duodenal bleeding ulcer can bleed distal
bleed with only clear succus   to the pylorus with the NGT sucking
back in the NGT?**   normal nonbloody gastric secretions! **If
                                        there is any question, perform EGD**

What would an algorithm for diagnosing and treating lower GI bleeding look like?

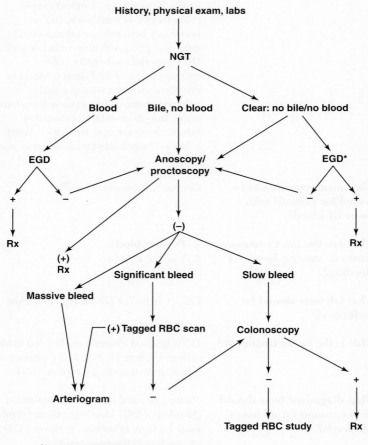

*Based on clinical suspicion

What is the diagnostic test of choice for localizing a slow to moderate lower GI bleeding source?

Colonoscopy

What test is performed to localize bleeding if there is too much active bleeding to see the source with a colonoscope?

A-gram (mesenteric angiography)

What is more sensitive for a slow, intermittent amount of blood loss: A-gram or tagged RBC study?

Radiolabeled RBC scan is more sensitive for blood loss at a rate of ≥0.5 mL/min or intermittent blood loss because it has a longer half-life (for arteriography, bleeding rate must be ≥1.0 mL/min)

What is the colonoscopic treatment option for bleeding vascular ectasia or polyp?

Laser or electrocoagulation; local epinephrine injection

What is the treatment if bleeding site is KNOWN and massive or recurrent lower GI bleeding continues?

Segmental resection of the bowel

What is the surgical treatment of massive lower GI bleeding WITHOUT localization?

Exploratory laparotomy with intraoperative enteroscopy and total abdominal colectomy as last resort

What percentage of cases spontaneously stop bleeding?

80%–90% stop bleeding with resuscitative measures only (at least temporarily)

What percentage of patients require emergent surgery for lower GI bleeding?

Only ≈10%

Does melena always signify active colonic bleeding?

NO—the colon is very good at storing material and often will store melena/maroon stools and pass them days later (follow patient, UO, HCT, and vital signs)

What is the therapeutic advantage of doing a colonoscopy?

Options of injecting substance (epinephrine) or coagulating vessels is an advantage with C-scope to control bleeding

What is the therapeutic advantage of doing an A-gram?

Ability to inject vasopressin and/or embolization, with at least temporary control of bleeding in >85%

Chapter 51

Inflammatory Bowel Disease: Crohn's Disease and Ulcerative Colitis

What is IBD?

Inflammatory Bowel Disease, inflammatory disease of the GI tract

What are the two inflammatory bowel diseases?

Crohn's disease and ulcerative colitis

What is another name for Crohn's disease?

Regional enteritis

What is ulcerative colitis often called?

UC

What is the cause of IBD?

No one knows, but probably an autoimmune process with environmental factors contributing

What is the differential diagnosis?

Crohn's versus ulcerative colitis, infectious colitis (e.g., *C. difficile,* amebiasis, shigellosis), ischemic colitis, irritable bowel syndrome, diverticulitis, Zollinger-Ellison syndrome (ZES), colon cancer, carcinoid, ischemic bowel

What are the extraintestinal manifestations seen in both types of IBD?

Ankylosing spondylitis, aphthous (oral) ulcers, iritis, pyoderma gangrenosum, erythema nodosum, clubbing of fingers, sclerosing cholangitis, arthritis, kidney disease (nephrotic syndrome, amyloid deposits)

How can these manifestations be remembered?

Think of the acronym **"A PIE SACK"**:

Aphthous ulcers

Pyoderma gangrenosum
Iritis
Erythema nodosum

Sclerosing cholangitis
Arthritis, **A**nkylosing spondylitis
Clubbing of fingers
Kidney (amyloid deposits, nephrotic syndrome)

COMPARISON OF CROHN'S DISEASE AND ULCERATIVE COLITIS

INCIDENCE

Crohn's disease:

Incidence	3–6/100,000
At-risk population	High in the Jewish population, low in the African black population, similar rates between African American and U.S. white population
Sex?	Female > male
Distribution?	Bimodal distribution (i.e., two peaks in incidence): peak incidence at 25 to 40 years of age; second bimodal distribution peak at 50 to 65 years of age

Ulcerative colitis:

Incidence?	10/100,000
At-risk population	High in the Jewish population, low in the African American population Positive family history in 20% of cases
Sex?	Male > female
Distribution?	Bimodal distribution at 20 to 35 and 50 to 65 years of age

INITIAL SYMPTOMS

Crohn's disease?	**Abdominal pain, diarrhea,** fever, weight loss, anal disease
Ulcerative colitis?	**Bloody diarrhea** (hallmark), fever, weight loss

ANATOMIC DISTRIBUTION

Crohn's disease?	Classic phrasing **"mouth to anus"**
	    Small bowel only (20%)
	    Small bowel and colon (40%)
	    Colon only (30%)

Ulcerative colitis?	Colon only (Think: ulcerative **COL**itis = **COL**on alone)

ROUTE OF SPREAD

Crohn's disease?	Small bowel, colon, or both **with "skip areas"** of normal bowel; hence, the name "regional enteritis"
Ulcerative colitis?	Almost always involves the rectum and spreads proximally always in a continuous route without "skip areas"
What is "backwash" ileitis?	Mild inflammation of the terminal ileum in ulcerative colitis; thought to be "backwash" of inflammatory mediators from the colon into the terminal ileum

BOWEL WALL INVOLVEMENT

Crohn's disease?	Full thickness (transmural involvement)
Ulcerative colitis?	Mucosa/submucosa only

ANAL INVOLVEMENT

Crohn's disease?	Common (fistulae, abscesses, fissures, ulcers)
Ulcerative colitis?	Uncommon

RECTAL INVOLVEMENT

Crohn's disease?	Rare
Ulcerative colitis?	100%

MUCOSAL FINDINGS

Crohn's disease (6)?
1. Aphthoid ulcers
2. Granulomas
3. Linear ulcers
4. Transverse fissures
5. Swollen mucosa
6. **Full-thickness wall involvement**

Ulcerative colitis (5)?
1. Granular, flat mucosa
2. Ulcers
3. **Crypt abscess**
4. Dilated mucosal vessels
5. **Pseudopolyps**

How can ulcerative colitis and Crohn's anal and wall involvement be remembered?

"CAT URP":
Crohn's = **A**nal–**T**ransmural
UC = **R**ectum–**P**artial wall thickness

DIAGNOSTIC TESTS

Crohn's disease?
Colonoscopy with biopsy, barium enema, UGI with small bowel follow-through, stool cultures

Ulcerative colitis?
Colonoscopy, barium enema, UGI with small bowel follow-through (to look for Crohn's disease), stool cultures

COMPLICATIONS

Crohn's disease?
Anal fistula/abscess, **fistula,** stricture, perforation, **abscesses,** toxic megacolon, colovesical fistula, enterovaginal fistula, hemorrhage, **obstruction,** cancer

Ulcerative colitis?
Cancer, toxic megacolon, colonic perforation, hemorrhage, strictures, obstruction, complications of surgery

CANCER RISK

Crohn's disease?	Overall increased risk, but about half that of ulcerative colitis
Ulcerative colitis?	≈5% risk of developing colon cancer at 10 years; then, risk increases ≈1% per year; thus, an incidence of ≈20% after 20 years of the disease (30% at 30 years)

INCIDENCE OF TOXIC MEGACOLON

Crohn's disease?	≈5%
Ulcerative colitis?	≈10%

INDICATIONS FOR SURGERY

Crohn's disease?	Obstruction, massive bleeding, fistula, perforation, suspicion of cancer, abscess (refractory to medical treatment), toxic megacolon (refractory to medical treatment), strictures, dysplasia
Ulcerative colitis?	Toxic megacolon (refractory to medical treatment); cancer prophylaxis; massive bleeding; failure of child to mature because of disease and steroids; perforation; suspicion of or documented cancer; acute severe symptoms refractory to medical treatment; inability to wean off of chronic steroids; obstruction; dysplasia; stricture
What are the common surgical options for ulcerative colitis?	1. Total proctocolectomy, distal rectal mucosectomy, and ileoanal pull through 2. Total proctocolectomy and Brooke ileostomy
What is "toxic megacolon"?	**Toxic** patient: sepsis, febrile, abdominal pain **Megacolon:** acutely and massively distended colon

What are the medication options for treating IBD?

Sulfasalazine, mesalamine (5-aminosalicylic acid)
Steroids, metronidazole (Flagyl®), azathioprine, 6-mercaptopurine (6-mp), infliximab

What is infliximab?

Antibody vs. TNF-α (tumor necrosis factor-alpha)

What is the active metabolite of sulfasalazine?

5'-aminosalicylate (5'-ASA), which is released in the colon

What is the medical treatment of choice for perianal Crohn's disease?

PO metronidazole (Flagyl®)

What are the treatment options for long-term remission of IBD?

6-mercaptopurine (6-mp), azathioprine, mesalamine

What medication is used for IBD "flare-ups"?

Steroids

What is a unique medication route option for ulcerative colitis?

Enemas (steroids, 5-ASA)

Which disease has "cobblestoning" more often on endoscopic exam?

Crohn's disease (Think: **C**rohn's = **C**obblestoning)

Which disease has pseudopolyps on colonoscopic exam?

Ulcerative colitis; pseudopolyps are polyps of hypertrophied mucosa surrounded by mucosal atrophy

Which disease has a "lead pipe" appearance on barium enema?

Chronic ulcerative colitis

Rectal bleeding/bloody diarrhea is a hallmark of which disease?

Ulcerative colitis (rare in Crohn's disease)

What is the most common indication for surgery in patients with Crohn's disease?

Small bowel obstruction (SBO)

What are the intraoperative findings of Crohn's disease?

Mesenteric **"fat creeping"** onto the antimesenteric border of the small bowel

Shortened (and thick) mesentery

Thick bowel wall

Fistula(e)

Abscess(es)

Why do you see fistulas and abscesses with Crohn's and not ulcerative colitis?

Crohn's disease is **transmural**

What is the operation for short strictures of the small bowel in Crohn's disease?

Stricturoplasty; basically a Heineke-Mikulicz pyloroplasty on the strictured segment (i.e., opened longitudinally and sewn closed in a transverse direction)

Should the appendix be removed during a laparotomy for abdominal pain if Crohn's disease is discovered?

Yes, if the cecum is not involved with active Crohn's disease

What is pouchitis?

Inflammation of the pouch of an ileoanal pull through; treat with metronidazole (Flagyl®)

Do you need a frozen section for margins during a bowel resection for Crohn's disease?

No, you need only grossly negative margins

What is it called when the entire colon is involved?

Pancolitis

Chapter 52   Liver

ANATOMY

What is the name of the liver capsule?

Glisson's capsule

What is the "bare" area?

Posterior section of the liver against the diaphragm that is "bare" without peritoneal covering

What is Cantle's line?

Line drawn from the gallbladder to a point just to the left of the inferior vena cava, which transects the liver into the right and left lobes

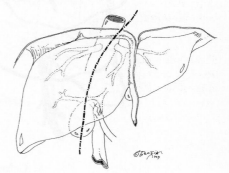

Which ligament goes from the anterior abdominal wall to the liver?

Falciform ligament

What does the falciform ligament contain?

Ligamentum teres (obliterated umbilical vein)

What is the coronary ligament?

Peritoneal reflection on top of the liver that crowns (hence "coronary") the liver and attaches it to the diaphragm

What are the triangular ligaments of the liver?

Right and left lateral extents of the coronary ligament, which form triangles

**What is the origin of the
hepatic arterial supply?**

From the proper hepatic artery off of the
celiac trunk (celiac trunk to common
hepatic artery to proper hepatic artery)

**Identify the arterial
branches of the celiac trunk:**

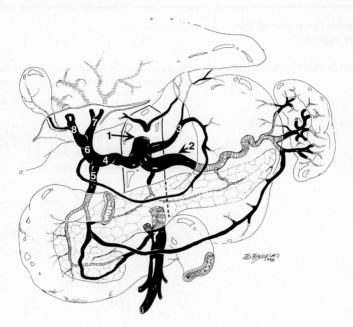

1. Celiac trunk
2. Splenic artery
3. Left gastric artery
4. Common hepatic artery
5. Gastroduodenal artery
6. Proper hepatic artery
7. Left hepatic artery
8. Right hepatic artery

What is the venous supply?

Portal vein (formed from the splenic
vein and the superior mesenteric vein)

**What is the hepatic venous
drainage?**

Via the hepatic veins, which drain into
the IVC (three veins: left, middle, and
right)

What sources provide oxygen to the liver?

Portal vein blood—50%
Hepatic artery blood—50%

From what sources does the liver receive blood?

Portal system—75%
Hepatic artery system—25%

Identify the segments of the liver (French system).

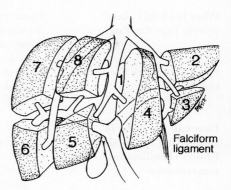

What is the overall arrangement of the segments in the liver?

Clockwise, starting at segment 1

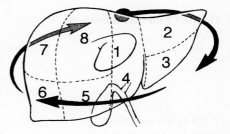

What is the maximum amount of liver that can be resected while retaining adequate liver function?

>80%; if given adequate recovery time, the original mass can be **regenerated** (Remember Prometheus!)

What are the signs/symptoms of liver disease?

Hepatomegaly, splenomegaly, icterus, pruritus (from bile salts in skin), blanching spider telangiectasia, gynecomastia, testicular atrophy, caput medusae, dark urine, clay-colored stools, bradycardia, edema, ascites, fever, fetor hepaticus (sweet musty smell), hemorrhoids, variceal bleeding, anemia, body hair loss, liver tenderness, palmar erythema

Which liver enzymes are made by hepatocytes?

AST and ALT (aspartate aminotransferase and alanine aminotransferase)

What is the source of alkaline phosphatase?

Ductal epithelium (thus, elevated with ductal obstruction)

What is Child's class? (Child-Turcotte-Pugh)

Classification system that estimates hepatic reserve in patients with hepatic failure and mortality

What comprises the Child's classification?

Laboratory: bilirubin, albumin
Clinical: encephalopathy, ascites, prothrombin time (PT)

How can the criteria comprising the modified Child's classification be remembered?

Use the acronym: **"A BEAP"**:
Ascites

Bilirubin
Encephalopathy
Albumin
PT (prothrombin time)

Define Child's classification:
A
B
C

Ascites	Bili	Enceph	ALB	PT INR
none	<2	none	>3.5	<1.7
controlled	2–3	minimal	2.8–3.5	1.7–2.2
uncontrolled	>3	severe	<2.8	>2.2

(Think: As in a letter grading system, A is better than B, B is better than C)

What is the operative mortality for a portocaval shunt vs. overall intra-abdominal operations with cirrhosis in the following Child's classes:
A?
B?
C?

<5% vs. overall = 10%
<15% vs. overall = 30%
≈33% vs. overall = 75%

What does the MELD score stand for?

Model for **E**nd-stage **L**iver **D**isease

What is measured in the MELD score?

INR, T.Bili, serum creatinine (SCR); find good MELD calculators online

What is the mortality in cirrhotic patients for nonemergent nontransplant surgery?	Increase in mortality by 1% per 1 point in the MELD score until 20, then 2% for each MELD point
What is the mortality in cirrhotic patients for emergent nontransplant surgery?	14% increase in mortality per 1 point of the MELD score

TUMORS OF THE LIVER

What is the most common liver cancer?	**Metastatic disease** outnumbers primary tumors 20:1; primary site is usually the GI tract
What is the most common primary malignant liver tumor?	Hepatocellular carcinoma (hepatoma)
What is the most common primary benign liver tumor?	Hemangioma
What lab tests comprise the workup for liver metastasis?	LFTs (AST and alkaline phosphatase are most useful), CEA for suspected primary colon cancer
What are the associated imaging studies?	CT scan, ultrasound, A-gram
What is a right hepatic lobectomy?	Removal of the right lobe of the liver (i.e., all tissue to the right of Cantle's line is removed)
What is a left hepatic lobectomy?	Removal of the left lobe of the liver (i.e., removal of all the liver tissue to the left of Cantle's line)
What is a right trisegmentectomy?	Removal of all the liver tissue to the right of the falciform ligament
What are the three common types of primary benign liver tumors?	1. Hemangioma 2. Hepatocellular adenoma 3. Focal nodular hyperplasia

What are the four common types of primary malignant liver tumors?	1. Hepatocellular carcinoma (hepatoma) 2. Cholangiocarcinoma (when intrahepatic) 3. Angiosarcoma (associated with chemical exposure) 4. Hepatoblastoma (most common in infants and children)
What chemical exposures are risk factors for angiosarcoma?	**Vinyl chloride,** arsenic, thorotrast contrast
What is a "hepatoma"?	Hepatocellular carcinoma
What are the other benign liver masses?	Benign liver cyst, bile duct hamartomas, bile duct adenoma
What is a liver "hamartoma"?	White hard nodule made up of normal liver cells

HEPATOCELLULAR ADENOMA

What is it?	Benign liver tumor
Describe the histology.	Normal hepatocytes without bile ducts
What are the associated risk factors?	Women, birth control pills (Think: **ABC** = **A**denoma **B**irth **C**ontrol), anabolic steroids, glycogen storage disease
What is the female:male ratio?	9:1
What is the average age of occurrence?	30–35 years of age
What are the signs/ symptoms?	RUQ pain/mass, RUQ fullness, bleeding (rare)
What are the possible complications?	Rupture with bleeding (33%), necrosis, pain, risk of hepatocellular carcinoma
How is the diagnosis made?	CT scan, U/S, +/– biopsy (rule out hemangioma with RBC-tagged scan!)

What is the treatment:
    Small?

Stop birth control pills—it may regress; if not, surgical resection is necessary

    Large (>5 cm), bleeding, painful, or ruptured?

Surgical resection

FOCAL NODULAR HYPERPLASIA (FNH)

What is it?

Benign liver tumor

Describe the histology.

Normal hepatocytes and **bile ducts (adenoma has no bile ducts)**

What is the average age of occurrence?

≈40 years

What are the associated risk factors?

Female gender

Are the tumors associated with birth control pills?

Yes, but not as clearly associated as with adenoma

How is the diagnosis made?

Nuclear technetium-99 study, U/S, CT scan, A-gram, biopsy

What is the classic CT scan finding?

Liver mass with **"central scar"** (Think: focal = central)

What are the possible complications?

Pain (no risk of cancer, very rarely hemorrhage)

Is there a cancer risk with FNH?

No (there is a cancer risk with adenoma)

What is the treatment?

Resection or **embolization** if patient is symptomatic; otherwise, follow if diagnosis is confirmed; stop birth control pills

Why does embolization work with FNH?

FNH tumors are usually fed by one major artery

HEPATIC HEMANGIOMA

What is it?	Benign vascular tumor of the liver
What is its claim to fame?	Most common primary benign liver tumor (up to 7% of population)
What are the signs/symptoms?	RUQ pain/mass, bruits
What are the possible complications?	Pain, congestive heart failure, coagulopathy, obstructive jaundice, gastric outlet obstruction, Kasabach-Merritt syndrome, hemorrhage (rare)
Define Kasabach-Merritt syndrome?	Hemangioma **and** thrombocytopenia and fibrinogenopenia
How is the diagnosis made?	CT scan with IV contrast, tagged red blood scan, MRI, ultrasound
Should biopsy be performed?	No (risk of hemorrhage with biopsy)
What is the treatment?	**Observation** (>90%)
What are the indications for resection?	Symptoms, hemorrhage, cannot make a diagnosis

HEPATOCELLULAR CARCINOMA

What is it?	Most common primary malignancy of the liver
By what name is it also known?	Hepatoma
What is its incidence?	Accounts for 80% of all primary malignant liver tumors
What are the geographic high-risk areas?	Africa and Asia
What are the associated risk factors?	**Hepatitis B virus, cirrhosis, aflatoxin** (fungi toxin of *Aspergillus flavus*); Other risk factors: α-1-antitrypsin deficiency, hemochromatosis, liver fluke (*Clonorchis sinensis*), anabolic steroids, polyvinyl chloride, glycogen storage disease (type I)

What percentage of patients with cirrhosis will develop hepatocellular carcinoma?

≈5%

What are the signs/ symptoms?

Dull RUQ pain, hepatomegaly (classic presentation: **painful hepatomegaly**), abdominal mass, weight loss, paraneoplastic syndromes, signs of portal hypertension, ascites, jaundice, fever, anemia, splenomegaly

What tests should be ordered?

Ultrasound, CT scan, angiography, tumor marker elevation

What is the tumor marker?

Elevated α-fetoprotein

What is the most common way to get a tissue diagnosis?

Needle biopsy with CT scan, ultrasound, or laparoscopic guidance

What is the most common site of metastasis?

Lungs

What is the treatment of hepatocellular carcinoma?

Surgical resection, if possible (e.g., lobectomy); liver transplant

What are the treatment options if the patient is not a surgical candidate?

Percutaneous ethanol tumor injection, cryotherapy, and intra-arterial chemotherapy

What are the indications for liver transplantation?

Cirrhosis and NO resection candidacy as well as no distant or lymph node metastases and no vascular invasion; the tumor must be single, <5-cm tumor or have three nodules, with none >3 cm

What is the prognosis under the following conditions:
Unresectable?

Almost none survive a year

Resectable?

≈35% are alive at 5 years

Which subtype has the best prognosis?

Fibrolamellar hepatoma (young adults)

ABSCESSES OF THE LIVER

What is a liver abscess?	Abscess (collection of pus) in the liver parenchyma
What are the types of liver abscess?	Pyogenic (bacterial), parasitic (amebic), fungal
What is the most common location of abscess in the liver?	Right lobe > left lobe
What are the sources?	Direct spread from biliary tract infection or Portal spread from GI infection (e.g., appendicitis, diverticulitis) Systemic source (bacteremia) Liver trauma (e.g., liver gunshot wound) Cryptogenic (unknown source)
What are the two most common types?	**Bacterial** (most common in the United States) and amebic (most common worldwide)

BACTERIAL LIVER ABSCESS

What are the three most common bacterial organisms affecting the liver?	Gram negatives: *E. coli, Klebsiella,* and *Proteus*
What are the most common sources/causes of bacterial liver abscesses?	Cholangitis, diverticulitis, liver cancer, liver metastasis
What are the signs/ symptoms?	**Fever, chills, RUQ pain,** leukocytosis, increased liver function tests (LFTs), jaundice, sepsis, weight loss
What is the treatment?	IV antibiotics (triple antibiotics with metronidazole), percutaneous drainage with CT scan or U/S guidance
What are the indications for operative drainage?	Multiple/loculated abscesses or if multiple percutaneous attempts have failed

AMEBIC LIVER ABSCESS

What is the etiology?	*Entamoeba histolytica* (typically reaches liver via portal vein from intestinal amebiasis)
How does it spread?	Fecal–oral transmission
What are the risk factors?	Patients from countries south of the U.S.–Mexican border, institutionalized patients, homosexual men, alcoholic patients
What are the signs/ symptoms?	RUQ pain, fever, hepatomegaly, diarrhea *Note:* chills are much less common with amebic abscesses than with pyogenic abscesses
Which lobe is most commonly involved?	Right lobe of the liver
Classic description of abscess contents?	"Anchovy paste" pus
How is the diagnosis made?	Lab tests, ultrasound, CT scan
What lab tests should be performed?	Indirect hemagglutination titers for *Entamoeba* antibodies elevated in >95% of cases, elevated LFTs
What is the treatment?	Metronidazole IV
What are the indications for percutaneous surgical drainage?	Refractory to metronidazole, bacterial co-infection, or peritoneal rupture
What are the possible complications of large left lobe liver amebic abscess?	Erosion into the pericardial sac (potentially fatal!)

HYDATID LIVER CYST

What is it?	Usually a right lobe cyst filled with *Echinococcus granulosus*

What are the risk factors?	Travel; exposure to dogs, sheep, and cattle (carriers)
What are the signs/ symptoms?	RUQ abdominal pain, jaundice, RUQ mass
How is the diagnosis made?	Indirect hemagglutination antibody test (serologic testing), Casoni skin test, ultrasound, CT, radiographic imaging
What are the findings on AXR?	Possible calcified outline of cyst
What are the major risks?	Erosion into the pleural cavity, pericardial sac, or biliary tree Rupture into the peritoneal cavity causing fatal anaphylaxis
What is the risk of surgical removal of echinococcal (hydatid) cysts?	Rupture or leakage of cyst contents into the abdomen may cause a fatal **anaphylactic** reaction
When should percutaneous drainage be performed?	Never; may cause leaking into the peritoneal cavity and anaphylaxis
What is the treatment?	**Mebendazole, followed by surgical resection;** large cysts can be drained and then injected with toxic irrigant (scoliocide) into the cyst unless aspirate is bilious (which means there is a biliary connection) followed by cyst removal
Which toxic irrigations are used?	Hypertonic saline, ethanol, or cetrimide

HEMOBILIA

What is it?	Blood draining via the common bile duct into the duodenum
What is the diagnostic triad?	Triad: 1. RUQ pain 2. Guaiac positive/upper GI bleeding 3. Jaundice
What are the causes?	Trauma with liver laceration, percutaneous transhepatic cholangiography (PTC), tumors

How is the diagnosis made?	EGD (blood out of the ampulla of Vater), A-gram
What is the treatment?	A-gram with embolization of the bleeding vessel

---

Chapter 53

Portal Hypertension

Identify the anatomy of the portal venous system:

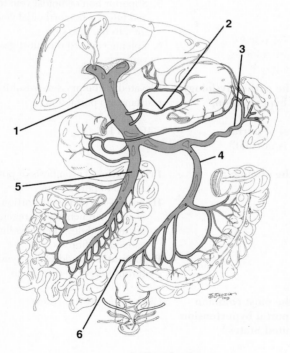

1. Portal vein
2. Coronary vein
3. Splenic vein
4. IMV (inferior mesenteric vein)
5. SMV (superior mesenteric vein)
6. Superior hemorrhoidal vein

Describe drainage of blood from the superior hemorrhoidal vein.

To the IMV, the splenic vein, and then the portal vein

Where does blood drain into from the IMV?

Into the splenic vein

Where does the portal vein begin?

At the confluence of the splenic vein and the SMV

What are the (6) potential routes of portal–systemic collateral blood flow (as seen with portal hypertension)?

1. Umbilical vein
2. Coronary vein to esophageal venous plexuses
3. Retroperitoneal veins (veins of Retzius)
4. Diaphragm veins (veins of Sappey)
5. Superior hemorrhoidal vein to middle and inferior hemorrhoidal veins and then to the iliac vein
6. Splenic veins to the short gastric veins

What is the pathophysiology of portal hypertension?

Elevated portal pressure resulting from resistance to portal flow

What level of portal pressure is normal?

<10 mm Hg

What is the etiology?

Prehepatic—Thrombosis of portal vein/ atresia of portal vein

Hepatic—**Cirrhosis** (distortion of normal parenchyma by regenerating hepatic nodules), hepatocellular carcinoma, fibrosis

Posthepatic—Budd-Chiari syndrome: thrombosis of hepatic veins

What is the most common cause of portal hypertension in the United States?

Cirrhosis (>90% of cases)

How many patients with alcoholism develop cirrhosis?

Surprisingly, <1 in 5

What percentage of patients with cirrhosis develop esophageal varices?

≈40%

How many patients with cirrhosis develop portal hypertension?

Approximately two thirds

What is the most common physical finding in patients with portal hypertension?

Splenomegaly (spleen enlargement)

What are the associated CLINICAL findings in portal hypertension (4)?

1. Esophageal varices
2. Splenomegaly
3. Caput medusae (engorgement of periumbilical veins)
4. Hemorrhoids

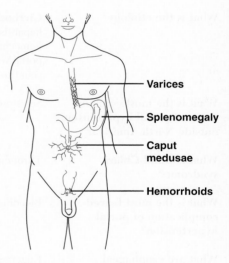

What other physical findings are associated with cirrhosis and portal hypertension?

Spider angioma, palmar erythema, ascites, truncal obesity and peripheral wasting, encephalopathy, asterixis (liver flap), gynecomastia, jaundice

What is the name of the periumbilical bruit heard with caput medusae?

Cruveilhier-Baumgarten bruit

**What constitutes the portal–
systemic collateral circulation
in portal hypertension in the
following conditions:**

Esophageal varices?

Coronary vein backing up into the
azygous system

Caput medusae?

Umbilical vein (via falciform ligament)
draining into the epigastric veins

Retroperitoneal varices?

Small mesenteric veins (veins of Retzius)
draining retroperitoneally into lumbar veins

Hemorrhoids?

Superior hemorrhoidal vein (which
normally drains into the inferior mesenteric vein) backing up into the middle
and inferior hemorrhoidal veins

What is the etiology?

Cirrhosis (90%), schistosomiasis,
hepatitis, Budd-Chiari syndrome,
hemochromatosis, Wilson's disease,
portal vein thrombosis, tumors, splenic
vein thrombosis

**What is the most common
cause of portal hypertension
outside North America?**

Schistosomiasis

**What is Budd-Chiari
syndrome?**

Thrombosis of the hepatic veins

**What is the most feared
complication of portal
hypertension?**

Bleeding from esophageal varices

**What are esophageal
varices?**

Engorgement of the esophageal venous
plexuses secondary to increased collateral
blood flow from the portal system as a
result of portal hypertension

**What is the "rule of 2/3" of
portal hypertension?**

2/3 of patients with cirrhosis will develop
portal hypertension
2/3 of patients with portal hypertension
will develop esophageal varices
2/3 of patients with esophageal varices
will bleed from the varices

In patients with cirrhosis and known varices who are suffering from upper GI bleeding, how often does that bleeding result from varices?

Only ≈50% of the time

What are the signs/symptoms?

Hematemesis, melena, hematochezia

What is the mortality rate from an acute esophageal variceal bleed?

≈50%

What is the initial treatment of variceal bleeding?

As with all upper GI bleeding: large bore IVs × 2, IV fluid, Foley catheter, type and cross blood, send labs, correct coagulopathy (vitamin K, fresh frozen plasma), +/− intubation to protect from aspiration

What is the diagnostic test of choice?

EGD (upper GI endoscopy)
Remember, **bleeding** is the result of varices only half the time; must rule out ulcers, gastritis, etc.

If esophageal varices cause bleeding, what are the EGD treatment options?

1. **Emergent endoscopic sclerotherapy:** a sclerosing substance is injected into the esophageal varices under direct endoscopic vision
2. **Endoscopic band ligation:** elastic band ligation of varices

What are the pharmacologic options?

Somatostatin (Octreotide) or **IV vasopressin** (and nitroglycerin, to avoid MI) to achieve vasoconstriction of the mesenteric vessels; if bleeding continues, consider balloon (**Sengstaken-Blakemore tube**) tamponade of the varices, β-blocker

What is a Sengstaken-Blakemore tube?

Tube with a gastric and esophageal balloon for tamponading an esophageal bleed (see page 268)

What is the next therapy after the bleeding is controlled?

Repeat endoscopic sclerotherapy/banding

What are the options if sclerotherapy and conservative methods fail to stop the variceal bleeding or bleeding recurs?

Repeat sclerotherapy/banding and treat conservatively
TIPS
Surgical shunt (selective or partial)
Liver transplantation

What is a "selective" shunt?

Shunt that selectively decompresses the varices without decompressing the portal vein

What does the acronym TIPS stand for?

Transjugular **I**ntrahepatic **P**ortosystemic **S**hunt

What is a TIPS procedure?

Angiographic radiologist places a small tube stent intrahepatically between the hepatic vein and a branch of the portal vein via a percutaneous jugular vein route

What is a "partial shunt"?

Shunt that directly decompresses the portal vein, but only partially

What is a Warren shunt?

Distal splenorenal shunt with ligation of the coronary vein—elective shunt procedure associated with low incidence of encephalopathy in patients postoperatively because only the splenic flow is diverted to decompress the varices

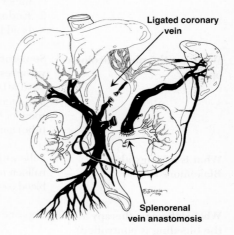

Ligated coronary vein

Splenorenal vein anastomosis

What is a contraindication to the Warren "selective" shunt?	Ascites
Define the following shunts:	
End-to-side portocaval shunt	"Total shunt"—portal vein (end) to IVC (side)
Side-to-side portocaval shunt	Side of portal vein anastomosed to side of IVC—partially preserves portal flow ("partial shunt")
Synthetic portocaval H-graft	"Partial shunt"—synthetic tube graft from the portal vein to the IVC (good option for patients with alcoholism; associated with lower incidence of encephalopathy and easier transplantation later)
Synthetic mesocaval H-graft	Synthetic graft from the SMV to the IVC
What is the most common perioperative cause of death following shunt procedure?	Hepatic failure, secondary to decreased blood flow (accounts for two thirds of deaths)
What is the major postoperative morbidity after a shunt procedure?	Increased incidence of hepatic encephalopathy because of decreased portal blood flow to the liver and decreased clearance of toxins/metabolites from the blood
What medication is infused to counteract the coronary artery vasoconstriction of IV vasopressin?	Nitroglycerin IV drip
What lab value roughly correlates with degree of encephalopathy?	Serum ammonia level (***Note:*** Thought to correlate with but not cause encephalopathy)
What medications are used to treat hepatic encephalopathy?	Lactulose PO, with or without neomycin PO

Chapter 54   Biliary Tract

ANATOMY

Name structures 1 through 8 (below) of the biliary tract:

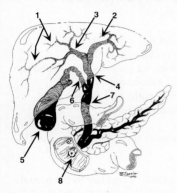

1. Intrahepatic ducts
2. Left hepatic duct
3. Right hepatic duct
4. Common hepatic duct
5. Gallbladder
6. Cystic duct
7. Common bile duct
8. Ampulla of Vater

Which is the proximal and which is the distal bile duct?

Proximal is close to the liver (bile and the liver is analogous to blood and the heart; they both flow distally)

What is the name of the node in Calot's triangle?

Calot's node

What are the small ducts that drain bile directly into the gallbladder from the liver?

Ducts of Luschka

Which artery is susceptible to injury during cholecystectomy?

Right hepatic artery, because of its proximity to the cystic artery and Calot's triangle

What is the name of the valves of the gallbladder?

Spiral valves of Heister

Where is the infundibulum of the gallbladder?

Near the cystic duct

Where is the fundus of the gallbladder?

At the end of the gallbladder

What is "Hartmann's pouch"?   Gallbladder infundibulum

What are the boundaries of   The **3 C's:**
the triangle of Calot?
1. **C**ystic duct
2. **C**ommon hepatic duct
3. **C**ystic artery

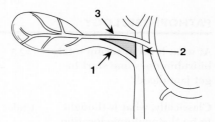

"Dr. Blackbourne, are you   Yes, look up *Gastroenterology*, 2002;
absolutely sure that the Trian-   123(5):1440
gle of Calot includes the cystic
artery and not the liver edge?"

PHYSIOLOGY

What is the source of   Bile duct epithelium; expect alkaline
alkaline phosphatase?   phosphatase to be elevated in bile duct
                             obstruction

What is in bile?   Cholesterol, lecithin (phospholipid), bile
                        acids, and bilirubin

What does bile do?   Emulsifies fats

What is the enterohepatic   Circulation of bile acids from liver to gut
circulation?   and back to the liver

Where are most of the bile   In the terminal ileum
acids absorbed?

What stimulates gallbladder   Cholecystokinin and vagal input
emptying?

What is the source of   Duodenal mucosal cells
cholecystokinin?

What stimulates the release   Fat, protein, amino acids, and HCl
of cholecystokinin?

What inhibits its release?	Trypsin and chymotrypsin
What are its actions?	Gallbladder emptying Opening of ampulla of Vater Slowing of gastric emptying Pancreas acinar cell growth and release of exocrine products

PATHOPHYSIOLOGY

At what level of serum total bilirubin does one start to get jaundiced?	>2.5
Classically, what is thought to be the anatomic location where one first finds evidence of jaundice?	Under the tongue
With good renal function, how high can the serum total bilirubin go?	Very rarely, >20
What are the signs and symptoms of obstructive jaundice?	Jaundice Dark urine Clay-colored stools (acholic stools) Pruritus (itching) Loss of appetite Nausea
What causes the itching in obstructive jaundice?	Bile salts in the dermis (not bilirubin!)
Define the following terms: **Cholelithiasis**	Gallstones in gallbladder

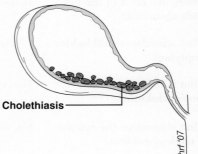

Cholethiasis

hrf '07

Choledocholithiasis   Gallstone in common bile duct

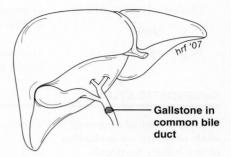

**Gallstone in
common bile
duct**

Cholecystitis   Inflammation of gallbladder

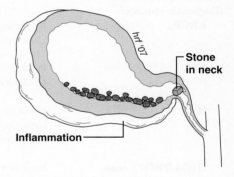

**Stone
in neck**

Inflammation

Cholangitis   Infection of biliary tract

Cholangiocarcinoma   Adenocarcinoma of bile ducts

Klatskin's tumor   Cholangiocarcinoma of bile duct at the
junction of the right and left hepatic
ducts

Biliary colic   Pain from gallstones, usually from a stone
at cystic duct: The pain is located in the
RUQ, epigastrium, or right subscapular
region of the back; it usually lasts minutes
to hours but eventually goes away; it
is often postprandial, especially after
fatty foods

Biloma	Intraperitoneal bile fluid collection
Choledochojejunostomy	Anastomosis between common bile duct and jejunum
Hepaticojejunostomy	Anastomosis of hepatic ducts or common hepatic duct to jejunum

DIAGNOSTIC STUDIES

What is the initial diagnostic study of choice for evaluation of the biliary tract/gall-bladder/cholelithiasis?	Ultrasound!
Define the following diagnostic studies:	
ERCP	**E**ndoscopic **R**etrograde **C**holangio**P**ancreatography
PTC	**P**ercutaneous **T**ranshepatic **C**holangiogram
IOC	**I**ntra**O**perative **C**holangiogram (done laparoscopically or open to rule out choledocholithiasis)
HIDA/PRIDA scan	Radioisotope study; isotope concentrated in liver and secreted into bile; will demonstrate cholecystitis, bile leak, or CBD obstruction
How does the HIDA scan reveal cholecystitis?	Non-opacification of the gallbladder from obstruction of the cystic duct
How often will plain x-ray films see gallstones?	10% to 15%

BILIARY SURGERY

What is a cholecystectomy?	Removal of the gallbladder laparoscopically or through a standard Kocher incision

What is a "lap chole"? LAParoscopic CHOLEcystectomy

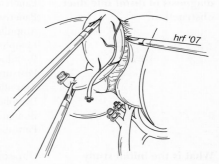

What is the Kocher incision? Right subcostal incision

What is a sphincterotomy? Cut through sphincter of Oddi to allow passage of gallstones from the common bile duct; most often done at ERCP; also known as papillotomy

How should postoperative biloma be treated after a lap chole?
1. Percutaneous drain bile collection
2. ERCP with placement of biliary stent past leak (usually cystic duct remnant leak)

What is the treatment of major CBD injury after a lap chole? Choledochojejunostomy

OBSTRUCTIVE JAUNDICE

What is it? Jaundice (hyperbilirubinemia >2.5) from obstruction of bile flow to the duodenum

What is the differential diagnosis of *proximal* bile duct obstruction?
Cholangiocarcinoma
Lymphadenopathy
Metastatic tumor
Gallbladder carcinoma
Sclerosing cholangitis
Gallstones
Tumor embolus
Parasites
Postsurgical stricture
Hepatoma
Benign bile duct tumor

What is the differential diagnosis of *distal* bile duct obstruction?	Choledocholithiasis **(gallstones)** Pancreatic carcinoma Pancreatitis Ampullary carcinoma Lymphadenopathy Pseudocyst Postsurgical stricture Ampulla of Vater dysfunction/stricture Lymphoma Benign bile duct tumor Parasites
What is the initial study of choice for obstructive jaundice?	Ultrasound
What lab results are associated with obstructive jaundice?	Elevated alkaline phosphatase, elevated bilirubin with or without elevated LFTs

CHOLELITHIASIS

What is it?	Formation of gallstones
What is the incidence?	≈10% of U.S. population will develop gallstones
What are the "Big 4" risk factors?	The **"four Fs":** **F**emale **F**at **F**orty **F**ertile (multiparity)
What are other less common risk factors for gallstones?	Oral contraceptives Bile stasis Chronic hemolysis (pigment stones) Cirrhosis Infection Native American heritage Rapid weight loss/gastric bypass Obesity Inflammatory bowel disease (IBD) Terminal ileal resection Total parenteral nutrition (TPN) Vagotomy Advanced age Hyperlipidemia Somatostatin therapy

What are the types of stones?	Cholesterol stones (75%) Pigment stones (25%)
What are the types of pigmented stones?	Black stones (contain calcium bilirubinate) Brown stones (associated with biliary tract infection)
What are the causes of black-pigmented stones?	Cirrhosis, hemolysis
What is the pathogenesis of cholesterol stones?	Secretion of bile **supersaturated** with cholesterol (relatively decreased amounts of lecithin and bile salts); then, cholesterol precipitates out and forms solid crystals, then gallstones
Is hypercholesterolemia a risk factor for gallstone formation?	No (but hyperlipidemia is)
What are the signs and symptoms?	Symptoms of: biliary colic, cholangitis, choledocholithiasis, gallstone, pancreatitis
Is biliary colic pain really "colic"?	No, symptoms usually last for hours; therefore, colic is a misnomer!
What percentage of patients with gallstones are *asymptomatic*?	80% of patients with cholelithiasis are asymptomatic!
What is thought to cause biliary colic?	Gallbladder contraction against a stone temporarily at the gallbladder/cystic duct junction; a stone in the cystic duct; or a stone passing through the cystic duct
What is Boas' sign?	Referred right subscapular pain of biliary colic
What are the five major complications of gallstones?	1. Acute cholecystitis 2. Choledocholithiasis 3. Gallstone pancreatitis 4. Gallstone ileus 5. Cholangitis

How is cholelithiasis diagnosed?

History
Physical examination
Ultrasound

How often does ultrasound detect cholelithiasis?

>98% of the time!

How often does ultrasound detect choledocholithiasis?

About 33% of the time . . . not a very good study for choledocholithiasis!

How are symptomatic or complicated cases of cholelithiasis treated?

By cholecystectomy

What are the possible complications of a lap chole?

Common bile duct injury; right hepatic duct/artery injury; cystic duct leak; biloma (collection of bile)

What are the indications for cholecystectomy in the asymptomatic patient?

Sickle-cell disease
Calcified gallbladder (porcelain gallbladder)
Patient is a child

Define IOC.

Intra**O**perative **C**holangiogram (dye in bile duct by way of the cystic duct with fluoro/x-ray)

What are the indications for an IOC (6)?

1. Jaundice
2. Hyperbilirubinemia
3. Gallstone pancreatitis (resolved)
4. Elevated alkaline phosphatase
5. Choledocholithiasis on ultrasound
6. To define anatomy

What is choledocholithiasis?

Gallstones in the common bile duct

What is the management of choledocholithiasis?

1. ERCP with papillotomy and basket/balloon retrieval of stones (pre- or postoperatively)
2. Laparoscopic transcystic duct or trans common bile duct retrieval
3. Open common bile duct exploration

What medication may dissolve a cholesterol gallstone?

Chenodeoxycholic acid, ursodeoxycholic acid (Actigall®); but if medication is stopped, gallstones often recur

What is the major feared complication of ERCP?	Pancreatitis

ACUTE CHOLECYSTITIS

What is the pathogenesis of acute cholecystitis?	Obstruction of cystic duct leads to inflammation of the gallbladder; ≈95% of cases result from calculi, and ≈5% from acalculous obstruction
What are the risk factors?	Gallstones
What are the signs and symptoms?	**Unrelenting** RUQ pain or tenderness **Fever** Nausea/vomiting Painful palpable gallbladder in 33% Positive Murphy's sign Right subscapular pain (referred) Epigastric discomfort (referred)
What is Murphy's sign?	Acute pain and **inspiratory arrest** elicited by palpation of the RUQ during inspiration
What are the complications of acute cholecystitis?	Abscess Perforation Choledocholithiasis Cholecystenteric fistula formation Gallstone ileus
What lab results are associated with acute cholecystitis?	Increased WBC; may have: Slight elevation in alkaline phosphatase, LFTs Slight elevation in amylase, T. Bili
What is the diagnostic test of choice for acute cholecystitis?	Ultrasound
What are the signs of acute cholecystitis on ultrasound?	Thickened gallbladder wall (>3 mm) Pericholecystic fluid Distended gallbladder Gallstones present/cystic duct stone Sonographic Murphy's sign (pain on inspiration after placement of ultrasound probe over gallbladder)

What is the difference between acute cholecystitis and biliary colic?

Biliary colic has temporary pain; acute cholecystitis has pain that does not resolve, usually with elevated WBCs, fever, and signs of acute inflammation on U/S

What is the treatment of acute cholecystitis?

IVFs, antibiotics, and cholecystectomy early

What are the steps in lap chole (6)?

1. Dissection of peritoneum overlying the cystic duct and artery
2. Clipping of cystic artery and transect
3. Division of cystic duct between clips
4. Dissection of gallbladder from the liver bed
5. Cauterization; irrigation; suction, to obtain hemostasis of the liver bed
6. Removal of the gallbladder through the umbilical trocar site

How is an IOC performed?

1. Place a clip on the cystic duct–gallbladder junction
2. Cut a small hole in the distal cystic duct to cannulate
3. Inject half-strength contrast and take an x-ray or fluoro

What percentage of patients has an accessory cystic artery?

10%

Why should the gallbladder specimen be opened in the operating room?

Looking for gallbladder cancer, anatomy

ACUTE ACALCULOUS CHOLECYSTITIS

What is it?

Acute cholecystitis without evidence of stones

What is the pathogenesis?

It is believed to result from sludge and gallbladder disuse and **biliary stasis,** perhaps secondary to absence of cholecystokinin stimulation (decreased contraction of gallbladder)

What are the risk factors?	Prolonged fasting TPN Trauma Multiple transfusions Dehydration Often occurs in prolonged postoperative or ICU setting
What are the diagnostic tests of choice?	1. **Ultrasound;** sludge and inflammation usually present with acute acalculous cholecystitis 2. HIDA scan
What are the findings on HIDA scan?	Nonfilling of the gallbladder
What is the management of acute acalculous cholecystitis?	Cholecystectomy, or cholecystostomy tube if the patient is unstable (placed percutaneously by radiology or open surgery)

CHOLANGITIS

What is it?	Bacterial infection of the biliary tract from obstruction (either partial or complete); potentially life-threatening
What are the common causes?	**Choledocholithiasis** Stricture (usually postoperative) Neoplasm (usually ampullary carcinoma) Extrinsic compression (pancreatic pseudocyst/pancreatitis) Instrumentation of the bile ducts (e.g., PTC/ERCP) Biliary stent
What is the most common cause of cholangitis?	Gallstones in common bile duct (choledocholithiasis)
What are the signs and symptoms?	**Charcot's triad:** fever/chills, RUQ pain, and jaundice **Reynold's pentad:** Charcot's triad plus altered mental status and shock
What lab results are associated with cholangitis?	Increased WBCs, bilirubin, and alkaline phosphatase, positive blood cultures

Which organisms are most commonly isolated with cholangitis?

Gram-negative organisms (*E. coli, Klebsiella, Pseudomonas, Enterobacter, Proteus, Serratia*) are the most common

Enterococci are the most common gram-positive bacteria

Anaerobes are less common (*B. fragilis* most frequent)

Fungi are even less common (*Candida*)

What are the diagnostic tests of choice?

Ultrasound and contrast study (e.g., ERCP or IOC) after patient has "cooled off" with IV antibiotics

What is suppurative cholangitis?

Severe infection with sepsis—"pus under pressure"

What is the management of cholangitis?

Nonsuppurative: IVF and antibiotics, with definitive treatment later (e.g., lap chole +/− ERCP)

Suppurative: IVF, antibiotics, and decompression; decompression can be obtained by ERCP with papillotomy, PTC with catheter drainage, or laparotomy with T-tube placement

SCLEROSING CHOLANGITIS

What is it?

Multiple inflammatory fibrous thickenings of bile duct walls resulting in biliary strictures

What is its natural history?

Progressive obstruction possibly leading to cirrhosis and liver failure; 10% of patients will develop cholangiocarcinoma

What is the etiology?

Unknown, but probably autoimmune

What is the major risk factor?

Inflammatory bowel disease

What type of IBD is the most common risk factor?

Ulcerative colitis (≈66%)

What are the signs and symptoms of sclerosing cholangitis?	Same as those for obstructive jaundice:
	  Jaundice
	  Itching (pruritus)
	  Dark urine
	  Clay-colored stools
	  Loss of energy
	  Weight loss
	  (Many patients are asymptomatic)

What are the complications?	Cirrhosis Cholangiocarcinoma (10%) Cholangitis Obstructive jaundice
How is it diagnosed?	Elevated alkaline phosphatase, and PTC or ERCP revealing "beads on a string" appearance on contrast study
What are the management options?	Hepatoenteric anastomosis (if primarily extrahepatic ducts are involved) and resection of extrahepatic bile ducts because of the risk of cholangiocarcinoma Transplant (if primarily intrahepatic disease or cirrhosis) Endoscopic balloon dilations
What percentage of patients with IBD develops sclerosing cholangitis?	<5%

GALLSTONE ILEUS

What is it?	Small bowel obstruction from a large gallstone (>2.5 cm) that has eroded through the gallbladder and into the duodenum/small bowel
What is the classic site of obstruction?	Ileocecal valve (but may cause obstruction in the duodenum, sigmoid colon)

What are the classic findings of gallstone ileus?

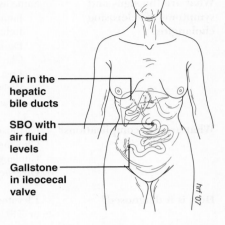

Air in the hepatic bile ducts

SBO with air fluid levels

Gallstone in ileocecal valve

What is the population at risk?

Gallstone ileus is most commonly seen in **women older than 70 years**

What are the signs/ symptoms?

Symptoms of SBO: distention, vomiting, hypovolemia, RUQ pain

Gallstone ileus causes what percentage of cases of SBO?

<1%

What are the diagnostic tests of choice?

Abdominal x-ray: occasionally reveals radiopaque gallstone in the bowel; **40% of patients show air in the biliary tract,** small bowel distention, and air fluid levels secondary to ileus

UGI: used if diagnosis is in question; will show cholecystenteric fistula and the obstruction

Abdominal CT: reveals air in biliary tract, SBO +/− gallstone in intestine

What is the management?

Surgery: enterotomy with removal of the stone ± interval cholecystectomy (interval-delayed)

CARCINOMA OF THE GALLBLADDER

What is it?

Malignant neoplasm arising in the gallbladder, vast majority are **adenocarcinoma (90%)**

What are the risk factors?	**Gallstones, porcelain gallbladder,** cholecystenteric fistula
What is the female:male ratio?	4:1
What is the most common site of gallbladder cancer in the gallbladder?	60% in fundus
What is a porcelain gallbladder?	Calcified gallbladder
What percentage of patients with a porcelain gallbladder will have gallbladder cancer?	≈50% (20%–60%)
What is the incidence?	**≈1% of all gallbladder specimens**
What are the symptoms?	Biliary colic, weight loss, anorexia; many patients are asymptomatic until late; may present as acute cholecystitis
What are the signs?	Jaundice (from invasion of the common duct or compression by involved pericholedochal lymph nodes), RUQ mass, palpable gallbladder (advanced disease)
What are the diagnostic tests of choice?	Ultrasound, abdominal CT, ERCP
What is the route of spread?	Contiguous spread to the liver is most common
What is the management under the following conditions?	
Confined to mucosa	Cholecystectomy
Confined to muscularis/serosa	Radical cholecystectomy: cholecystectomy and wedge resection of overlying liver, and lymph node dissection ± chemotherapy/XRT
What is the main complication of a lap chole for gallbladder cancer?	Trocar site tumor implants (***Note:*** if known preoperatively, perform open cholecystectomy)

What is the prognosis for gallbladder cancer?

Dismal overall: <5% 5-year survival as most are unresectable at diagnosis

T1 with cholecystectomy: 95% 5-year survival

CHOLANGIOCARCINOMA

What is it?

Malignancy of the extrahepatic or intrahepatic ducts—**primary bile duct cancer**

What is the histology?

Almost all are adenocarcinomas

Average age at diagnosis?

≈65 years, equally affects male/female

What are the signs and symptoms?

Those of biliary obstruction: jaundice, **pruritus, dark urine, clay-colored stools, cholangitis**

What is the most common location?

Proximal bile duct

What are the risk factors?

Choledochal cysts
Ulcerative colitis
Thorotrast contrast dye (used in 1950s)
Sclerosing cholangitis
Liver flukes (clonorchiasis)
Toxin exposures (e.g., Agent Orange)

What is a Klatskin tumor?

Tumor that involves the junction of the right and left hepatic ducts

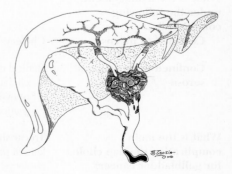

What are the diagnostic tests of choice?	Ultrasound, CT scan, ERCP/PTC with biopsy/brushings for cytology, MRCP
What is an MRCP?	MRI with visualization of pancreatic and bile ducts
What is the management of proximal bile duct cholangiocarcinoma?	Resection with Roux-en-Y hepaticoje-junostomy (anastomose bile ducts to jejunum) ± unilateral hepatic lobectomy
What is the management of distal common bile duct cholangiocarcinoma?	Whipple procedure

MISCELLANEOUS CONDITIONS

What is a porcelain gallbladder?	**Calcified gallbladder** seen on abdominal x-ray; results from chronic cholelithiasis/cholecystitis with calcified scar tissue in gallbladder wall; **cholecystectomy** required because of the strong association of **gallbladder carcinoma** with this condition
What is hydrops of the gallbladder?	Complete obstruction of the cystic duct by a gallstone, with filling of the gallbladder with fluid (not bile) from the gallbladder mucosa
What is Gilbert's syndrome?	Inborn error in liver bilirubin uptake and glucuronyl transferase resulting in hyperbilirubinemia (Think: **G**ilbert's = **G**lucuronyl)
What is Courvoisier's gallbladder?	Palpable, **nontender** gallbladder (unlike gallstone disease) associated with cancer of the head of the pancreas; able to distend because it has not been "scarred down" by gallstones
What is Mirizzi's syndrome?	Common hepatic duct obstruction as a result of **extrinsic** compression from a gallstone impacted in the cystic duct

Chapter 55   Pancreas

Identify the regions of the pancreas:

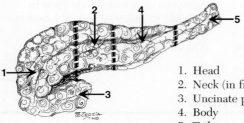

1. Head
2. Neck (in front of the SMV)
3. Uncinate process
4. Body
5. Tail

What structure is the tail of the pancreas said to "tickle"?	Spleen
Name the two pancreatic ducts.	1. Wirsung duct 2. Santorini duct
Which duct is the main duct?	Duct of Wirsung is the major duct (Think: **S**antorini = **S**mall duct)

How is blood supplied to the head of the pancreas?	1. Celiac trunk → gastroduodenal →
	   Anterior superior pancreaticoduodenal
	      artery
	   Posterior superior pancreaticoduodenal
	      artery
	2. Superior mesenteric artery →
	   Anterior inferior pancreaticoduodenal
	      artery
	   Posterior inferior pancreaticoduodenal
	      artery
	3. Splenic artery →
	   Dorsal pancreatic artery

Why must the duodenum be removed if the head of the pancreas is removed?	They share the same blood supply (gastroduodenal artery)

What is the endocrine function of the pancreas?	Islets of Langerhans: α-cells: glucagon β-cells: insulin

What is the exocrine function of the pancreas? Digestive enzymes: amylase, lipase, trypsin, chymotrypsin, carboxypeptidase

What maneuver is used to mobilize the duodenum and pancreas and evaluate the entire pancreas? Kocher maneuver: Incise the lateral attachments of the duodenum and then lift the pancreas to examine the posterior surface

PANCREATITIS

ACUTE PANCREATITIS

What is it? Inflammation of the pancreas

What are the most common etiologies in the United States?
1. Alcohol abuse (50%)
2. Gallstones (30%)
3. Idiopathic (10%)

What is the acronym to remember all of the causes of pancreatitis? "I GET SMASHED":
Idiopathic

Gallstones
Ethanol
Trauma

Scorpion bite
Mumps (viruses)
Autoimmune
Steroids
Hyperlipidemia
ERCP
Drugs

What are the symptoms? Epigastric pain (frequently radiates to back); nausea and vomiting

What are the signs of pancreatitis? Epigastric tenderness
Diffuse abdominal tenderness
Decreased bowel sounds (adynamic ileus)
Fever
Dehydration/shock

What is the differential diagnosis?	Gastritis/PUD Perforated viscus Acute cholecystitis SBO Mesenteric ischemia/infarction Ruptured AAA Biliary colic Inferior MI/pneumonia
What lab tests should be ordered?	CBC LFT Amylase/lipase Type and cross ABG Calcium Chemistry Coags Serum lipids
What are the associated diagnostic findings?	Lab—High amylase, high lipase, high WBC AXR—Sentinel loop, colon cutoff, possibly gallstones (only 10% visible on x-ray) U/S—Phlegmon, cholelithiasis CT—Phlegmon, pancreatic necrosis
What is the most common sign of pancreatitis on AXR?	Sentinel loop(s)
What is the treatment?	NPO IVF NGT if vomiting +/– TPN vs. postpyloric tube feeds H_2 blocker/PPI Analgesia (Demerol®, not morphine—less sphincter of Oddi spasm) Correction of coags/electrolytes +/– Alcohol withdrawal prophylaxis "Tincture of time"

What are the possible complications?

Pseudocyst
Abscess/infection
Pancreatic necrosis
Splenic/mesenteric/portal vessel rupture or thrombosis
Pancreatic ascites/pancreatic pleural effusion
Diabetes
ARDS/sepsis/MOF
Coagulopathy/DIC
Encephalopathy
Severe hypocalcemia

What is the prognosis?

Based on Ranson's criteria

Are postpyloric tube feeds safe in acute pancreatitis?

YES

What are Ranson's criteria for the following stages:
    At presentation?

1. Age >55
2. WBC >16,000
3. Glc >200
4. AST >250
5. LDH >350

    During the initial 48 hours?

1. Base deficit >4
2. BUN increase >5 mg/dL
3. Fluid sequestration >6 L
4. Serum Ca^{2+} <8
5. Hct decrease >10%
6. PO_2 (ABG) <60 mm Hg
   (Amylase value is NOT one of Ranson's criteria!)

What is the mortality per positive criteria:
    0 to 2?

<5%

    3 to 4?

≈15%

    5 to 6?

≈40%

    7 to 8?

≈100%

How can the admission Ranson criteria be remembered?	**"GA LAW** (Georgia law)": **G**lucose >200 **A**ge >55 **L**DH >350 **A**ST >250 **W**BC >16,000 ("Don't mess with the pancreas and don't mess with the Georgia law")
How can Ranson's criteria at less than 48 hours be remembered?	**"C HOBBS** (Calvin and Hobbes)": **C**alcium <8 mg/dL **H**ct drop of >10% **O**$_2$ <60 (Pao$_2$) **B**ase deficit >4 **B**un >5 increase **S**equestration >6 L
How can the AST versus LDH values in Ranson's criteria be remembered?	Alphabetically and numerically: A before L and 250 before 350 Therefore, AST >250 and LDH >350
What is the etiology of hypocalcemia with pancreatitis?	Fat saponification: fat necrosis binds to calcium
What complication is associated with splenic vein thrombosis?	Gastric varices (treatment with splenectomy)
Can TPN with lipids be given to a patient with pancreatitis?	Yes, if the patient does not suffer from hyperlipidemia (triglycerides <300)
What is the least common cause of acute pancreatitis (and possibly the most commonly asked cause on rounds!)	Scorpion bite (found on the island of Trinidad)

CHRONIC PANCREATITIS

What is it?

Chronic inflammation of the pancreas region causing destruction of the parenchyma, fibrosis, and calcification, resulting in loss of endocrine and exocrine tissue

What are the subtypes?

1. Chronic calcific pancreatitis
2. Chronic obstructive pancreatitis (5%)

What are the causes?

Alcohol abuse (most common; 70% of cases)
Idiopathic (15%)
Hypercalcemia (hyperparathyroidism)
Hyperlipidemia
Familial (found in families without any other risk factors)
Trauma
Iatrogenic
Gallstones

What are the symptoms?

Epigastric and/or back pain, weight loss, steatorrhea

What are the associated signs?

Type 1 diabetes mellitus (up to one third)
Steatorrhea (up to one fourth), weight loss

What are the signs of pancreatic exocrine insufficiency?

Steatorrhea (fat malabsorption from lipase insufficiency—stools float in water)
Malnutrition

What are the signs of pancreatic endocrine insufficiency?

Diabetes (glucose intolerance)

What are the common pain patterns?

Unrelenting pain
Recurrent pain

What is the differential diagnosis?

PUD, biliary tract disease, AAA, pancreatic cancer, angina

What percentage of patients with chronic pancreatitis have or will develop pancreatic cancer?

≈2%

What are the appropriate lab tests?

Amylase/lipase
72-hour fecal fat analysis
Glc tolerance test (IDDM)

Why may amylase/lipase be normal in a patient with chronic pancreatitis?

Because of extensive pancreatic tissue loss ("burned-out pancreas")

What radiographic tests should be performed?

CT—Has greatest sensitivity for gland enlargement/atrophy, calcifications, masses, pseudocysts
KUB—Calcification in the pancreas
ERCP—Ductal irregularities with dilation and stenosis (Chain of Lakes), pseudocysts

What is the medical treatment?

Discontinuation of alcohol use—can reduce attacks, though parenchymal damage continues secondary to ductal obstruction and fibrosis
Insulin for type 1 diabetes mellitus
Pancreatic enzyme replacement
Narcotics for pain

What is the surgical treatment?

Puestow—longitudinal pancreaticojejunostomy (pancreatic duct **must be dilated**)
Duval—distal pancreaticojejunostomy
Near-total pancreatectomy

What is the Frey procedure?

Longitudinal pancreaticojejunostomy with core resection of the pancreatic head

What is the indication for surgical treatment of chronic pancreatitis?

Severe, prolonged/refractory pain

What are the possible complications of chronic pancreatitis?

Insulin dependent diabetes mellitus
Steatorrhea
Malnutrition
Biliary obstruction
Splenic vein thrombosis
Gastric varices
Pancreatic pseudocyst/abscess
Narcotic addiction
Pancreatic ascites/pleural effusion
Splenic artery aneurysm

GALLSTONE PANCREATITIS

What is it?	Acute pancreatitis from a gallstone in or passing through the ampulla of Vater (the exact mechanism is unknown)
How is the diagnosis made?	Acute pancreatitis and cholelithiasis and/or choledocholithiasis and no other cause of pancreatitis (e.g., no history of alcohol abuse)
What radiologic tests should be performed?	U/S to look for gallstones CT to look at the pancreas, if symptoms are severe
What is the treatment?	Conservative measures and early interval cholecystectomy (laparoscopic cholecystectomy or open cholecystectomy) and intraoperative cholangiogram (IOC) 3 to 5 days (after pancreatic inflammation resolves)
Why should early interval cholecystectomy be performed on patients with gallstone pancreatitis?	Pancreatitis will recur in ≈33% of patients within 8 weeks (so always perform early interval cholecystectomy and IOC in 3 to 5 days when pancreatitis resolves)
What is the role of ERCP?	1. Cholangitis 2. Refractory choledocholithiasis

HEMORRHAGIC PANCREATITIS

What is it?	Bleeding into the parenchyma and retroperitoneal structures with extensive pancreatic necrosis
What are the signs?	Abdominal pain, shock/ARDS, Cullen's sign, Grey Turner's sign, Fox's sign
Define the following terms: **Cullen's sign**	**Bluish discoloration of the periumbilical area** from retroperitoneal hemorrhage tracking around to the anterior abdominal wall through fascial planes

Grey Turner's sign	**Ecchymosis or discoloration of the flank** in patients with retroperitoneal hemorrhage from dissecting blood from the retroperitoneum (Think: Grey **TURN**er = **TURN** side to side = flank [side] hematoma)
Fox's sign	**Ecchymosis of the inguinal ligament** from blood tracking from the retroperitoneum and collecting at the inguinal ligament
What are the significant lab values?	Increased amylase/lipase Decreased Hct Decreased calcium levels
What radiologic test should be performed?	CT scan with IV contrast

PANCREATIC ABSCESS

What is it?	Infected peripancreatic purulent fluid collection
What are the signs/ symptoms?	Fever, unresolving pancreatitis, epigastric mass
What radiographic tests should be performed?	Abdominal CT with needle aspiration → send for Gram stain/culture
What are the associated lab findings?	Positive Gram stain and culture of bacteria
Which organisms are found in pancreatic abscesses?	Gram negative (most common): *Escherichia coli, Pseudomonas, Klebsiella* Gram positive: *Staphylococcus aureus, Candida*
What is the treatment?	Antibiotics and percutaneous drain placement or operative débridement and placement of drains

PANCREATIC NECROSIS

What is it?
Dead pancreatic tissue, usually following acute pancreatitis

How is the diagnosis made?
Abdominal CT with IV contrast; dead pancreatic tissue does not take up IV contrast and is not enhanced on CT scan (i.e., doesn't "light up")

What is the treatment:
    Sterile?
Medical management

    Suspicious of infection?
CT-guided FNA

    Toxic, hypotensive?
Operative débridement

PANCREATIC PSEUDOCYST

What is it?
Encapsulated collection of pancreatic fluid

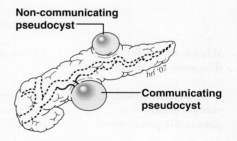

What makes it a "pseudo" cyst?
Wall is formed by inflammatory fibrosis, NOT epithelial cell lining

What is the incidence?
≈1 in 10 after alcoholic pancreatitis

What are the associated risk factors?
Acute pancreatitis < chronic pancreatitis from alcohol

What is the most common cause of pancreatic pseudocyst in the United States?
Chronic alcoholic pancreatitis

What are the symptoms?

Epigastric pain/mass
Emesis
Mild fever
Weight loss
Note: Should be suspected when a
patient with acute pancreatitis fails to
resolve pain

What are the signs?

Palpable epigastric mass, tender
epigastrium, ileus

What lab tests should be performed?

Amylase/lipase
Bilirubin
CBC

What are the diagnostic findings?

Lab—High amylase, leukocytosis, high
bilirubin (if there is obstruction)
U/S—Fluid-filled mass
CT—Fluid-filled mass, good for showing
multiple cysts
ERCP—Radiopaque contrast material
fills cyst if there is a communicating
pseudocyst (i.e., pancreatic duct
communicates with pseudocyst)

What is the differential diagnosis of a pseudocyst?

Cystadenocarcinoma, cystadenoma

What are the possible complications of a pancreatic pseudocyst?

Infection, bleeding into the cyst, fistula,
pancreatic ascites, gastric outlet
obstruction, SBO, biliary obstruction

What is the treatment?

Drainage of the cyst or observation

What is the waiting period before a pseudocyst should be drained?

It takes 6 weeks for pseudocyst walls to
"mature" or become firm enough to hold
sutures and most will resolve in this
period of time if they are going to

What percentage of pseudocysts resolve spontaneously?

≈50%

What is the treatment for pseudocyst with bleeding into cyst?

Angiogram amd embolization

What is the treatment for pseudocyst with infection?

Percutaneous external drainage/ IV antibiotics

What size pseudocyst should be drained?

Most experts say:
  Pseudocysts larger than 5 cm have a
    small chance of resolving and have
    a higher chance of complications
  Calcified cyst wall
  Thick cyst wall

What are three treatment options for pancreatic pseudocyst?

1. Percutaneous aspiration/drain
2. Operative drainage
3. Transpapillary stent via ERCP
   (pseudocyst must communicate with
   pancreatic duct)

What are the surgical options for the following conditions:

Pseudocyst adherent to the stomach?

Cystogastrostomy (drain into the stomach)

Pseudocyst adherent to the duodenum?

Cystoduodenostomy (drain into the duodenum)

Pseudocyst not adherent to the stomach or duodenum?

Roux-en-Y cystojejunostomy (drain into the Roux limb of the jejunum)

Pseudocyst in the tail of the pancreas?

Resection of the pancreatic tail with the pseudocyst

What is an endoscopic option for drainage of a pseudocyst?

Endoscopic cystogastrostomy

What must be done during a surgical drainage procedure for a pancreatic pseudocyst?

Biopsy of the cyst wall to rule out a cystic carcinoma (e.g., cystadenocarcinoma)

What is the most common cause of death due to pancreatic pseudocyst?

Massive hemorrhage into the pseudocyst

PANCREATIC CARCINOMA

What is it?	Adenocarcinoma of the pancreas arising from duct cells
What are the associated risk factors?	**Smoking 3× risk,** diabetes mellitus, heavy alcohol use, chronic pancreatitis, diet high in fried meats, previous gastrectomy
What is the male to female ratio?	3:2
What is the African American to white ratio?	2:1
What is the average age?	>60 years
What are the different types?	>80% are duct cell adenocarcinomas; other types include cystadenocarcinoma and acinar cell carcinoma
What percentage arise in the pancreatic head?	**66%** arise in the pancreatic **head; 33%** arise in the **body and tail**
Why are most pancreatic cancers in the tail nonresectable?	These tumors grow without symptoms until it is too late and they have already spread—head of the pancreas tumors draw attention earlier because of biliary obstruction
What are the signs/ symptoms of tumors based on location:	
Head of the pancreas?	**Painless jaundice** from obstruction of common bile duct; weight loss; abdominal pain; back pain; weakness; **pruritus** from bile salts in skin; anorexia; **Courvoisier's sign;** acholic stools; dark urine; diabetes
Body or tail?	Weight loss and pain (90%); migratory thrombophlebitis (10%); jaundice (<10%); nausea and vomiting; fatigue
What are the most common symptoms of cancer of the pancreatic HEAD?	1. Weight loss (90%) 2. Pain (75%) 3. Jaundice (70%)

What is "Courvoisier's sign"?	Palpable, nontender, distended gallbladder
What percentage of patients with cancers of the pancreatic HEAD have Courvoisier's sign?	33%
What is the classic presentation of pancreatic cancer in the head of the pancreas?	Painless jaundice
What metastatic lymph nodes described classically for gastric cancer can be found with metastatic pancreatic cancer?	Virchow's node; Sister Mary Joseph's nodule
What are the associated lab findings?	Increased direct bilirubin and alkaline phosphatase (as a result of biliary obstruction) Increased LFTs Elevated pancreatic tumor markers
Which tumor markers are associated with pancreatic cancer?	CA-19-9
What does CA-19-9 stand for?	**C**arbohydrate **A**ntigen 19-9
What diagnostic studies are performed?	Abdominal CT, U/S, cholangiography (ERCP to rule out choledocholithiasis and cell brushings), endoscopic U/S with biopsy
What are the pancreatic cancer STAGES:	
Stage I?	Tumor is limited to pancreas, with no nodes or metastases
Stage II?	Tumor extends into bile duct, peripancreatic tissues, or duodenum; there are no nodes or metastases
Stage III?	Same findings as stage II plus **positive nodes** or celiac or SMA involvement

Stage IVA? Tumor extends to stomach, colon, spleen, or major vessels, with any nodal status and no distant metastases

Stage IVB? **Distant metastases** (any nodal status, any tumor size) are found

What is the treatment based on location:
Head of the pancreas? Whipple procedure (pancreaticoduodenectomy)

Body or tail? Distal resection

What factors signify inoperability? Vascular encasement (SMA, hepatic artery)
Liver metastasis
Peritoneal implants
Distant lymph node metastasis (periaortic/celiac nodes)
Distant metastasis
Malignant ascites

Is portal vein or SMV involvement an absolute contraindication for resection? No—can be resected and reconstructed with vein interposition graft at some centers

Should patients undergo preoperative biliary drainage (e.g., ERCP)? No (exceptions for symptoms/ preoperative XRT, trials, etc.)

Define the Whipple procedure (pancreaticoduodenectomy). Cholecystectomy
Truncal vagotomy
Antrectomy
Pancreaticoduodenectomy—removal of head of pancreas and duodenum
Choledochojejunostomy—anastomosis of common bile duct to jejunum
Pancreaticojejunostomy—anastomosis of distal pancreas remnant to jejunum
Gastrojejunostomy—anastomosis of stomach to jejunum

What is the complication rate after a Whipple procedure? ≈25%

What mortality rate is associated with a Whipple procedure?

<5% at busy centers

What is the "pylorus-preserving Whipple"?

No antrectomy; anastomose duodenum to jejunum

What are the possible post-Whipple complications?

Delayed gastric emptying (if antrectomy is performed); **anastomotic leak** (from the bile duct or pancreatic anastomosis), causing pancreatic/biliary fistula; wound infection; postgastrectomy syndromes; sepsis; pancreatitis

Why must the duodenum be removed if the head of the pancreas is resected?

They share the same blood supply

What is the postoperative adjuvant therapy?

Chemotherapy +/− XRT

What is the palliative treatment if the tumor is inoperable and biliary obstruction is present?

PTC or ERCP and placement of stent across obstruction

What is the prognosis at 1 year after diagnosis?

Dismal; 90% of patients die within 1 year of diagnosis

What is the survival rate at 5 years after resection?

20%

MISCELLANEOUS

What is an annular pancreas?

Pancreas encircling the duodenum; if obstruction is present, bypass, **do not resect**

What is pancreatic divisum?

Failure of the two pancreatic ducts to fuse; the normally small duct (**S**mall = **S**antorini) of Santorini acts as the main duct in pancreatic divisum (Think: the two pancreatic ducts are **D**ivided = **D**ivisum)

What is heterotopic pancreatic tissue?	Heterotopic pancreatic tissue usually found in the stomach, intestine, duodenum
What is a Puestow procedure?	Longitudinal filleting of the pancreas/pancreatic duct with a side-to-side anastomosis with the small bowel
What medication decreases output from a pancreatic fistula?	Somatostatin (GI-inhibitory hormone)
Which has a longer half-life: amylase or lipase?	Lipase; therefore, amylase may be normal and lipase will remain elevated longer
What is the WDHA syndrome?	Pancreatic **VIP**oma (**V**asoactive **I**ntestinal **P**olypeptide tumor) Also known as Verner-Morrison syndrome Tumor secretes VIP, which causes: **W**atery **D**iarrhea **H**ypokalemia **A**chlorhydria (inhibits gastric acid secretion)
What is the Whipple triad of pancreatic insulinoma?	1. Hypoglycemia (Glc <50) 2. Symptoms of hypoglycemia: mental status changes/vasomotor instability 3. Relief of symptoms with administration of glucose
What is the most common islet cell tumor?	Insulinoma
What pancreatic tumor is associated with gallstone formation?	Somatostatinoma (inhibits gallbladder contraction)
What is the triad found with pancreatic somatostatinoma tumor?	1. Gallstones 2. Diabetes 3. Steatorrhea
What are the two classic findings with pancreatic glucagonoma tumors?	1. Diabetes 2. Dermatitis/rash (necrotizing migratory erythema)

Chapter 56   **Breast**

ANATOMY OF THE BREAST AND AXILLA

Name the boundaries of the axilla for dissection:

Superior boundary
: Axillary vein

Posterior boundary
: Long thoracic nerve

Lateral boundary
: Latissimus dorsi muscle

Medial boundary
: Lateral to, deep to, or medial to pectoral minor muscle, depending on level of nodes taken

What four nerves must the surgeon be aware of during an axillary dissection?

1. **Long thoracic nerve**
2. **Thoracodorsal nerve**
3. Medial pectoral nerve
4. Lateral pectoral nerve

Describe the location of these nerves and the muscle each innervates:

Long thoracic nerve
: Courses along lateral chest wall in midaxillary line on serratus anterior muscle; innervates serratus anterior muscle

Thoracodorsal nerve
: Courses lateral to long thoracic nerve on latissimus dorsi muscle; innervates latissimus dorsi muscle

Medial pectoral nerve
: Runs **lateral** to or through the pectoral minor muscle, actually **lateral** to the lateral pectoral nerve; innervates the pectoral minor and pectoral major muscles

Lateral pectoral nerve
: Runs **medial** to the medial pectoral nerve (names describe orientation from the brachial plexus!); innervates the pectoral major

Identify the nerves in the axilla on the illustration below:

1. Thoracodorsal nerve
2. Long thoracic nerve
3. Medial pectoral nerve
4. Lateral pectoral nerve
5. Axillary vein

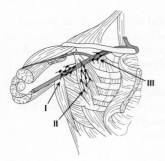

What is the name of the deformity if you cut the long thoracic nerve in this area?

"Winged scapula"

What is the name of the CUTANEOUS nerve that crosses the axilla in a transverse fashion? (Many surgeons try to preserve this nerve.)

Intercostobrachial nerve

What is the name of the large vein that marks the upper limit of the axilla?

Axillary vein

What is the lymphatic drainage of the breast?

Lateral: axillary lymph nodes
Medial: parasternal nodes that run with internal mammary artery

What are the levels of axillary lymph nodes?

Level I (low): lateral to pectoral minor
Level II (middle): deep to pectoral minor
Level III (high): medial to pectoral minor
In breast cancer, a higher level of involvement has a worse prognosis, but the level of involvement is less important than the number of positive nodes (Think: Levels I, II, and III are in the same inferior–superior anatomic order as the Le Fort facial fractures and the trauma neck zones; *I dare you to forget!*)

What are Rotter's nodes?	Nodes between the pectoralis major and minor muscles; not usually removed unless they are enlarged or feel suspicious intraoperatively
What are the suspensory breast ligaments called?	Cooper's ligaments
What is the mammary "milk line"?	Embryological line from shoulder to thigh where "supernumerary" breast areolar and/or nipples can be found
What is the "tail of Spence"?	"Tail" of breast tissue that tapers into the axilla
Which hormone is mainly responsible for breast milk production?	Prolactin

BREAST CANCER

What is the incidence of breast cancer?	**12% lifetime risk**
What percentage of women with breast cancer have no known risk factor?	75%!
What percentage of all breast cancers occur in women younger than 30 years?	≈2%
What percentage of all breast cancers occur in women older than 70 years?	33%
What are the major breast cancer susceptibility genes?	**BRCA1** and **BRCA2** (easily remembered: **BR** = **BR**east and **CA** = **CA**ncer)
What option exists to decrease the risk of breast cancer in women with BRCA?	Prophylactic bilateral mastectomy
What is the most common motivation for medicolegal cases involving the breast?	Failure to diagnose a breast carcinoma

What is the "TRIAD OF ERROR" for misdiagnosed breast cancer?	1. Age <45 years 2. Self-diagnosed mass 3. Negative mammogram ***Note:*** >75% of cases of **MISDIAGNOSED** breast cancer have these three characteristics
What are the history risk factors for breast cancer?	**"NAACP":** 　**N**ulliparity 　**A**ge at menarche (younger than 13 years) 　**A**ge at menopause (older than 55 years) 　**C**ancer of the breast (in self or family) 　**P**regnancy with first child (>30 years)
What are physical/anatomic risk factors for breast cancer?	**"CHAFED LIPS":** 　**C**ancer in the breast (3% synchronous contralateral cancer) 　**H**yperplasia (moderate/florid) (2× risk) 　**A**typical hyperplasia (4×) 　**F**emale (100× male risk) 　**E**lderly 　**D**CIS 　**L**CIS 　**I**nherited genes (BRCA I and II) 　**P**apilloma (1.5×) 　**S**clerosing adenosis (1.5×)
What is the relative risk of hormone replacement therapy?	1–1.5
Is "run of the mill" fibrocystic disease a risk factor for breast cancer?	No
What are the possible symptoms of breast cancer?	No symptoms Mass in the breast Pain (**most are painless**) Nipple discharge Local edema Nipple retraction Dimple Nipple rash

Why does skin retraction occur?

Tumor involvement of Cooper's ligaments and subsequent traction on ligaments pull skin inward

What are the signs of breast cancer?

Mass (1 cm is usually the smallest lesion that can be palpated on examination)
Dimple
Nipple rash
Edema
Axillary/supraclavicular nodes

What is the most common site of breast cancer?

Approximately one half of cancers develop in the upper outer quadrants

What are the different types of invasive breast cancer?

Infiltrating ductal carcinoma ($\approx$75%)
Medullary carcinoma ($\approx$15%)
Infiltrating lobular carcinoma ($\approx$5%)
Tubular carcinoma ($\approx$2%)
Mucinous carcinoma (colloid) ($\approx$1%)
Inflammatory breast cancer ($\approx$1%)

What is the most common type of breast cancer?

Infiltrating ductal carcinoma

What is the differential diagnosis?

Fibrocystic disease of the breast
Fibroadenoma
Intraductal papilloma
Duct ectasia
Fat necrosis
Abscess
Radial scar
Simple cyst

Describe the appearance of the edema of the dermis in inflammatory carcinoma of the breast.

Peau d'orange (orange peel)

What are the screening recommendations for breast cancer:
    Breast exam recommendations?

Self-exam of breasts monthly
Ages 20 to 40 years: breast exam every 2 to 3 years by a physician
>40 years: annual breast exam by physician

Mammograms?

Recommendations are controversial, but most experts say:

Baseline mammogram between 35 and 40 years

Mammogram every year or every other year for ages 40 to 50

Mammogram yearly after age 50

When is the best time for breast self-exams?

1 week after menstrual period

Why is mammography a more useful diagnostic tool in older women than in younger?

Breast tissue undergoes fatty replacement with age, making masses more visible; younger women have more fibrous tissue, which makes mammograms harder to interpret

What are the radiographic tests for breast cancer?

Mammography and breast ultrasound, MRI

What is the classic picture of breast cancer on mammogram?

Spiculated mass

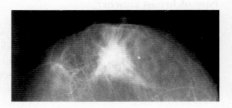

Which option is best to evaluate a breast mass in a woman younger than 30 years?

Breast ultrasound

What are the methods for obtaining tissue for pathologic examination?

Fine needle aspiration (FNA), core biopsy (larger needle core sample), mammotome stereotactic biopsy, and open biopsy, which can be incisional (cutting a **piece** of the mass) or excisional (cutting out the **entire** mass)

What are the indications for biopsy?

Persistent mass after aspiration
Solid mass
Blood in cyst aspirate
Suspicious lesion by mammography/ultrasound/MRI
Bloody nipple discharge
Ulcer or dermatitis of nipple
Patient's concern of persistent breast abnormality

What is the process for performing a biopsy when a nonpalpable mass is seen on mammogram?

Stereotactic (mammotome) biopsy or needle localization biopsy

What is a needle loc biopsy (NLB)?

Needle localization by radiologist, followed by biopsy; removed breast tissue must be checked by mammogram to ensure all of the suspicious lesion has been excised

What is a mammotome biopsy?

Mammogram-guided computerized stereotatic core biopsies

What is obtained first, the mammogram or the biopsy?

Mammogram is obtained first; otherwise, tissue extraction (core or open) may alter the mammographic findings (fine needle aspiration may be done prior to the mammogram because the fine needle usually will not affect the mammographic findings)

What would be suspicious mammographic findings?

Mass, microcalcifications, stellate/spiculated mass

What is a "radial scar" seen on mammogram?

Spiculated mass with central lucency, +/– microcalcifications

What tumor is associated with a radial scar?

Tubular carcinoma; thus, biopsy is indicated

What is the "workup" for a breast mass?

1. Clinical breast exam
2. Mammogram or breast ultrasound
3. Fine needle aspiration, core biopsy, or open biopsy

How do you proceed if the mass appears to be a cyst?

Aspirate it with a needle

Is the fluid from a breast cyst sent for cytology?

Not routinely; bloody fluid should be sent for cytology

When do you proceed to open biopsy for a breast cyst?

1. In the case of a second cyst recurrence
2. Bloody fluid in the cyst
3. Palpable mass after aspiration

What is the preoperative staging workup in a patient with breast cancer?

Bilateral mammogram (cancer in one breast is a risk factor for cancer in the contralateral breast!)

CXR (to check for lung metastasis)

LFTs (to check for liver metastasis)

Serum calcium level, alkaline phosphatase (if these tests indicate bone metastasis/"bone pain," proceed to bone scan)

Other tests, depending on signs/ symptoms (e.g., head CT if patient has focal neurologic deficit, to look for brain metastasis)

What hormone receptors must be checked for in the biopsy specimen?

Estrogen and progesterone receptors—this is **key for determining adjuvant treatment**; this information must be obtained on all specimens (including fine needle aspirates)

What staging system is used for breast cancer?

TMN: Tumor/**M**etastases/**N**odes (AJCC)

Describe the staging (simplified):

Stage I

Tumor ≤2 cm in diameter without metastases, **no nodes**

Stage IIA

Tumor ≤2 cm in diameter with mobile axillary nodes **or**
Tumor 2 to 5 cm in diameter, no nodes

Stage IIB

Tumor 2 to 5 cm in diameter with mobile axillary nodes **or**
Tumor >5 cm **with no nodes**

Stage IIIA	Tumor >5 cm with mobile axillary nodes **or** Any size tumor with **fixed** axillary nodes, no metastases
Stage IIIB	Peau d'orange (skin edema) or Chest wall invasion/fixation or Inflammatory cancer or Breast skin ulceration or Breast skin satellite metastases or Any tumor and + ipsilateral **internal mammary** lymph nodes
Stage IIIC	Any size tumor, no distant mets POSITIVE: supraclavicular, infraclavicular, or internal mammary lymph nodes
Stage IV	**Distant metastases** (including ipsilateral supraclavicular nodes)
What are the sites of metastases?	Lymph nodes (most common) Lung/pleura Liver Bones Brain
What are the major treatments of breast cancer?	Modified radical mastectomy Lumpectomy and radiation + sentinel lymph node dissection (Both treatments either +/– postop chemotherapy/tamoxifen)
What are the indications for radiation therapy after a modified radical mastectomy?	Stage IIIA Stage IIIB Pectoral muscle/fascia invasion Positive internal mammary LN Positive surgical margins ≥4 positive axillary LNs postmenopausal
What breast carcinomas are candidates for lumpectomy and radiation (breast-conserving therapy)?	Stage I and stage II (tumors <5 cm)

What approach may allow a patient with stage IIIA cancer to have breast-conserving surgery?

NEOadjuvant chemotherapy—if the preop chemo shrinks the tumor

What is the treatment of inflammatory carcinoma of the breast?

Chemotherapy first! Then often followed by radiation, mastectomy, or both

What is a "lumpectomy and radiation"?

Lumpectomy (segmental mastectomy: removal of a **part** of the breast); axillary node dissection; and a course of radiation therapy **after** operation, over a period of several weeks

What is the major absolute contraindication to lumpectomy and radiation?

Pregnancy

What are other contraindications to lumpectomy and radiation?

Previous radiation to the chest
Positive margins
Collagen vascular disease (e.g., scleroderma)
Extensive DCIS (often seen as diffuse microcalcification)
Relative contraindications:
  Lesion that cannot be seen on the mammograms (i.e., early recurrence will be missed on follow-up mammograms)
  Very small breast (no cosmetic advantage)

What is a modified radical mastectomy?

Breast, axillary nodes (level II, I), and nipple–areolar complex are removed
Pectoralis major and minor muscles are **not** removed (Auchincloss modification)
Drains are placed to drain lymph fluid

Where are the drains placed with an MRM?

1. Axilla
2. Chest wall (breast bed)

When should the drains be removed?

<30 cc/day drainage

What are the potential complications after a modified radical mastectomy?

Ipsilateral arm lymphedema, infection, injury to nerves, skin flap necrosis, hematoma/seroma, phantom breast syndrome

During an axillary dissection, should the patient be paralyzed?

NO, because the nerves (long thoracic/thoracodorsal) are stimulated with resultant muscle contraction to help identify them

How can the long thoracic and thoracodorsal nerves be identified during an axillary dissection?

Nerves can be stimulated with a forceps, which results in contraction of the latissimus dorsi (thoracodorsal nerve) or anterior serratus (long thoracic nerve)

When do you remove the drains after an axillary dissection?

When there is <30 cc of drainage per day, or on POD #14 (whichever comes first)

What is a sentinel node biopsy?

Instead of removing all the axillary lymph nodes, the **primary** draining or "sentinel" lymph node is removed

How is the sentinel lymph node found?

Inject blue dye and/or technetium-labeled sulfur colloid (best results with both)

What follows a positive sentinel node biopsy?

Removal of the rest of the axillary lymph nodes

What is now considered the standard of care for lymph node evaluation in women with T1 or T2 tumors (stages I and IIA) and clinically negative axillary lymph nodes?

Sentinel lymph node dissection

What do you do with a mammotome biopsy that returns as "atypical hyperplasia"?

Open needle loc biopsy as many will have DCIS or invasive cancer

How does tamoxifen work?

It binds estrogen receptors

What is the treatment for local recurrence in breast after lumpectomy and radiation?

"Salvage" mastectomy

Can tamoxifen prevent breast cancer?

Yes. In the Breast Cancer Prevention Trial of 13,000 women at increased risk of developing breast cancer, tamoxifen reduced risk by ≈50% across all ages

What are common options for breast reconstruction?

TRAM flap, implant, latissimus dorsi flap

What is a TRAM flap?

Transverse **R**ectus **A**bdominis **M**yocutaneous flap

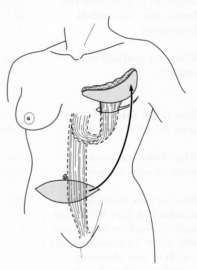

What are side effects of tamoxifen?

Endometrial cancer (2.5× relative risk), DVT, pulmonary embolus, cataracts, hot flashes, mood swings

In high-risk women, is there a way to reduce the risk of developing breast cancer?

Yes, tamoxifen for 5 years will lower the risk by up to 50%, but, with an increased risk of endometrial cancer and clots, it must be an individual patient determination

Give the common adjuvant
therapy for the following
patients with breast cancer.
(These are rough guidelines;
check for current uidelines,
as they are always changing.)
(ER = estrogen receptor):

Premenopausal, node +, ER −	Chemotherapy
Premenopausal, node +, ER +	Chemotherapy and tamoxifen
Premenopausal, node −, ER +	Tamoxifen
Postmenopausal, node +, ER +	Tamoxifen, +/− chemotherapy
Postmenopausal, node +, ER −	Chemotherapy, +/− tamoxifen

What type of chemotherapy is usually used for breast cancer?

CMF (**C**yclophosphamide, **M**ethotrexate, 5-**F**luorouracil) or **CAF** (**C**yclophosphamide, **A**driamycin, 5-**F**luorouracil)

Chemotherapy for high-risk tumors with negative lymph nodes should be considered. What makes a tumor "HIGH RISK"?

High risk:
>1 cm in size
Lymphatic/vascular invasion
Nuclear grade (high)
S phase (high)
ER negative
HER-2/neu overexpression

DCIS

What does DCIS stand for?   **D**uctal **C**arcinoma **I**n **S**itu

What is DCIS also known as?   Intraductal carcinoma

Describe DCIS.   Cancer cells in the duct without invasion (In situ: Cells do not penetrate the basement membrane)

What are the signs/symptoms? Usually none; usually nonpalpable

What are the mammographic findings? Microcalcifications

How is the diagnosis made? Core or open biopsy

What is the most aggressive histologic type? Comedo

What is the risk of lymph node metastasis with DCIS? <2% (usually when microinvasion is seen)

What is the major risk with DCIS? Subsequent development of infiltrating ductal carcinoma in the **same breast**

What is the treatment for DCIS in the following cases:

Tumor <1 cm (low grade)? Remove with 1 cm margins +/− XRT

Tumor >1 cm? Perform lumpectomy with 1 cm margins and radiation **or** total mastectomy (**no** axillary dissection)

What is a total (simple) mastectomy? Removal of the breast and nipple without removal of the axillary nodes (always remove nodes with invasive cancer)

When must a simple mastectomy be performed for DCIS? Diffuse breast involvement (e.g., diffuse microcalcifications), >1 cm and contraindication to radiation

What is the role of axillary node dissection with DCIS? No role in true DCIS (i.e., without microinvasion); some perform a sentinel lymph node dissection for high-grade DCIS

What is adjuvant for DCIS?
1. Tamoxifen
2. Postlumpectomy XRT

What is the role of tamoxifen in DCIS? Tamoxifen for 5 years will lower the risk up to 50%, but with increased risk of endometrial cancer and clots; it must be an individual patient determination

What is a memory aid for the breast in which DCIS breast cancer arises?	Cancer arises in the **same** breast as DCIS (Think: **D**CIS = **D**irectly in same breast)

LCIS

What is LCIS?	**L**obular **C**arcinoma **I**n **S**itu (carcinoma cells in the lobules of the breast without invasion)
What are the signs/ symptoms?	There are none
What are the mammographic findings?	There are none
How is the diagnosis made?	LCIS is found **incidentally** on biopsy
What is the major risk?	Carcinoma of **either** breast
Which breast is most at risk for developing an invasive carcinoma?	Equal risk in both breasts! (Think of LCIS as a **risk marker** for future development of cancer in either breast)
What percentage of women with LCIS develop an invasive breast carcinoma?	≈30% in the 20 years after diagnosis of LCIS!
What type of invasive breast cancer do patients with LCIS develop?	Most commonly, **infiltrating ductal carcinoma, with equal distribution** in the contralateral and ipsilateral breasts
What medication may lower the risk of developing breast cancer in LCIS?	Tamoxifen for 5 years will lower the risk up to 50%, but with an increased risk of endometrial cancer and clots; it must be an individual patient determination
What is the treatment of LCIS?	Close follow-up (or bilateral simple mastectomy in high-risk patients)
What is the major difference in the subsequent development of invasive breast cancer with DCIS and LCIS?	LCIS cancer develops in *either* breast; DCIS cancer develops in the ipsilateral breast

How do you remember which breast is at risk for invasive cancers in patients with LCIS?

Think: **LCIS** = **L**iberally in either breast

MISCELLANEOUS

What is the most common cause of bloody nipple discharge in a young woman?

Intraductal papilloma

What is the most common breast tumor in patients younger than 30 years?

Fibroadenoma

What is Paget's disease of the breast?

Scaling rash/dermatitis of the nipple caused by invasion of skin by cells from a ductal carcinoma

What are the common options for breast reconstruction after a mastectomy?

Saline implant
TRAM flap

MALE BREAST CANCER

What is the incidence of breast cancer in men?

<1% of all breast cancer cases (1/150)

What is the average age at diagnosis?

65 years of age

What are the risk factors?

Increased estrogen
Radiation
Gynecomastia from increased estrogen
Estrogen therapy
Klinefelter's syndrome (XXY)
BRCA2 carriers

Is benign gynecomastia a risk factor for male breast cancer?

No

What type of breast cancer do men develop?

Nearly 100% of cases are ductal carcinoma (men do not usually have breast lobules)

What are the signs/symptoms of breast cancer in men?	Breast mass (most are painless), breast skin changes (ulcers, retraction), and nipple discharge (usually blood or a blood-tinged discharge)
What is the most common presentation?	Painless breast mass
How is breast cancer in men diagnosed?	Biopsy and mammogram
What is the treatment?	1. Mastectomy 2. Sentinel LN dissection of clinically negative axilla 3. Axillary dissection if clinically positive axillary LN

BENIGN BREAST DISEASE

What is the most common cause of green, straw-colored, or brown nipple discharge?	Fibrocystic disease
What is the most common cause of breast mass after breast trauma?	Fat necrosis
What is Mondor's disease?	Thrombophlebitis of superficial breast veins
What must be ruled out with spontaneous galactorrhea (+/− amenorrhea)?	Prolactinoma (check pregnancy test and prolactin level)

CYSTOSARCOMA PHYLLODES

What is it?	Mesenchymal tumor arising from breast lobular tissue; most are benign (***Note:*** "sarcoma" is a misnomer, as the vast majority are benign; 1% of breast cancers)
What is the usual age of the patient with this tumor?	35–55 years (usually older than the patient with fibroadenoma)

What are the signs/ symptoms?	Mobile, smooth breast mass that resembles a fibroadenoma on exam, mammogram/ultrasound findings
How is it diagnosed?	Through core biopsy or excision
What is the treatment?	If benign, wide local excision; if malignant, simple total mastectomy
What is the role of axillary dissection with cystosarcoma phyllodes tumor?	Only if clinically palpable axillary nodes, as the malignant form rarely spreads to nodes (most common site of metastasis is the lung)
Is there a role for chemotherapy with cystosarcoma phyllodes?	Consider chemotherapy if large tumor >5 cm and "stromal overgrowth"

FIBROADENOMA

What is it?	Benign tumor of the breast consisting of stromal overgrowth, collagen arranged in "swirls"
What is the clinical presentation of a fibroadenoma?	Solid, mobile, **well-circumscribed** round breast mass, usually <40 years of age
How is fibroadenoma diagnosed?	Negative needle aspiration looking for fluid; ultrasound; core biopsy
What is the treatment?	Surgical resection for large or growing lesions; small fibroadenomas can be observed closely
What is this tumor's claim to fame?	Most common breast tumor in women <30 years

FIBROCYSTIC DISEASE

What is it?	Common benign breast condition consisting of fibrous (rubbery) and cystic changes in the breast
What are the signs/ symptoms?	Breast pain or tenderness that varies with the menstrual cycle; cysts; and fibrous ("nodular") fullness

How is it diagnosed?	Through breast exam, history, and aspirated cysts (usually straw-colored or green fluid)
What is the treatment for symptomatic fibrocystic disease?	**Stop caffeine** Pain medications (NSAIDs) Vitamin E, evening primrose oil (danazol and OCP as last resort)
What is done if the patient has a breast cyst?	Needle drainage: If aspirate is bloody or a palpable mass remains after aspiration, an open biopsy is performed If the aspirate is straw colored or green, the patient is followed closely; then, if there is recurrence, a second aspiration is performed Re-recurrence usually requires open biopsy

MASTITIS

What is it?	Superficial infection of the breast (cellulitis)
In what circumstance does it most often occur?	Breast-feeding
What bacteria are most commonly the cause?	*Staphylococcus aureus*
How is mastitis treated?	Stop breast-feeding and use a breast pump instead; apply heat; administer antibiotics
Why must the patient with mastitis have close follow-up?	To make sure that she does not have inflammatory breast cancer!

BREAST ABSCESS

What are the causes?	Mammary ductal ectasia (stenosis of breast duct) and mastitis
What is the most common bacteria?	Nursing = *Staphylococcus aureus* Nonlactating = mixed infection
What is the treatment of breast abscess?	Antibiotics (e.g., dicloxacillin) Needle or open drainage with cultures taken Resection of involved ducts if recurrent Breast pump if breast-feeding

What is lactational mastitis?
Infection of the breast during breast-feeding—most commonly caused by *S. aureus;* treat with antibiotics and follow for abscess formation

What must be ruled out with a breast abscess in a nonlactating woman?
Breast cancer!

MALE GYNECOMASTIA

What is it?
Enlargement of the male breast

What are the causes?
Medications
Illicit drugs (marijuana)
Liver failure
Increased estrogen
Decreased testosterone

What is the major differential diagnosis in the older patient?
Male breast cancer

What is the treatment?
Stop or change medications; correct underlying cause if there is a hormonal imbalance; and perform biopsy or subcutaneous mastectomy (i.e., leave nipple) if refractory to conservative measures and time

Chapter 57 Endocrine

ADRENAL GLAND

ANATOMY

Where is the drainage of the *left* adrenal vein?
Left renal vein

Where is the drainage of the *right* adrenal vein?
Inferior vena cava (IVC)

NORMAL ADRENAL PHYSIOLOGY

What is CRH?	Corticotropin-**R**eleasing **H**ormone: released from anterior hypothalamus and causes release of ACTH from anterior pituitary
What is ACTH?	**A**dreno**C**ortico**T**ropic **H**ormone: released normally by anterior pituitary, which in turn causes adrenal gland to release cortisol
What feeds back to inhibit ACTH secretion?	Cortisol

CUSHING'S SYNDROME

What is Cushing's syndrome?	Excessive **cortisol** production (Think: **C**ushing's = **C**ortisol
What is the most common cause?	Iatrogenic (i.e., prescribed prednisone)
What is the second most common cause?	Cushing's disease (most common noniatrogenic cause)
What is Cushing's disease?	Cushing's syndrome caused by excess production of ACTH by anterior **pituitary**
What is an ectopic ACTH source?	Tumor not found in the pituitary that secretes ACTH, which in turn causes adrenal gland to release cortisol without the normal negative feedback loop
What are the signs/ symptoms of Cushing's syndrome?	Truncal obesity, hirsutism, "moon" facies, acne, "buffalo hump," purple striae, hypertension, diabetes, weakness, depression, easy bruising, myopathy
How can cortisol levels be indirectly measured over a short duration?	By measuring urine cortisol or the breakdown product of cortisol, 17 hydroxycorticosteroid (**17-OHCS**), in the urine
What is a direct test of serum cortisol?	Serum cortisol level (highest in the morning and lowest at night in healthy patients)

What initial tests should be performed in Cushing's syndrome?

Electrolytes
Serum cortisol
Urine-free cortisol, urine 17-OHCS
Low-dose dexamethasone suppression test

What is the low-dose dexamethasone suppression test?

Dexamethasone is a synthetic cortisol that results in negative feedback on ACTH secretion and subsequent cortisol secretion in healthy patients; patients with **Cushing's syndrome** do **not** suppress their cortisol secretion

After the dexamethasone test, what is next?

Check ACTH levels

Can plasma ACTH levels be checked directly?

Yes

What is the workup in a patient suspected of having Cushing's syndrome?

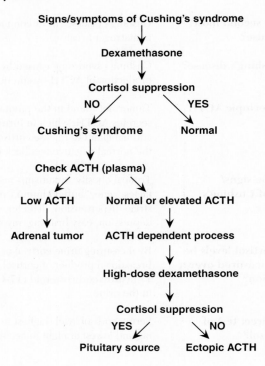

Signs/symptoms of Cushing's syndrome
↓
Dexamethasone
↓
Cortisol suppression
NO ↙   ↘ YES
Cushing's syndrome   Normal
↓
Check ACTH (plasma)
↙   ↘
Low ACTH   Normal or elevated ACTH
↓   ↓
Adrenal tumor   ACTH dependent process
↓
High-dose dexamethasone
↓
Cortisol suppression
YES ↙   ↘ NO
Pituitary source   Ectopic ACTH

In ACTH-dependent Cushing's syndrome, how do you differentiate between a pituitary vs. an ectopic ACTH source?

High-dose dexamethasone test:
Pituitary source—cortisol is suppressed
Ectopic ACTH source—no cortisol suppression

Summarize the "Cushing's syndrome" lab values found in the majority of patients with the following conditions:
Healthy patients

Normal cortisol and ACTH, suppression with low-dose or high-dose dexamethasone (<1/2)

Cushing's disease (pituitary ACTH hypersecretion)

High cortisol and ACTH, no suppression with low-dose dexamethasone, suppression with high-dose dexamethasone

Adrenal tumor

High cortisol, low ACTH, no suppression with low-dose or high-dose dexamethasone

Ectopic ACTH-producing tumor

High cortisol and ACTH, no suppression with low-dose or high-dose dexamethasone

What is the test for equivocal results for differentiating pituitary vs. ectopic ACTH tumor?

Bilateral petrosal vein sampling, especially with CRH infusion

What is the most common site of ectopic ACTH-producing tumor?

>66% are oat cell tumors of the lung (#2 is carcinoid)

How are the following tumors treated:
Adrenal adenoma?

Adrenalectomy (almost always **unilateral**)

Adrenal carcinoma?

Surgical excision (only 33% of cases are operable)

Ectopic ACTH-producing tumor?

Surgical excision, if feasible

Cushing's *disease*?

Transphenoidal adenomectomy

What medication must be given to a patient who is undergoing surgical correction of Cushing's syndrome?	Cortisol (usually hydrocortisone until PO is resumed)
What medications inhibit cortisol production?	1. Ketoconazole 2. Metyrapone 3. Aminoglutethimide 4. Mitotane
Give the mechanism of action: **Ketoconazole (an antifungal)**	Inhibits 11 β-hydroxylase, c17-20 lyase, and cholesterol side-chain cleavage
Aminoglutethimide (an anticonvulsant)	Inhibits cleavage of cholesterol side chains
Mitotane	Inhibits 11 β-hydroxylase and cholesterol side-chain cleavage; causes irreversible adrenocortical cells (and thus can be used for "medical adrenalectomy")
Metyrapone	Inhibits 11 β-hydroxylase
What is a complication of BILATERAL adrenalectomy?	Nelson's syndrome—occurs in 10% of patients after bilateral adrenalectomy
What is Nelson's syndrome?	Functional pituitary adenoma producing excessive ACTH and mass effect producing visual disturbances, hyperpigmentation, amenorrhea, with elevated ACTH levels Think: **N**elson = **N**uclear reaction in the pituitary

ADRENAL INCIDENTALOMA

What is an incidentaloma?	Tumor found in the adrenal gland **incidentally** on a CT scan performed for an unrelated reason
What is the incidence of incidentalomas?	4% of all CT scans (9% of autopsies)

What is the most common cause of incidentaloma?	Nonfunctioning adenoma (>75% of cases)
What is the differential diagnosis of incidentaloma?	Nonfunctioning adenoma Pheochromocytoma Adrenocortical carcinoma Aldosteronoma Metastatic disease Nodular hyperplasia
What is the risk factor for carcinoma?	Solid tumor >6 cm in diameter
What is the treatment?	Controversial for smaller/medium-sized tumors, but almost all surgeons would agree that resection is indicated for solid incidentalomas >6 cm in diameter because of risk of cancer
What are the indications for removal of adrenal incidentaloma less than 6 cm?	MRI T2 signal >2 **Hormonally active** = hyperfunctioning tumor Enlarging cystic lesion Does not look like an adenoma
What tumor must be ruled out prior to biopsy or surgery for any adrenal mass?	Pheochromocytoma (24-hour urine for catecholamine, VMA, metanephrines)

PHEOCHROMOCYTOMA

What is it?	Tumor of the adrenal **MEDULLA** and sympathetic ganglion (from chromaffin cell lines) that produces **catecholamines** (norepinephrine > epinephrine)
What is the incidence?	Cause of hypertension in ≈1/500 hypertensive patients (≈10% of U.S. population has hypertension)
Which age group is most likely to be affected?	Any age (children and adults); average age is 40 to 60 years
What are the associated risk factors?	MEN-II, family history, von Recklinghausen disease, von Hippel-Lindau disease

What are the signs/ symptoms?	"Classic" triad: **1. Palpitations** **2. Headache** **3. Episodic diaphoresis** Also, hypertension (50%), pallor → flushing, anxiety, weight loss, tachycardia, hyperglycemia
How can the pheochromocytoma SYMPTOMS triad be remembered?	Think of the first three letters in the word **PHE**ochromocytoma: **P**alpitations **H**eadache **E**pisodic diaphoresis
What is the most common sign of pheochromocytoma?	Hypertension
What is the differential diagnosis?	Renovascular hypertension, menopause, migraine headache, carcinoid syndrome, preeclampsia, neuroblastoma, anxiety disorder with panic attacks, hyperthyroidism, insulinoma
What diagnostic tests should be performed?	Urine screen: **V**anillyl**M**andelic **A**cid **(VMA), metanephrine,** and normetanephrine (all breakdown products of the catechols) Urine/serum **epinephrine/ norepinephrine** levels
What are the other common lab findings?	Hyperglycemia (epinephrine increases glucose, norepinephrine decreases insulin) Polycythemia (resulting from intravascular volume depletion)
What is the most common site of a pheochromocytoma?	**Adrenal** >90%
What are the other sites for pheochromocytoma?	Organ of Zuckerkandl, thorax (mediastinum), bladder, scrotum
What are the tumor localization tests?	CT scan, MRI, ^{131}**I-MIBG**, PET scan, OctreoScan (^{111}In-pentetreotide scan)

What does ^{131}I-MIBG stand for?

Iodine^{131}**M**eta**I**odo**B**enzyl**G**uanidine

How to remember MIBG and pheochromocytoma?

Think: **MIBG** = **My Big** = and thus "My Big Pheo" = **MIBG Pheo**

How does the ^{131}I-MIBG scan work?

^{131}I-MIBG is a norepinephrine analog that collects in adrenergic vesicles and, thus, in pheochromocytomas

What is the role of PET scan?

Positron **E**mission **T**omography is helpful in localizing pheochromocytomas that do not accumulate MIBG

What is the scan for imaging adrenal cortical pheochromocytoma?

NP-59 (a cholesterol analog)

What is the localizing option if a tumor is not seen on CT, MRI, or I-MIBG?

IVC venous sampling for catecholamines (gradient will help localize the tumor)

What is the tumor site if epinephrine is elevated?

Must be adrenal or near the adrenal gland (e.g., organ of Zuckerkandl), because nonadrenal tumors lack the capability to methylate norepinephrine to epinephrine

What percentage of patients have malignant tumors?

≈10%

Can histology be used to determine malignancy?

No; only distant metastasis or invasion can determine malignancy

What is the classic pheochromocytoma "rule of 10's"?

10% malignant
10% bilateral
10% in children
10% multiple tumors
10% extra-adrenal

What is the preoperative/ medical treatment?

Increase intravascular volume with α-blockade (e.g., phenoxybenzamine or prazosin) to allow reduction in catecholamine-induced vasoconstriction and resulting volume depletion; treatment should start as soon as diagnosis is made +/− β-blockers

How can you remember phenoxybenzamine as a medical treatment of pheochromocytoma?

PHEochromocytoma = **PHE**noxybenzamine

What is the surgical treatment?

Tumor resection with early ligation of venous drainage (lower possibility of catecholamine release/crisis by tying off drainage) and minimal manipulation

What are the possible perioperative complications?

Anesthetic challenge: hypertensive crisis with manipulation (treat with nitroprusside), hypotension with total removal of the tumor, cardiac dysrhythmias

In the patient with pheochromocytoma, what must be ruled out?

MEN type II (almost all cases are bilateral)

What is the organ of Zuckerkandl?

Body of embryonic chromaffin cells around the abdominal aorta (near the inferior mesenteric artery); normally atrophies during childhood, but is the most common site of extra-adrenal pheochromocytoma

CONN'S SYNDROME

What is it?

Primary hyper**aldosteronism** due to high aldosterone production

How do you remember what Conn's syndrome is?

CONn's disease = **HYPERAL**dosterone = "**CON HYPER AL**"

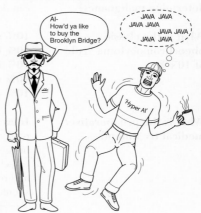

What are the common sources?

Adrenal adenoma or **adrenal hyperplasia;** aldosterone is abnormally secreted by an adrenal adenoma (66%) > hyperplasia > carcinoma

What is the normal physiology for aldosterone secretion?

BP in the renal afferent arteriole is low
Low sodium and hyperkalemia cause
    renin secretion from juxtaglomerular
    cells
Renin then converts angiotensinogen to
    angiotensin I
Angiotensin converting enzyme in the
    lung then converts angiotensin I to
    angiotensin II
Angiotensin II then causes the adrenal
    glomerulosa cells to secrete
    aldosterone

What is the normal physiologic effect of aldosterone?

Aldosterone causes sodium retention for exchange of potassium in the kidney, result-ing in fluid retention and increased BP

What are the signs/ symptoms?

Hypertension, headache, polyuria, weakness

What are the two classic clues of Conn's syndrome?

1. Hypertension
2. Hypokalemia

Classically, what kind of hypertension?

Diastolic hypertension

What are the renin levels with Conn's syndrome?

Normal or decreased!

What percentage of all patients with hypertension have Conn's syndrome?

1%

What diagnostic tests should be ordered?

1. Plasma aldosterone concentration
2. Plasma renin activity

What ratio of these diagnostic tests is associated with primary hyperaldosteronism?

Aldosterone to renin ratio of >30

What is secondary hyperaldosteronism?	Hyperaldosteronism resulting from abnormally high renin levels (renin increases angiotensin/aldosterone)
What diagnostic tests should be performed?	CT scan, adrenal venous sampling for aldosterone levels, saline infusion
What is the saline infusion test?	Saline infusion will decrease aldosterone levels in normal patients but not in Conn's syndrome
What is the preoperative treatment?	Spironolactone, K^+ supplementation
What is spironolactone?	Antialdosterone medication (works at the kidney tubule)
What are the causes of Conn's syndrome?	Adrenal adenoma (66%) Bilateral idiopathic adrenal hyperplasia (30%) Adrenal cancer (<1%)
What is the treatment of the following conditions:	
Adenoma?	Unilateral adrenalectomy (laparoscopic)
Unilateral hyperplasia?	Unilateral adrenalectomy (laparoscopic)
Bilateral hyperplasia?	Spironolactone (usually no surgery)
What are the renin levels in patients with PRIMARY hyperaldosteronism?	Normal or low (key point!)

ADDISON'S DISEASE

What is it?	Acute adrenal insufficiency
What are the electrolyte findings?	HYPERkalemia, hyponatremia
How do you remember what ADDISON's disease is?	Think: **ADD**ison's disease = **AD**renal **D**own

INSULINOMA

What is it?	Insulin-producing tumor arising from β cells

What is the incidence?

#1 Islet cell neoplasm; half of β cell tumors of the pancreas produce insulin

What are the associated risks?

Associated with MEN-I syndrome (**PPP** = **P**ituitary, **P**ancreas, **P**arathyroid tumors)

What are the signs/ symptoms?

Sympathetic nervous system symptoms resulting from hypoglycemia: palpitations, diaphoresis, tremulousness, irritability, weakness

What are the neurologic symptoms?

Personality changes, confusion, obtundation, seizures, coma

What is Whipple's triad?

1. Hypoglycemic symptoms produced by fasting
2. Blood glucose <50 mg/dL during symptomatic attack
3. Relief of symptoms by administration of glucose

What is the differential diagnosis?

Reactive hypoglycemia
Functional hypoglycemia with gastrectomy
Adrenal insufficiency
Hypopituitarism
Hepatic insufficiency
Munchausen syndrome (insulin self-injections)
Nonislet cell tumor causing hypoglycemia
Surreptitious administration of insulin or OHAs

What lab tests should be performed?

Glucose and insulin levels during fast; C-peptide and proinsulin levels (if self-injection of insulin is a concern, as insulin injections have **no** proinsulin or C-peptides)

What diagnostic tests should be performed?

Fasting hypoglycemia with inappropriately high levels of insulin
72-hour fast, then check glucose and insulin levels every 6 hours (monitor very closely because patient can develop hypoglycemic crisis)

What is the diagnostic fasting insulin to glucose ratio?	>0.4
What localizing tests should be performed?	CT scan, A-gram, endoscopic U/S, venous catheterization (to sample blood along portal and splenic veins to measure insulin and localize tumor), intraoperative U/S
What is the medical treatment?	Diazoxide, to suppress insulin release
What is the surgical treatment?	Surgical resection
What is the prognosis?	≈80% of patients have a benign solitary adenoma that is cured by surgical resection

GLUCAGONOMA

What is it?	Glucagon-producing tumor
Where is it located?	Pancreas (usually in the tail)
What are the symptoms?	**Necrotizing migratory erythema** (usually below the waist), glossitis, stomatitis, diabetes
What are the skin findings?	Necrotizing migratory erythema is a red, often psoriatic-appearing rash with serpiginous borders over the trunk and limbs
What are the associated lab findings?	Hyperglycemia, low amino acid levels, high glucagon levels
What is the classic finding on CBC?	Anemia
What is the classic nutritional finding?	Low amino acid levels
What stimulation test is used for glucagonoma?	Tolbutamide stimulation test: IV tolbutamide results in elevated glucagon levels
What test is used for localization?	CT scan

What is the medical treatment of necrotizing migratory erythema?	Somatostatin, IV amino acids
What is the treatment?	Surgical resection

SOMATOSTATINOMA

What is it?	Pancreatic tumor that secretes somatostatin
What is the diagnostic triad?	**DDD:** 1. **D**iabetes 2. **D**iarrhea (steatorrhea) 3. **D**ilation of the gallbladder with gallstones
What is used to make the diagnosis?	CT scan and somatostatin level
What is the treatment?	Resection (do not enucleate)
What is the medical treatment if the tumor is unresectable?	Streptozocin, dacarbazine, or doxorubicin

ZOLLINGER-ELLISON SYNDROME (ZES)

What is it?	**Gastrinoma:** non-β islet cell tumor of the pancreas (or other locale) that produces gastrin, causing gastric hypersecretion of HCl acid, resulting in GI **ulcers**
What is the incidence?	1/1000 in patients with peptic ulcer disease, but nearly 2% in patients with **recurrent ulcers**
What is the associated syndrome?	MEN-I syndrome
What percentage of patients with ZES have MEN-I syndrome?	≈25% (75% of cases of Z-E syndrome are "sporadic")
What percentage of patients with MEN-I will have ZES?	≈50%

With gastrinoma, what lab tests should be ordered to screen for MEN-I?

1. Calcium level
2. Parathyroid hormone level

What are the signs/ symptoms?

Peptic ulcers, diarrhea, weight loss, abdominal pain

What causes the diarrhea?

Massive acid hypersecretion and destruction of digestive enzymes

What are the signs?

PUD (epigastric pain, hematemesis, melena, hematochezia), GERD, diarrhea, **recurrent ulcers,** ulcers in unusual locations (e.g., proximal jejunum)

What are the possible complications?

GI hemorrhage/perforation, gastric outlet obstruction/stricture, metastatic disease

What is the differential diagnosis of increased gastrin?

Postvagotomy
Gastric outlet obstruction
G-cell hyperplasia
Pernicious anemia
Atrophic gastritis
Short gut syndrome
Renal failure
H_2 blocker, PPI

Which patients should have a gastrin level checked?

Those with recurrent ulcer; ulcer in unusual position (e.g., jejunum) or refractory to medical management; before any operation for ulcer

What lab tests should be performed?

Fasting gastrin level
Postsecretin challenge gastrin level
Calcium (screen for MEN-I)
Chem 7

What are the associated gastrin levels?

NL fasting = 100 pg/ml
ZES fasting = 200–1000 pg/ml
Basal acid secretion; (ZES >15 mEq/hr, nl <10mEq/hr)

What is the secretin stimulation test?

IV secretin is administered and the gastrin level is determined; patients with ZES have a paradoxic increase in gastrin

What are the classic secretin stimulation results?

Lab results with secretin challenge:
NL—Decreased gastrin
ZES—Increased gastrin (increased by >200 pg/ml)

How can you remember the diagnostic stimulation test for Z-E syndrome?

Think: **"Secret Z-E GAS": SECRET**in = **Z-E GAS**trin

What tests are used to evaluate ulcers?

EGD, UGI, or both

What tests are used to localize the tumor?

Octreotide scan (somatostatin receptor scan), abdominal CT, MRI, endoscopic ultrasonography (EUS)

What is the most common site?

Pancreas

What is the most common NONpancreatic site?

Duodenum

What are some other sites?

Stomach, lymph nodes, liver, kidney, ovary

Define "Passaro's triangle."

A.k.a. "gastrinoma triangle," a triangle drawn from the following points:
1. Cystic duct/CBD junction
2. Junction of the second and third portions of the duodenum
3. Neck of the pancreas

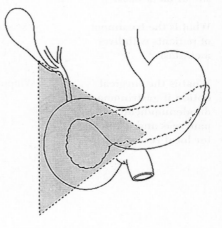

What percentage of gastrinomas are in Passaro's triangle?

≈80%

What is the next step if the tumor cannot be localized?

Exploratory surgery (if tumor is not in pancreas, open duodenum and look), proximal gastric vagotomy if not found

What is the medical treatment?

H_2 blockers, omeprazole, somatostatin

What is the surgical treatment needed for each of the following:
    Tumor in head of pancreas?

1. Enucleation of tumor
2. Whipple procedure if main pancreatic duct is involved

    Tumor in body or tail of pancreas?

Distal pancreatectomy

    Tumor in duodenum?

Local resection

    Unresectable tumor?

High selective vagotomy

What percentage have malignant tumors?

66%

What is the most common site of metastasis?

Liver

What is the treatment of patients with liver metastasis?

Excision, if technically feasible

What is the surgical option if gastrinoma is in duodenum/head of pancreas and is too large for local resection?

Whipple procedure

What is the prognosis with the following procedures:	
Complete excision?	90% 10-year survival
Incomplete excision?	25% 10-year survival

MULTIPLE ENDOCRINE NEOPLASIA

What is it also known as?	MEN syndrome
What is it?	Inherited condition of propensity to develop multiple endocrine tumors
How is it inherited?	Autosomal dominant (but with a significant degree of variation in penetrance)
Which patients should be screened for MEN?	All family members of patients diagnosed with MEN

MEN TYPE I

What is the common eponym?	Wermer's syndrome (Think: **W**ermer = **W**inner = **#1** = type **1**)
What is the gene defect in MEN type I?	Chromosome 11 (Think: 11 = 1)
What are the most common tumors and their incidences?	"PPP": **P**arathyroid hyperplasia ($\approx$90%) **P**ancreatic islet cell tumors ($\approx$66%) Gastrinoma: ZES (50%) Insulinoma (20%) **P**ituitary tumors ($\approx$50%)
How can tumors for MEN-I be remembered?	Think: type **1** = **P**rimary, **P**rimary, **P**rimary = **PPP** = **P**arathyroid, **P**ancreas, **P**ituitary
How can the P's associated with MEN-I be remembered?	All the P's are followed by a vowel: PA, PA, PI
What percentage of patients with MEN-I have parathyroid hyperplasia?	$\approx$90%

What percentage of patients with MEN-I have a gastrinoma?	≈50%
What other tumors (in addition to PPP) are associated with MEN-I?	Adrenal (30%) and thyroid (15%) adenomas

MEN TYPE IIa

What is the common eponym?	Sipple's syndrome (Think: **S**ipple = **S**econd = **#2** = type **2**)
What is the gene defect in MEN type IIa?	RET (Think: re**T** = **T**wo)
What are the most common tumors and their incidences?	"MPH": **M**edullary thyroid carcinoma (100%); Calcitonin secreted **P**heochromocytoma (>33%); Catecholamine excess **H**yperparathyroidism (≈50%); Hypercalcemia
How can the tumors involved with MEN-IIa be remembered?	Think: type **2** = **2 MPH** or **2 M**iles **P**er **H**our = **MPH** = **M**edullary, **P**heochromocytoma, **H**yperparathyroid
How can the P of MPH be remembered?	Followed by the consonant "H"— PHEOCHROMOCYTOMA (remember, the P's of MEN-I are followed by vowels)
What percentage of patients with MEN-IIa have medullary carcinoma of the thyroid?	100%

MEN TYPE IIb

What are the most common abnormalities, their incidences, and symptoms?	"MMMP": **M**ucosal neuromas (100%)—in the nasopharynx, oropharynx, larynx, and conjunctiva **M**edullary thyroid carcinoma (≈85%)— more aggressive than in MEN-IIa **M**arfanoid body habitus (long/lanky) **P**heochromocytoma (≈50%) and found bilaterally

How can the features of MEN-IIb be remembered?	**MMMP** (Think: **3M P**lastics)
How can you remember that MEN-IIb is marfanoid habitus?	Think: "**TO BE** marfanoid" = **II B** marfanoid
What is the anatomic distribution of medullary thyroid carcinoma in MEN-II?	**Almost always bilateral** (non–MEN-II cases are almost always **unilateral!**)
What are the physical findings/signs of MEN-IIb?	Mucosal neuromas (e.g., mouth, eyes) Marfanoid body habitus Pes cavus/planum (large arch of foot/flatfooted) Constipation
What is the most common GI complaint of patients with MEN-IIb?	**Constipation** resulting from ganglioneuromatosis of GI tract
What percentage of pheochromocytomas in MEN-IIa/b are bilateral?	≈70% (but found bilaterally in only 10% of all patients diagnosed with pheochromocytoma)
What is the major difference between MEN-IIa and MEN-IIb?	MEN-IIa = parathyroid hyperplasia MEN-IIb = **no** parathyroid hyperplasia (and neuromas, marfanoid habitus, pes cavus [extensive arch of foot], etc.)
What type of parathyroid disease is associated with MEN-I and MEN-IIa?	**Hyperplasia** (treat with removal of all parathyroid tissue with autotransplant of some of the parathyroid tissue to the forearm)
What percentage of patients with Z-E syndrome have MEN-I?	≈25%

Chapter 58   **Thyroid Gland**

THYROID DISEASE

ANATOMY

Identify the following structures:

1. Pyramidal lobe
2. Right lobe
3. Isthmus
4. Left lobe

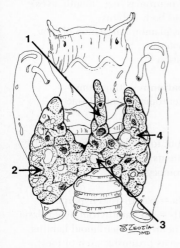

Define the arterial blood supply to the thyroid.

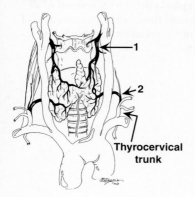

Thyrocervical trunk

Two arteries:

1. Superior thyroid artery (first branch of the external carotid artery)
2. Inferior thyroid artery (branch of the thyrocervical trunk) (IMA artery rare)

What is the venous drainage of the thyroid?

Three veins:
1. Superior thyroid vein
2. **Middle** thyroid vein
3. Inferior thyroid vein

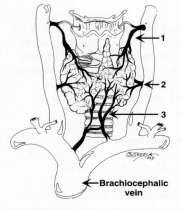

1

2

3

← **Brachiocephalic vein**

Name the thyroid lobe appendage coursing toward the hyoid bone from around the thyroid isthmus.

Pyramidal lobe

What percentage of patients have a pyramidal lobe?

≈50%

What veins do you first see after opening the platysma muscle when performing a thyroidectomy?

Anterior jugular veins

Name the lymph node group around the pyramidal thyroid lobe.

Delphian lymph node group

What is the thyroid isthmus?

Midline tissue border between the left and right thyroid lobes

Which ligament connects the thyroid to the trachea?

Ligament of Berry

What is the IMA (not I.M.A.) artery?

Small inferior artery to the thyroid from the aorta or innominate artery

What percentage of patients have an IMA artery?

≈3%

Name the most posterior extension of the lateral thyroid lobes.	Tubercle of Zuckerkandl
Which paired nerves must be carefully identified during a thyroidectomy?	**Recurrent laryngeal nerves,** which are found in the tracheoesophageal grooves and dive behind the cricothyroid muscle; damage to these nerves paralyzes laryngeal abductors and causes hoarseness if unilateral, and airway obstruction if bilateral
What other nerve is at risk during a thyroidectomy and what are the symptoms?	**Superior laryngeal nerve;** if damaged, patient will have a deeper and quieter voice (unable to hit high pitches)
What is the name of the famous opera singer whose superior laryngeal nerve was injured during thyroidectomy?	**Urban legend** has it that it was Amelita Galli-Curci, but no objective data support such a claim (*Ann Surg* 233:588, April 2001)

PHYSIOLOGY

What is TRH?	**T**hyrotropin-**R**eleasing **H**ormone released from the hypothalamus; causes release of TSH
What is TSH?	**T**hyroid-**S**timulating **H**ormone released by the anterior pituitary; causes release of thyroid hormone from the thyroid
What are the thyroid hormones?	T3 and T4
What is the most active form of thyroid hormone?	T3
What is a negative feedback loop?	T3 and T4 feed back negatively on the anterior pituitary (causing decreased release of TSH in response to TRH)
What is the most common site of conversion of T4 to T3?	Peripheral (e.g., liver)

What is Synthroid® (levothyroxine): T3 or T4?	T4
What is the half-life of Synthroid® (levothyroxine)?	7 days
What do parafollicular cells secrete?	Calcitonin

THYROID NODULE

What percentage of people have a thyroid nodule?	≈5%
What is the differential diagnosis of a thyroid nodule?	Multinodular goiter Adenoma Hyperfunctioning adenoma Cyst Thyroiditis Carcinoma/lymphoma Parathyroid carcinoma
Name three types of nonthyroidal neck masses.	1. Inflammatory lesions (e.g., abscess, lymphadenitis) 2. Congenital lesions (i.e., thyroglossal duct [midline], branchial cleft cyst [lateral]) 3. Malignant lesions: lymphoma, metastases, squamous cell carcinoma
What studies can be used to evaluate a thyroid nodule?	U/S—solid or cystic nodule Fine Needle Aspirate (**FNA**) → cytology ^{123}I scintiscan—hot or cold nodule
What is the DIAGNOSTIC test of choice for thyroid nodule?	FNA
What is the percentage of false negative results on FNA for thyroid nodule?	≈5%

What is meant by a hot versus a cold nodule?

Nodule uptake of IV ^{131}I or ^{99}mT
Hot—Increased ^{123}I uptake = functioning/hyperfunctioning nodule
Cold—Decreased ^{123}I uptake = nonfunctioning nodule

What are the indications for a ^{123}I scintiscan?

1. Nodule with multiple "nondiagnostic" FNAs with low TSH
2. Nodule with thyrotoxicosis and low TSH

What is the role of thyroid suppression of a thyroid nodule?

Diagnostic and therapeutic; administration of thyroid hormone suppresses TSH secretion, and up to half of the benign thyroid nodules will disappear!

In evaluating a thyroid nodule, which of the following suggest thyroid carcinoma:
History?

1. Neck radiation
2. Family history (thyroid cancer, MEN-II)
3. Young age (especially children)
4. Male > female

Signs?

1. Single nodule
2. Cold nodule
3. Increased calcitonin levels
4. Lymphadenopathy
5. Hard, immobile nodule

Symptoms?

1. Voice change (vocal cord paralysis)
2. Dysphagia
3. Discomfort (in neck)
4. Rapid enlargement

What is the most common cause of thyroid enlargement?

Multinodular goiter

What are indications for surgery with multinodular goiter?

Cosmetic deformity, compressive symptoms, cannot rule out cancer

What is Plummer's disease?

Toxic multinodular goiter

MALIGNANT THYROID NODULES

What percentage of cold thyroid nodules are malignant?	≈25% in adults
What percentage of multinodular masses are malignant?	≈1%
What is the treatment of a patient with a history of radiation exposure, thyroid nodule, and negative FNA?	Most experts would remove the nodule surgically (because of the high risk of radiation)
What should be done with thyroid cyst aspirate?	Send to cytopathology

THYROID CARCINOMA

Name the FIVE main types of thyroid carcinoma and their relative percentages.	1. Papillary carcinoma: 80% (**P**opular = **P**apillary) 2. Follicular carcinoma: 10% 3. Medullary carcinoma: 5% 4. Hürthle cell carcinoma: 4% 5. Anaplastic/undifferentiated carcinoma: 1% to 2%
What are the signs/ symptoms?	Mass/nodule, lymphadenopathy; most are **euthyroid**
What comprises the workup?	**FNA,** thyroid U/S, TSH, calcium level, CXR, +/− scintiscan ^{123}I
What oncogenes are associated with thyroid cancers?	*Ras* gene family and RET proto-oncogene

PAPILLARY ADENOCARCINOMA

What is papillary carcinoma's claim to faim?	Most common thyroid cancer (Think: **P**apillary = **P**opular) = 80% of all thyroid cancers
What is the environmental risk?	Radiation exposure

What is the average age?	30–40 years
What is the sex distribution?	Female > male; 2:1
What are the associated histologic findings?	Psammoma bodies (Remember, **P** = **P**sammoma = **P**apillary)
Describe the route and rate of spread.	Most spread via lymphatics (cervical adenopathy); spread occurs slowly
^{131}I uptake?	Good uptake
What is the 10-year survival rate?	≈95%
What is the treatment for: <1.5 cm and no history of neck radiation exposure?	Options: 1. Thyroid lobectomy and isthmectomy 2. Near-total thyroidectomy 3. Total thyroidectomy
>1.5 cm, bilateral, + cervical node metastasis OR a history of radiation exposure?	Total thyroidectomy
What is the treatment for: Lateral palpable cervical lymph nodes?	Modified neck dissection (ipsilateral)
Central?	Central neck dissection
Do positive cervical nodes affect the prognosis?	NO!
What is a "lateral aberrant thyroid" in papillary cancer?	Misnomer—it is metastatic papillary carcinoma to a lymph node
What postoperative medication should be administered?	Thyroid hormone replacement, to suppress TSH
What is a postoperative treatment option for papillary carcinoma?	Postoperative ^{131}I scan can locate residual tumor and distant metastasis that can be treated with ablative doses of ^{131}I

What is the most common site of distant metastases?	Pulmonary (lungs)
What are the "P's" of papillary thyroid cancer (7)?	**P**apillary cancer: **P**opular (most common) **P**sammoma bodies **P**alpable lymph nodes (spreads most commonly by lymphatics, seen in ≈33% of patients) **P**ositive ^{131}I uptake **P**ositive prognosis **P**ostoperative ^{131}I scan to diagnose/treat metastases **P**ulmonary metastases

FOLLICULAR ADENOCARCINOMA

What percentage of thyroid cancers does it comprise?	≈10%
Describe the nodule consistency.	Rubbery, encapsulated
What is the route of spread?	Hematogenous, more aggressive than papillary adenocarcinoma
What is the male:female ratio?	1:3
^{131}I uptake?	Good uptake
What is the overall 10-year survival rate?	≈85%
Can the diagnosis be made by FNA?	No; tissue structure is needed for a diagnosis of cancer
What histologic findings define malignancy in follicular cancer?	Capsular or blood vessel invasion
What is the most common site of distant metastasis?	Bone
What is the treatment for follicular cancer?	Total thyroidectomy

What is the postoperative treatment option if malignant?	Postoperative ^{131}I scan for diagnosis/treatment
What are the 4 "F's" of follicular cancer?	Follicular cancer: Far-away metastasis (spreads hematogenously) Female (3 to 1 ratio) FNA ... NOT (FNA CANNOT diagnose cancer) Favorable prognosis

HÜRTHLE CELL THYROID CANCER

What is it?	Thyroid cancer of the Hürthle cells
What percentage of thyroid cancers does it comprise?	≈5%
What is the cell of origin?	Follicular cells
^{131}I uptake?	No uptake
How is the diagnosis made?	FNA can identify cells, but malignancy can be determined only by tissue histology (like follicular cancer)
What is the route of metastasis?	Lymphatic > hematogenous
What is the treatment?	Total thyroidectomy
What is the 10-year survival rate?	80%

MEDULLARY CARCINOMA

What percentage of all thyroid cancers does it comprise?	≈5%
With what other conditions is it associated?	MEN type II; autosomal-dominant genetic transmission
Histology?	Amyloid (aMyloid = Medullary)
What does it secrete?	Calcitonin (tumor marker)

What is the appropriate stimulation test?	Pentagastrin (causes an increase in calcitonin)
Describe the route of spread.	Lymphatic and hematogenous distant metastasis
How is the diagnosis made?	FNA
^{131}I uptake?	Poor uptake
What is the associated genetic mutation?	RET proto-oncogene
What is the female/male ratio?	Female > male; 1.5:1
What is the 10-year survival rate?	80% without LN involvement 45% with LN spread
What should all patients with medullary thyroid cancer also be screened for?	MEN II: pheochromocytoma, hyperparathyroidism
If medullary thyroid carcinoma and pheochromocytoma are found, which one is operated on first?	Pheochromocytoma
What is the treatment?	Total thyroidectomy and **median lymph node dissection** Modified neck dissection, if lateral cervical nodes are positive

What are the "M's" of medullary carcinoma?	Medullary cancer:
	    MEN II
	    a**M**yloid
	    Median lymph node dissection
	    Modified neck dissection if lateral nodes are positive

ANAPLASTIC CARCINOMA

What is it also known as?	Undifferentiated carcinoma
What is it?	Undifferentiated cancer arising in ≈75% of previously differentiated thyroid cancers (most commonly, follicular carcinoma)

What percentage of all thyroid cancers does it comprise?	$\approx 2\%$
What is the gender preference?	Women > men
What are the associated histologic findings?	Giant cells, spindle cells
^{131}I uptake?	Very poor uptake
How is the diagnosis made?	FNA (large tumor)
What is the major differential diagnosis?	Thyroid lymphoma (much better prognosis!)
What is the treatment of the following disorders:	
Small tumors?	Total thyroidectomy + XRT/chemotherapy
Airway compromise?	Debulking surgery and tracheostomy, XRT/chemotherapy
What is the prognosis?	Dismal, because most patients are at stage IV at presentation (3% alive at 5 years)

MISCELLANEOUS

What laboratory value must be followed postoperatively after a thyroidectomy?	**Calcium** decreased secondary to parathyroid damage; during lobectomy, the parathyroids must be spared and their blood supply protected; if blood supply is compromised intraoperatively, they can be autografted into the sternocleidomastoid muscle or forearm
What is the differential diagnosis of postoperative dyspnea after a thyroidectomy?	Neck hematoma (remove sutures and clot at the **bedside**) **Bilateral** recurrent laryngeal nerve damage
What is a "lateral aberrant rest" of the thyroid?	Misnomer: It is **papillary** cancer of a lymph node from metastasis

BENIGN THYROID DISEASE

What is the most common cause of hyperthyroidism?	Graves' disease
What is Graves' disease?	Diffuse goiter with hyperthyroidism, exophthalmos, and pretibial myxedema
What is the etiology?	Caused by circulating **antibodies** that stimulate TSH receptors on follicular cells of the thyroid and cause deregulated production of thyroid hormones (i.e., hyperthyroidism)
What is the female:male ratio?	6:1
What specific physical finding is associated with Graves'?	Exophthalmos
How is the diagnosis made?	Increased T3, T4, and anti-TSH receptor antibodies, decreased TSH, global uptake of ^{131}I radionuclide
Name treatment option modalities for Graves' disease.	1. **Medical blockade:** iodide, propranolol, propylthiouracil (PTU), methimazole, Lugol's solution (potassium iodide) 2. **Radioiodide ablation:** most popular therapy 3. **Surgical resection** (bilateral subtotal thyroidectomy)
What are the possible indications for surgical resection?	Suspicious nodule; if patient is noncompliant or refractory to medicines, pregnant, a child, or if patient refuses radioiodide therapy
What is the major complication of radioiodide or surgery for Graves' disease?	Hypothyroidism
What does PTU stand for?	**P**ropyl**T**hio**U**racil

How does PTU work?

1. Inhibits incorporation of iodine into T4/T3 (by blocking peroxidase oxidation of iodide to iodine)
2. Inhibits peripheral conversion of T4 to T3

How does methimazole work?

Inhibits incorporation of iodine into T4/T3 **only** (by blocking peroxidase oxidation of iodide to iodine)

TOXIC MULTINODULAR GOITER

What is it also known as?

Plummer's disease

What is it?

Multiple thyroid nodules with one or more nodules producing thyroid hormone, resulting in hyperfunctioning thyroid (hyperthyroidism or a "toxic" thyroid state)

What medication may bring on hyperthyroidism with a multinodular goiter?

Amiodarone (or any iodine-containing medication/contrast)

How is the hyperfunctioning nodule(s) localized?

^{131}I radionuclide scan

What is the treatment?

Surgically remove hyperfunctioning nodule(s) with lobectomy or near total thyroidectomy

What is Pemberton's sign?

Large goiter causes plethora of head with raising of both arms

THYROIDITIS

What are the features of ACUTE thyroiditis?

Painful, swollen thyroid; fever; overlying skin erythema; dysphagia

What is the cause of ACUTE thyroiditis?

Bacteria (usually *Streptococcus* or *Staphylococcus*), usually caused by a thyroglossal fistula or anatomic variant

What is the treatment of ACUTE thyroiditis?

Antibiotics, drainage of abscess, needle aspiration for culture; most patients need definitive surgery later to remove the fistula

What are the features of SUBACUTE thyroiditis?

Glandular swelling, tenderness, often follows URI, elevated ESR

What is the cause of SUBACUTE thyroiditis?

Viral infection

What is the treatment of SUBACUTE thyroiditis?

Supportive: NSAIDS, ± steroids

What is De Quervain's thyroiditis?

Just another name for SUBACUTE thyroiditis caused by a virus (Think: De QuerVain = **V**irus)

How can the differences between etiologies of ACUTE and SUBACUTE thyroiditis be remembered?

Alphabetically: **A** before **S**, **B** before **V** (i.e., **A**cute before **S**ubacute and **B**acterial before **V**iral and thus: **A**cute = **B**acterial and **S**ubacute = **V**iral)

What are the common causative bacteria in acute suppurative thyroiditis?

Streptococcus or *Staphylococcus*

What are the two types of chronic thyroiditis?

1. Hashimoto's thyroiditis
2. Riedel's thyroiditis

What are the features of Hashimoto's (chronic) thyroiditis?

Firm and rubbery gland, 95% in women, lymphocyte invasion

What is the claim to fame of Hashimoto's disease?

Most common cause of hypothyroidism in the United States

What is the etiology of Hashimoto's disease?

Autoimmune (Think: Hashim**OTO** = **AUTO**; thus, Hashimoto = autoimmune)

What lab tests should be performed to diagnose Hashimoto's disease?

Antithyroglobulin and microsomal antibodies

What is the medical treatment for Hashimoto's thyroiditis?

Thyroid hormone replacement if hypothyroid (surgery is reserved for compressive symptoms and/or if cancer needs to be ruled out)

What is Riedel's thyroiditis?	Benign inflammatory thyroid enlargement **with fibrosis** of thyroid Patients present with painless, large thyroid Fibrosis may involve surrounding tissues
What is the treatment for Riedel's thyroiditis?	Surgical tracheal decompression, thyroid hormone replacement as needed— possibly steroids/tamoxifen if refractory

Chapter 59   Parathyroid

ANATOMY

How many parathyroids are there?	Usually **four** (two superior and two inferior)
What percentage of patients have five parathyroid glands?	≈5% (Think: 5 = 5)
What percentage of patients have three parathyroid glands?	≈10%
What is the usual position of the inferior parathyroid glands?	Posterior and lateral behind the thyroid and below the inferior thyroid artery
What is the most common site of an "extra" gland?	Thymus gland
What percentage of patients have a parathyroid gland in the mediastinum?	≈1%
If only three parathyroid glands are found at surgery, where can the fourth one be hiding?	Thyroid gland Thymus/mediastinum Carotid sheath Tracheoesophageal groove Behind the esophagus

What is the embryologic origin of the following structures:

Superior parathyroid glands?	Fourth pharyngeal pouch
Inferior parathyroid glands?	Third pharyngeal pouch (counterintuitive)

What supplies blood to the parathyroid glands?

Inferior thyroid artery

What percentage of patients have all four parathyroid glands supplied by the inferior thyroid arteries exclusively?

≈80%

What is DiGeorge's syndrome?

Congenital absence of the parathyroid glands and the thymus

What is the most common cause of hypercalcemia in hospitalized patients?

Cancer

What is the most common cause of hypercalcemia in outpatients?

Hyperparathyroidism

PHYSIOLOGY

What cell type produces PTH?

Chief cells produce **P**ara**T**hyroid **H**ormone (**PTH**)

What are the major actions of PTH?

Increases blood **calcium** levels (takes from bone breakdown, GI absorption, increased resorption from kidney, excretion of phosphate by kidney), **decreases** serum phosphate

How does vitamin D work?

Increases intestinal absorption of calcium and phosphate

Where is calcium absorbed?

Duodenum and proximal jejunum

HYPERPARATHYROIDISM (HPTH)

Define primary HPTH.	Increased secretion of PTH by parathyroid gland(s); marked by elevated calcium, low phosphorus
Define secondary HPTH.	Increased serum PTH resulting from calcium wasting caused by **renal failure or decreased GI calcium absorption,** rickets or osteomalacia; calcium levels are usually **low**
Define tertiary HPTH.	Persistent HPTH after correction of secondary hyperparathyroidism; results from autonomous PTH secretion not responsive to the normal negative feedback due to elevated Ca^{++} levels
What are the methods of imaging the parathyroids?	Surgical operation Ultrasound **Sestamibi scan** ^{201}TI (technetium)–thallium subtraction scan CT/MRI A-gram (rare) Venous sampling for PTH (rare)
What are the indications for a localizing preoperative study?	**Reoperation** for recurrent hyperparathyroidism
What is the most common cause of primary HPTH?	Adenoma (>85%)
What are the etiologies of primary HPTH and percentages?	**Adenoma** (≈85%) Hyperplasia (≈10%) Carcinoma (≈1%)
What is the incidence of primary HPTH in the United States?	≈1/1000–4000
What are the risk factors for primary HPTH?	Family history, MEN-I and MEN-IIa, irradiation

What are the signs/ symptoms of primary HPTH hypercalcemia?

"Stones, bones, groans, and psychiatric overtones":
  Stones: Kidney stones
  Bones: Bone pain, pathologic fractures, subperiosteal resorption
  Groans: Muscle pain and weakness, pancreatitis, gout, constipation
  Psychiatric overtones: Depression, anorexia, anxiety
  Other symptoms: Polydipsia, weight loss, HTN (10%), polyuria, lethargy

What is the "33 to 1" rule?

Most patients with primary HPTH have a ratio of serum (Cl^-) to phosphate ≥ 33

What plain x-ray findings are classic for HPTH?

Subperiosteal bone resorption (usually in hand digits; said to be "pathognomonic" for HPTH!)

How is primary HPTH diagnosed?

Labs—elevated PTH (hypercalcemia, ↓ phosphorus, ↑ chloride); urine calcium should be checked for familial hypocalciuric hypercalcemia

What is familial hypocalciuric hypercalcemia?

Familial (autosomal-dominant) inheritance of a condition of **asymptomatic** hypercalcemia and low urine calcium, with or without elevated PTH; in contrast, hypercalcemia from HPTH results in high levels of urine calcium
Note: Surgery to remove parathyroid glands is not indicated for this diagnosis

How many of the glands are USUALLY affected by the following conditions:
  Hyperplasia?   4

  Adenoma?   1

  Carcinoma?   1

What percentage of adenomas are not single but found in more than one gland?

$\approx 5\%$

What is the differential diagnosis of hypercalcemia?

"CHIMPANZEES":

    Calcium overdose

    Hyperparathyroidism (1°/2°/3°),

    Hyperthyroidism, **H**ypocalciuric **H**ypercalcemia (familial)

    Immobility/**I**atrogenic (thiazide diuretics)

    Metastasis/**M**ilk alkali syndrome (rare)

    Paget's disease (bone)

    Addison's disease/acromegaly

    Neoplasm (colon, lung, breast, prostate, multiple myeloma)

    Zollinger-Ellison syndrome

    Excessive vitamin D

    Excessive vitamin A

    Sarcoid

What is the initial medical treatment of hypercalcemia (1° HPTH)?

Medical—IV fluids, furosemide—**NOT** thiazide diuretics

What is the definitive treatment of HPTH in the following cases:

Primary HPTH resulting from HYPERPLASIA?

Neck exploration removing all parathyroid glands and leaving at least 30 mg of parathyroid tissue placed in the forearm muscles (nondominant arm, of course!)

Primary HPTH resulting from parathyroid ADENOMA?

Surgically remove adenoma (send for frozen section) and biopsy all abnormally enlarged parathyroid glands (some experts biopsy all glands)

Primary HPTH resulting from parathyroid CARCINOMA?

Remove carcinoma, ipsilateral thyroid lobe, and all enlarged lymph nodes (modified radical neck dissection for LN metastases)

Secondary HPTH?

Correct calcium and phosphate; perform renal transplantation (no role for parathyroid surgery)

Tertiary HPTH?	Correct calcium and phosphate; perform surgical operation to remove all parathyroid glands and reimplant 30 to 40 mg in the forearm if **REFRACTORY** to medical management
Why place 30 to 40 mg of sliced parathyroid gland in the forearm?	To retain parathyroid function; if HPTH recurs, remove some of the parathyroid gland from the easily accessible forearm
What must be ruled out in the patient with HPTH from hyperplasia?	MEN type I and MEN type IIa
What carcinomas are commonly associated with hypercalcemia?	**Breast cancer metastases,** prostate cancer, kidney cancer, lung cancer, pancreatic cancer, multiple myeloma
What is the most likely diagnosis if a patient has a PALPABLE neck mass, hypercalcemia, and elevated PTH?	Parathyroid carcinoma (vast majority of other causes of primary HPTH have nonpalpable parathyroids)

PARATHYROID CARCINOMA

What is it?	Primary carcinoma of the parathyroid gland
What is the number of glands usually affected?	1
What are the signs/ symptoms?	Hypercalcemia, elevated PTH, **PALPABLE** parathyroid gland (50%), pain in neck, recurrent laryngeal nerve paralysis (change in voice), hypercalcemic crisis (usually associated with calcium levels >14)
What is the common tumor marker?	**H**uman **C**horionic **G**onadotropin (**HCG**)
What is the treatment?	Surgical resection of parathyroid mass with ipsilateral thyroid lobectomy, ipsilateral lymph node resection

What percentage of all cases of primary HPTH are caused by parathyroid carcinoma?	1%

POSTOPERATIVE COMPLICATIONS OF PARATHYROIDECTOMY

What are the possible postoperative complications after a parathyroidectomy?	Recurrent nerve injury (unilateral: voice change; bilateral: airway obstruction), neck hematoma (open at bedside if breathing is compromised), hypocalcemia, superior laryngeal nerve injury
What is "hungry bone syndrome"?	Severe hypocalcemia seen after surgical correction of HPTH as chronically calcium-deprived bone aggressively absorbs calcium
What are the signs/ symptoms of postoperative hypocalcemia?	Perioral tingling, paresthesia, +Chvostek's sign, +Trousseau's sign, +tetany
What is the treatment of hypoparathyroidism?	Acute: IV calcium Chronic: PO calcium, and vitamin D
What is parathyromatosis?	Multiple small hyperfunctioning parathyroid tissue masses found over the neck and mediastinum—thought to be from congenital rests or spillage during surgery—remove surgically (RARE)

Chapter 60

Spleen and Splenectomy

Which arteries supply the spleen?	Splenic artery (a branch of the celiac trunk) and the short gastric arteries that arise from the gastroepiploic arteries
What is the venous drainage of the spleen?	**Portal** vein, via the splenic vein and the left gastroepiploic vein

What is said to "tickle" the spleen?

Tail of the pancreas

What percentage of people have an accessory spleen?

≈20%

What percentage of the total body platelets are stored in the spleen?

33%

What are the functions of the human spleen?

Filters abnormal RBCs (does NOT store RBCs like canine spleen!), stores platelets, produces tuftsin and properdin (opsins), produces antibodies (especially IGM) and is site of phagocytosis

What is "delayed splenic rupture"?

Subcapsular hematoma or pseudoaneurysm may rupture some time after blunt trauma, causing "delayed splenic rupture"; rupture classically occurs about 2 weeks after the injury and presents with shock/abdominal pain

What are the signs/symptoms of ruptured/injured spleen?

Hemoperitoneum and Kehr's sign, LUQ abdominal pain, Ballance's sign

What is Kehr's sign?

Left shoulder pain seen with splenic rupture

What is Ballance's sign?

LUQ dullness to percussion

What is Seagesser's sign?

Phrenic nerve compression causing neck tenderness in splenic rupture

How is a spleen injury diagnosed?

Abdominal CT, **if the patient is stable;** DPL or FAST exam if the patient is unstable

What is the treatment?

1. Nonoperative in a stable patient with an isolated splenic injury without hilar involvement/complete rupture
2. If patient is unstable, DPL/FAST laparotomy with splenorrhaphy or splenectomy
3. Embolization is an option in selected patients

What is a splenorrhaphy?

Splenic salvage operation: wrapping vicral mesh, aid of topical hemostatic agents or partial splenectomy, sutures (buttressed)

What are the other indications for splenectomy:
Malignant diseases?

Hodgkin's staging not conclusive by CT scan (rare)
Splenic tumors (primary/metastatic/locally invasive)
Hypersplenism caused by other leukemias/non-Hodgkin's lymphomas

Anemias?

Medullary fibrosis with myeloid metaplasia
Hereditary elliptocytosis
Sickle cell anemia (rare, most autosplenectomize)
Pyruvate kinase deficiency
Autoimmune hemolytic anemia
Hereditary spherocytosis
Thalassemias (e.g., β-thalassemia major a.k.a. Cooley's)

Thrombocytopenia?

ITP (**I**diopathic **T**hrombocytopenic **P**urpura)
TTP (**T**hrombotic **T**hrombocytopenic **P**urpura)

Miscellaneous indications?

Variceal bleeding with splenic vein thrombosis, Gaucher's disease, splenic abscess, refractory splenic cysts, hypersplenism, Felty's syndrome

Is G6PD deficiency an indication for splenectomy?

NO

What are the possible postsplenectomy complications?

Thrombocytosis, subphrenic abscess, atelectasis, pancreatitis gastric dilation, and **O**verwhelming **P**ost**S**plenectomy **S**epsis (**OPSS**)

What causes OPSS?

Increased susceptibility to fulminant bacteremia, meningitis, or pneumonia because of loss of splenic function

What is the incidence of OPSS in adults?	<1%
What is the incidence and overall mortality of OPSS in children?	1% to 2% with 50% mortality rate
What is the typical presentation of OPSS?	Fever, lethargy, common cold, sore throat, URI followed by confusion, shock, and coma with death ensuing within 24 hours in up to 50% of patients
What are the common organisms associated with OPSS?	**Encapsulated:** *Streptococcus pneumoniae, Neisseria meningitides, H. influenzae*
What is the most common bacteria in OPSS?	*Streptococcus pneumoniae*
What is the preventive treatment of OPSS?	Vaccinations for pneumococcus, *H. influenzae,* and meningococcus Prophylactic penicillin for all minor infections/illnesses and immediate medical care if febrile illness develops
What is the best time to give immunizations to splenectomy patients?	**Preoperatively,** if at all possible If emergent, then *2 weeks* postoperatively
What lab tests are abnormal after splenectomy?	WBC count increases by 50% over the baseline; marked **thrombocytosis** occurs; RBC smear is abnormal
What are the findings on postsplenectomy RBC smear?	Peripheral smear will show Pappenheimer bodies, Howell-Jolly bodies, and Heinz bodies
When and how should thrombocytosis be treated?	When platelet count is >1 million, most surgeons will treat with **aspirin**
What is the most common cause of splenic vein thrombosis?	Pancreatitis
What opsonins does the spleen produce?	**PRO**perdin, **TUF**tsin (Think: "**PRO**fessionally **TUF** spleen")

What is the most common cause of ISOLATED GASTRIC varices?

Splenic vein thrombosis (usually from pancreatitis)

What is the treatment of gastric varices caused by splenic vein thrombosis?

Splenectomy

Which patients develop hyposplenism?

Patients with ulcerative colitis

What vaccinations should every patient with a splenectomy receive?

Pneumococcus
Meningococcus
Haemophilus influenzae type B

Define hypersplenism.

Hyperfunctioning spleen
Documented loss of blood elements
    (WBC, Hct, platelets)
Large spleen (splenomegaly)
Hyperactive bone marrow (trying to keep
    up with loss of blood elements)

Define splenomegaly.

Enlarged spleen

What is idiopathic thrombocytopenic purpura (ITP)?

Autoimmune (antiplatelet antibodies IgG in >90% of patients) platelet destruction leading to troublesome bleeding and purpura

What is the most common cause of failure to correct thrombocytopenia after splenectomy for ITP?

Missed accessory spleen

What are the "I's" of ITP?

Immune etiology (**I**gG antiplatelets ABs)
Immunosuppressive treatment (initially
    treated with steroids)
Immune globulin
Improvement with splenectomy (75% of
    patients have improved platelet counts
    after splenectomy)

What is TTP?

Thrombotic **T**hrombocytopenic **P**urpura

What is the treatment of choice for TTP?	Plasmapheresis (splenectomy reserved as a last resort—very rare)
What is the most common physical finding of portal hypertension?	Splenomegaly

---

Chapter 61

Surgically Correctable HTN

What is it?	Hypertension caused by conditions that are amenable to surgical correction
What percentage of patients with HTN have a surgically correctable cause?	≈7%
What diseases that cause HTN are surgically correctable?	Think **"CAN I CHURP?"**: **C**ushing's syndrome **A**ortic coarctation **N**euroblastoma/neoplasia **I**ncreased intracranial pressure **C**onn's syndrome (primary hyperaldosteronism) **H**yperparathyroidism/hyperthyroidism **U**nilateral renal parenchymal disease **R**enal artery stenosis **P**heochromocytoma
What is the formula for pressure?	Pressure = flow × resistance or **P = F × R** (Think: **P**ower **FoR**ward); thus, an increase in flow, resistance, or both, results in an increase in pressure

Chapter 62

Soft Tissue Sarcomas and Lymphomas

SOFT TISSUE SARCOMAS

What are they?	Soft tissue tumors, derived from mesoderm
Sarcoma **means what in GREEK?**	"Fish flesh"
Sarcomas are more common in upper or lower extremities?	50% of sarcomas are in the extremities and are 3.5× **more** common in the **lower** extremity (thigh)
How common are they?	0.6% of malignant tumors
What is the median age at diagnosis?	55 years
What are the risk factors?	"RALES": **R**adiation **A**IDS (Immunosuppression) **L**ymphedema **E**xposure to chemicals **S**yndromes (e.g., Gardner's/Li-Fraumeni)

Name the following types of malignant sarcoma:

Fat	Liposarcoma
Gastrointestinal	**GIST** (**G**astro**I**ntestinal **S**tromal **T**umor)
Myofibroblast	Malignant fibrous histiocytoma
Striated muscle	Rhabdomyosarcoma
Vascular endothelium	Angiosarcoma
Fibroblast	Fibrosarcoma

Lymph vessel	Lymphangiosarcoma
Peripheral nerve	Malignant neurilemmoma or schwannoma
AIDS	Kaposi's sarcoma
Lymphedema	Lymphangiosarcoma
What are the signs/ symptoms?	Soft tissue mass; pain from compression of adjacent structures, often noticed after minor trauma to area of mass
How do most sarcomas metastasize?	Hematogenously (i.e., via blood)
What is the most common location and route of metastasis?	**Lungs** via hematogenous route
What tests should be done in the preoperative workup?	CXR, ± chest CT, LFTs
What are the three most common malignant sarcomas in adults?	Fibrous histiocytoma (25%) Liposarcoma (20%) Leiomyosarcoma (15%)
What are the two most common in children?	Rhabdomyosarcoma (about 50%), fibrosarcoma (20%)
What is the most common type to metastasize to the lymph nodes?	Malignant fibrous histiocytoma
What is the most common sarcoma of the retroperitoneum?	Liposarcoma
How do sarcomas locally invade?	Usually along anatomic planes such as fascia, vessels, etc.
How is the diagnosis made?	Imaging workup—MRI is superior to CT at distinguishing the tumor from adjacent structures Mass <3 cm: excisional biopsy **Mass >3 cm:** incisional biopsy or **core biopsy**

Define excisional biopsy.

Biopsy by removing the **entire** mass

Define incisional biopsy.

Biopsy by removing a **piece** of the mass

What is the orientation of incision for incisional biopsy of a suspected extremity sarcoma?

Longitudinal, not transverse, so that the incision can be incorporated in a future resection if biopsy for sarcoma is positive

Define core biopsy.

Large-bore needle that takes a core of tissue (like a soil sample)

What determines histologic grade of sarcomas?

1. Differentiation
2. Mitotic count
3. Tumor necrosis
Grade 1 = well differentiated
Grade 2 = moderately differentiated
Grade 3 = poorly differentiated

Define the following American Joint Committee for Cancer Staging (AJCC) Sarcoma Stages:

Stage I

Well differentiated (**grade 1**), any size, no nodes, no metastases

Stage IIA

<5 cm, **grade 2 or grade 3**

Stage IIB

>5 cm, **grade 2**

Stage III

Positive nodes or >5 cm and **grade 3**

Stage IV

Distant metastases

What is a pseudocapsule and what is its importance?

Outer layer of a sarcoma that represents compressed malignant cells; microscopic extensions of tumor cells invade through the pseudocapsule into adjacent structures—thus, definitive therapy must include a wide margin of resection to account for this phenomenon and not just be "shelled-out" like a benign growth

What is the most important factor in the prognosis?

Histologic grade of the primary lesion

What is the treatment?	Surgical resection and radiation (with or without chemotherapy)
What surgical margins are obtained?	2 cm (1 cm minimum)
What is the "limb-sparing" surgery for extremity sarcoma?	Avoidance of amputation with local resection and chemoradiation
What is the treatment of pulmonary metastasis?	Surgical resection for isolated lesions
What tests should be done in the follow-up?	Physical examination, CXR, repeat CT/ MRI of the area of resection to look for recurrence
What syndrome of lymphan-giosarcoma arises in chronic lymphedema after axillary dissection for breast cancer?	Stewart-Treves syndrome
What syndrome is associated with breast cancer and soft tissue sarcoma?	Li-Fraumeni syndrome (p53 tumor suppressor gene mutation)

LYMPHOMA

How is the diagnosis made?	Cervical or axillary node excisional biopsy
What cell type is associated with the histology of Hodgkin's disease?	Reed-Sternberg cells
What are the four histopathologic types of Hodgkin's disease?	1. Nodular sclerosing (most common; ≈50% of cases) 2. Mixed cellularity 3. Lymphocyte predominant (best prognosis) 4. Lymphocyte depleted
What are the indications for a "staging laparotomy" in Hodgkin's disease?	Rarely performed Most experts rely on CT scans, PET scans, bone marrow biopsy, and other directed imaging and biopsies

Define the stages (Ann Arbor) of Hodgkin's disease:

Stage I

Single lymph node region (Think: Stage **1** = **1** region)

Stage II

Two or more lymph node regions on **the same side of the diaphragm** (Think: Stage **2** = >**2** regions)

Stage III

Involvement on **both** sides of the diaphragm

Stage IV

Diffuse and/or disseminated involvement

What is stage A Hodgkin's?

Asymptomatic (Think: **A**symptomatic = stage **A**)

What is stage B Hodgkin's?

Symptomatic: weight loss, fever, night sweats, etc. (Think: Stage **B** = **B**ad)

What is the "E" on the staging?

Extralymphatic site involvement (**E** = **E**xtralymphatic)

What treatments are used for low versus advanced stage Hodgkin's lymphoma?

Low stage: radiotherapy
Advanced stage: chemotherapy

What percentage of patients with Hodgkin's disease can be cured?

≈80%

GI LYMPHOMA

What is it?

Non-Hodgkin's lymphoma arising in the GI tract

What is the risk factor for gastric lymphoma?

Helicobacter pylori

What are the signs/ symptoms?

Abdominal pain, obstruction, GI hemorrhage, GI tract perforation, fatigue

What is the treatment of intestinal lymphoma?

Surgical resection with removal of draining lymph nodes and chemotherapy

What is the most common site of primary GI tract lymphoma?

Stomach (66%) (see *Maltoma*, p. 281)

Chapter 63   Skin Lesions

**What are the most common
skin cancers?**

1. Basal cell carcinoma (75%)
2. Squamous cell carcinoma (20%)
3. Melanoma (4%)

**What is the most common
fatal skin cancer?**

Melanoma

**What is malignant
melanoma?**

A redundancy! All melanomas are
considered malignant!

SQUAMOUS CELL CARCINOMA

What is it?

Carcinoma arising from epidermal cells

**What are the most common
sites?**

Head, neck, and hands

What are the risk factors?

Sun exposure, pale skin, chronic
inflammatory process, immunosuppression,
xeroderma pigmentosum, arsenic

**What is a precursor skin
lesion?**

Actinic keratosis

What are the signs/symptoms?

Raised, slightly pigmented skin lesion;
ulceration/exudate; chronic scab; itching

How is the diagnosis made?

Small lesion—excisional biopsy
Large lesions—incisional biopsy

What is the treatment?

Small lesion (<1 cm): Excise with 0.5-cm
  margin
Large lesion (>1 cm): Resect with 1- to
  2-cm margins of normal tissue (large
  lesions may require skin graft/flap)

**What is the dreaded sign of
metastasis?**

Palpable lymph nodes (remove involved
lymph nodes)

What is Marjolin's ulcer?

Squamous cell carcinoma that arises in an
area of chronic inflammation (e.g., chronic
fistula, burn wound, osteomyelitis)

What is the prognosis?	Excellent if totally excised (95% cure rate); most patients with positive lymph node metastasis eventually die from metastatic disease
What is the treatment for solitary metastasis?	Surgical resection

BASAL CELL CARCINOMA

What is it?	Carcinoma arising in the germinating basal cell layer of epithelial cells
What are the risk factors?	Sun exposure, fair skin, radiation, chronic dermatitis, xeroderma pigmentosum
What are the most common sites?	Head, neck, and hands
What are the signs/ symptoms?	Slow-growing skin mass (chronic, scaly); scab; ulceration, with or without pigmentation, often described as "pearl-like"
How is the diagnosis made?	Excisional or incisional biopsy
What is the treatment?	Resection with 5-mm margins (2-mm margin in cosmetically sensitive areas)
What is the risk of metastasis?	Very low (recur locally)

MISCELLANEOUS SKIN LESIONS

What is an Epidermal Inclusion Cyst?	**EIC** = Benign subcutaneous cyst filled with epidermal cells (should be removed surgically) filled with waxy material; no clinical difference from a sebaceous cyst
What is a sebaceous cyst?	Benign subcutaneous cyst filled with sebum (waxy, paste-like substance) from a blocked sweat gland (should be removed with a small area of skin that includes the blocked gland); may become infected; much less common than EIC

What is actinic keratosis?

Premalignant skin lesion from sun exposure; seen as a scaly skin lesion (surgical removal eliminates the 20% risk of cancer transformation)

What is seborrheic keratosis?

Benign pigmented lesion in the elderly; observe or treat by excision (especially if there is any question of melanoma), curettage, or topical agents

How to remember actinic keratosis vs. seborrheic keratosis malignant potential?

Actinic **K**eratosis = **AK** = **A**sset **K**icker = premalignant
Seborrheic **K**eratosis = **SK** = **S**oft **K**icker = benign

What is Bowen's disease of the skin?

Squamous carcinoma in situ (should be removed or destroyed, thereby removing the problem)

What is "Mohs" surgery?

Mohs technique or surgery: repeats thin excision until margins are clear by microscopic review (named after Dr. Mohs)—used to minimize collateral skin excision (e.g., on the face)

Chapter 64   Melanoma

What is it?

Neoplastic disorder produced by malignant transformation of the melanocyte; melanocytes are derived from neural crest cells

Which patients are at greatest risk?

White patients with blonde/red hair, fair skin, freckling, a history of blistering sunburns, blue/green eyes, actinic keratosis
Male > female

What are the most common sites (3)?

1. Skin
2. Eyes
3. Anus
(Think: **SEA** = **S**kin, **E**yes, **A**nus)

What is the most common site in African Americans?	Palms of the hands, soles of the feet (acral lentiginous melanoma)
What characteristics are suggestive of melanoma?	Usually a pigmented lesion with an irregular border, irregular surface, or irregular coloration Other clues: darkening of a pigmented lesion, development of pigmented satellite lesions, irregular margins or surface elevations, notching, recent or rapid enlargement, erosion or ulceration of surface, pruritus
What are the "ABCDs" of melanoma?	**A**symmetry **B**order irregularity **C**olor variation **D**iameter >6 mm and **D**ark lesion
What are the associated risk factors?	Severe sunburn before age 18, giant congenital nevi, family history, race (White), ultraviolet radiation (sun), multiple dysplastic nevi
How does location differ in men and women?	Men get more lesions on the trunk; women on the extremities
Which locations are unusual?	Noncutaneous regions, such as mucous membranes of the vulva/vagina, anorectum, esophagus, and choroidal layer of the eye
What is the most common site of melanoma in men?	Back (33%)
What is the most common site of melanoma in women?	Legs (33%)
What are the four major histologic types?	1. Superficial spreading 2. Lentigo maligna 3. Acral lentiginous 4. Nodular
Define the following terms: **Superficial spreading melanoma**	Occurs in both sun-exposed and non-exposed areas; **most common** of all melanomas (75%)

Lentigo maligna melanoma	Malignant cells that are superficial, found usually in elderly patients on the head or neck Called "Hutchinson's freckle" if noninvasive Least aggressive type; very good prognosis Accounts for <10% of all melanomas
Acral lentiginous melanoma	Occurs on the palms, soles, subungual areas, and mucous membranes Accounts for ≈5% of all melanomas (most common melanoma in African American patients; ≈50%)
Nodular melanoma	Vertical growth predominates Lesions are usually dark Most aggressive type/worst prognosis Accounts for ≈15% of all melanomas
Amelanotic melanoma	Melanoma from melanocytes but with obvious lack of pigment
What is the most common type of melanoma?	Superficial spreading (≈75%) (Think: **SUPER**ficial = **SUPER**ior)
What type of melanoma arises in Hutchinson's freckle?	Lentigo maligna melanoma
What is Hutchinson's freckle?	Lentigo maligna melanoma in the radial growth phase without vertical extension (noninvasive); usually occurs on the faces of elderly women

STAGING

What are the American Joint Committee on Cancer (AJCC) stages simplified:	
IA?	<1 mm without ulceration
IB?	<1 mm with ulceration or 1–2 mm without ulceration

IIA?	1–2 mm with ulceration or 2–4 mm without ulceration
IIB?	2–4 mm with ulceration or >4 mm without ulceration
IIC?	>4 mm with ulceration
III?	Positive nodes
IV?	Distant metastases
What are the common sites of metastasis?	Nodes (local) Distant: lung, liver, bone, heart, and brain Melanoma has a specific attraction for small bowel mucosa and distant cutaneous sites Brain metastases are a common cause of death
What are the metastatic routes?	Both lymphatic and hematogenous
How is the diagnosis made?	Excisional biopsy (complete removal leaving only normal tissue) or incisioned biopsy for very large lesions (***Note:*** Early diagnosis is crucial)
What is the role of shave biopsy?	No role
What is the "sentinel node" biopsy?	Inject Lymphazurin® blue dye, colloid with a radiolabel, or both around the melanoma; the first LN in the draining chain is identified as the "sentinel lymph node" and reflects the metastatic status of the group of lymph nodes
When is elective lymph node dissection recommended?	Controversial—possible advantage in melanomas 1 to 2 mm in depth but jury still out; sentinel node biopsy if >1 mm is becoming very common

What is the recommended size of the surgical margin for depth of invasion:

    Melanoma in situ?   0.5-cm margin

    ≤1 mm thick?   1-cm margin

    1–4 mm thick?   2-cm margin

    >4 mm thick?   3-cm margin

What is the treatment for digital melanoma?

Amputation

What is the treatment of palpable lymph node metastasis?

Lymphadenectomy

What factors determine the prognosis?

Depth of invasion and metastasis are the most important factors (Superficial spreading and lentigo maligna have a better prognosis because they have a longer horizontal phase of growth and are thus diagnosed at an earlier stage; nodular has the worst prognosis because it grows predominantly vertically and metastasizes earlier)

What is the workup to survey for metastasis in the patient with melanoma?

Physical exam, LFTs, CXR (bone scan/CT/MRI reserved for symptoms)

What is the treatment of intestinal metastasis?

Surgical resection to prevent bleeding/obstruction

Which malignancy is most likely to metastasize to the bowel?

Melanoma

What is the surgical treatment of nodal metastasis?

Lymphadenectomy

What is FDA-approved adjuvant therapy?

Interferon alpha-2b (for stages IIB/III)

What is the treatment of unresectable brain metastasis?	Radiation
What is the treatment of isolated adrenal metastasis?	Surgical resection
What is the treatment of isolated lung metastasis?	Surgical resection
What is the most common symptom of anal melanoma?	Bleeding
What is the treatment of anal melanoma?	APR or wide excision (no survival benefit from APR, but better local control)
What other experimental therapy is available for metastatic disease?	1. Monoclonal antibodies 2. Chemotherapy (e.g., dacarbazine) 3. Vaccinations
What is the median survival with distant metastasis?	≈6 months

Chapter 65 Surgical Intensive Care

INTENSIVE CARE UNIT (ICU) BASICS

How is an ICU note written?	By **systems:** Neurologic (e.g., GCS, MAE, pain control) Pulmonary (e.g., vent settings) CVS (e.g., pressors, Swan numbers) GI (gastrointestinal) Heme (CBC) FEN (e.g., Chem 10, nutrition) Renal (e.g., urine output, BUN, Cr) ID (e.g., T_{max}, WBC, antibiotics) Assessment Plan (***Note:*** physical exam included in each section)

What is the best way to report urine output in the ICU?

24 hrs/last shift/last 3 hourly rate = "urine output has been 2 liters over last 24 hrs, 350 last shift, and 45, 35, 40 cc over the last 3 hours"

What are the possible causes of fever in the ICU?

Central line infection
Pneumonia/atelectasis
UTI, urosepsis
Intra-abdominal abscess
Sinusitis
DVT
Thrombophlebitis
Drug fever
Fungal infection, meningitis, wound infection
Endocarditis

What is the most common bacteria in ICU pneumonia?

Gram-negative rods

What is the acronym for the basic ICU care checklist (Dr. Vincent)?

"FAST HUG":
Feeding
Analgesia
Sedation
Thromboembolic prophylaxis

Head-of-bed elevation (pneumonia prevention)
Ulcer prevention
Glucose control

INTENSIVE CARE UNIT FORMULAS AND TERMS YOU SHOULD KNOW

What is CO?

Cardiac Output: HR (heart rate) × SV (stroke volume)

What is the normal CO?

4–8 L/min

What factors increase CO?

Increased contractility, heart rate, and preload; decreased afterload

What is CI?

Cardiac Index: CO/BSA (body surface area)

What is the normal CI?	2.5–3.5 L/min/M$_2$
What is SV?	**S**troke **V**olume: the amount of blood pumped out of the ventricle each beat; simply, end diastolic volume minus the end systolic volume **or** CO/HR
What is the normal SV?	60–100 cc
What is CVP?	**C**entral **V**enous **P**ressure: indirect measurement of intravascular volume status
What is the normal CVP?	4–11
What is PCWP?	**P**ulmonary **C**apillary **W**edge **P**ressure: indirectly measures left atrial pressure, which is an estimate of intravascular volume (LV filling pressure)
What is the normal PCWP?	5–15
What is anion gap?	$Na^+ - (Cl^- + HCO_3^-)$
What are the normal values for anion gap?	10–14
Why do you get an increased anion gap?	Unmeasured acids are unmeasured anions in the equation that are part of the "counterbalance" to the sodium cation
What are the causes of increased anion gap acidosis in surgical patients?	Think **"SALUD"**: **S**tarvation **A**lcohol (ethanol/methanol) **L**actic acidosis **U**remia (renal failure) **D**KA
Define MODS.	**M**ultiple **O**rgan **D**ysfunction **S**yndrome
What is SVR?	**S**ystemic **V**ascular **R**esistance: MAP – CVP / CO × 80 (remember, P = F × R, **P**ower **F**o**R**ward; and calculating resistance: **R = P/F**)
What is SVRI?	**S**ystemic **V**ascular **R**esistance **I**ndex: SVR/BSA

What is the normal SVRI?	1500–2400
What is MAP?	**M**ean **A**rterial **P**ressure: diastolic blood pressure + **1/3 (systolic–diastolic pressure)** (***Note:*** Not the mean between diastolic and systolic blood pressure because diastole lasts longer than systole)
What is PVR?	**P**ulmonary **V**ascular **R**esistance: PA(MEAN) – PCWP / CO × 80 (PA is pulmonary artery pressure and LA is left atrial or PCWP pressure)
What is the normal PVR value?	100 ± 50
What is the formula for arterial oxygen content?	Hemoglobin × O_2 saturation (SaO_2) × 1.34
What is the basic formula for oxygen delivery?	CO × (oxygen content)
What is the full formula for oxygen delivery?	CO × (1.34 × Hgb × SaO_2) × 10
What factors can increase oxygen delivery?	Increased CO by increasing SV, HR, or both; increased O_2 content by increasing the hemoglobin content, SaO_2, or both
What is mixed venous oxygen saturation?	SvO_2; simply, the O_2 saturation of the blood in the right ventricle or pulmonary artery; an indirect measure of peripheral oxygen supply and demand
Which lab values help assess adequate oxygen delivery?	SvO_2 (low with inadequate delivery), lactic acid (elevated with inadequate delivery), pH (acidosis with inadequate delivery), base deficit
What is FENa?	**F**ractional **E**xcretion of Sodium (**Na$^+$**): (U_{Na^+} × P_{cr} / P_{Na^+} × U_{cr}) × 100
What is the memory aid for calculating FENa?	Think: YOU NEED PEE = **U** (**U**rine) **N** (**Na$^+$**) **P** (**P**lasma); U_{Na^+} × P_{cr}; for the denominator, switch everything, P_{Na^+} × U_{cr} (cr = creatinine)

What is the prerenal FENa value?	<1.0; renal failure from decreased renal blood flow (e.g., cardiogenic, hypovolemia, arterial obstruction, etc.)
How long does Lasix® effect last?	6 hours = **LASIX** = **LA**sts **SIX** hours
What is the formula for flow/pressure/resistance?	Remember **P**ower **F**o**R**ward: **P**ressure = **F**low × **R**esistance
What is the "10 for 0.08 rule" of acid-base?	For every increase of $PaCO_2$ by **10** mm Hg, the pH falls by **0.08**
What is the "40, 50, 60 for 70, 80, 90 rule" for O_2 sats?	PaO_2 of **40, 50, 60** corresponds roughly to an O_2 sat of **70, 80, 90,** respectively
One liter of O_2 via nasal cannula raises FiO_2 by how much?	≈3%
What is pure respiratory acidosis?	Low pH (acidosis), increased $PaCO_2$, normal bicarbonate
What is pure respiratory alkalosis?	High pH (alkalosis), decreased $PaCO_2$, normal bicarbonate
What is pure metabolic acidosis?	Low pH, low bicarbonate, normal $PaCO_2$
What is pure metabolic alkalosis?	High pH, high bicarbonate, normal $PaCO_2$
List how the body compensates for each of the following:	
Respiratory acidosis	Increased bicarbonate
Respiratory alkalosis	Decreased bicarbonate
Metabolic acidosis	Decreased $PaCO_2$
Metabolic alkalosis	Increased $PaCO_2$
What does MOF stand for?	**M**ultiple **O**rgan **F**ailure
What does SIRS stand for?	**S**ystemic **I**nflammatory **R**esponse **S**yndrome

SICU DRUGS

DOPAMINE

What is the site of action and effect at the following levels:

Low dose (1–3 μg/kg/min)? ++ dopa agonist; **renal vasodilation** (a.k.a. "renal dose dopamine")

Intermediate dose (4–10 μg/kg/min)? + α_1, ++ β_1; positive inotropy and some vasoconstriction

High dose (>10 μg/kg/min)? +++ α_1 agonist; marked afterload increase from arteriolar vasoconstriction

Has "renal dose" dopamine been shown to decrease renal failure? NO

DOBUTAMINE

What is the site of action? +++ β_1 agonist, ++ β_2

What is the effect? ↑ inotropy; ↑ chronotropy, **decrease in systemic vascular resistance**

ISOPROTERENOL

What is the site of action? +++ β_1 and β_2 agonist

What is the effect? ↑ inotropy; ↑ chronotropy; (+ vasodilation of skeletal and mesenteric vascular beds)

EPINEPHRINE (EPI)

What is the site of action? ++ α_1, α_2, ++++ β_1, and β_2 agonist

What is the effect? ↑ inotropy; ↑ chronotropy

What is the effect at high doses? Vasoconstriction

NOREPINEPHRINE (NE)

What is the site of action? +++ α_1, α_2, +++ β_1, and β_1 agonist

What is the effect? ↑ inotropy; ↑ chronotropy; ++ increase in blood pressure

What is the effect at high doses?	Severe vasoconstriction

VASOPRESSIN

What is the action?	Vasoconstriction (increases MAP, SVR)
What are the indications?	Hypotension, especially refractory to other vasopressors (low-dose infusion—0.01–0.04 units per minute) or as a bolus during ACLS (40 u)

NITROGLYCERINE (NTG)

What is the site of action?	+++ venodilation; + arteriolar dilation
What is the effect?	Increased venous capacitance, decreased preload, coronary arteriole vasodilation

SODIUM NITROPRUSSIDE (SNP)

What is the site of action?	+++ venodilation; +++ arteriolar dilation
What is the effect?	Decreased preload and afterload (allowing blood pressure titration)
What is the major toxicity of SNP?	**Cyanide** toxicity

INTENSIVE CARE PHYSIOLOGY

Define the following terms:	
Preload	Load on the heart muscle that stretches it to end-diastolic volume (end-diastolic pressure) = intravascular volume
Afterload	Load or resistance the heart must pump against = vascular tone = SVR
Contractility	Force of heart muscle contraction
Compliance	Distensibility of heart by the preload
What is the Frank-Starling curve?	Cardiac output increases with increasing preload up to a point

What is the clinical significance of the steep slope of the Starling curve relating end-diastolic volume to cardiac output?	Demonstrates the importance of preload in determining cardiac output
What factors influence the oxygen content of whole blood?	Oxygen content is composed largely of that oxygen bound to hemoglobin, and is thus determined by the hemoglobin concentration and the arterial oxygen saturation; the partial pressure of oxygen dissolved in plasma plays a minor role
What factors influence mixed venous oxygen saturation?	Oxygen **delivery** (hemoglobin concentration, arterial oxygen saturation, cardiac output) and oxygen **extraction** by the peripheral tissues
What lab test for tissue ischemia is based on the shift from aerobic to anaerobic metabolism?	Serum lactic acid levels
Define the following terms: **Dead space**	That part of the inspired air that does not participate in gas exchange (e.g., the gas in the large airways/ET tube not in contact with capillaries) Think: space = air
Shunt fraction	That fraction of pulmonary venous blood that does not participate in gas exchange Think: shunt = blood
What causes increased dead space?	Overventilation (emphysema, excessive PEEP) or underperfusion (pulmonary embolus, low cardiac output, pulmonary artery vasoconstriction)
At high shunt fractions, what is the effect of increasing FiO_2 on arterial PO_2?	At high shunt fractions (>50%), changes in FiO_2 have almost no effect on arterial PO_2 because the blood that does "see" the O_2 is already at maximal O_2 absorption; thus, increasing the FiO_2 has no effect (FiO_2 can be minimized to prevent oxygen toxicity)

Define ARDS.

Acute **R**espiratory **D**istress **S**yndrome: lung inflammation causing respiratory failure

What is the ARDS diagnostic triad?

"CXR":
   Capillary wedge pressure <18
   X-ray of chest with bilateral infiltrates
   Ratio of PaO_2 to FiO_2 <200

What does the classic chest x-ray look like with ARDS?

Bilateral fluffy infiltrates

How can you remember the PaO_2 to FiO_2, or PF, ratio?

Think: "**PUFF**" ratio: **PF** ratio = **P**aO_2: **F**iO_2 ratio

At what concentration does O_2 toxicity occur?

FiO_2 of >60% × 48 hours; thus, try to keep FiO_2 below 60% at all times

What are the ONLY ventilatory parameters that have been shown to decrease mortality in ARDS patients?

Low tidal volumes (≤6 cc/kg) and low plateau pressures <30

What are the main causes of carbon dioxide retention?

Hypoventilation, increased dead space ventilation, and increased carbon dioxide production (as in hypermetabolic states)

Why are carbohydrates minimized in the diet/TPN of patients having difficulty with hypercapnia?

Respiratory **Q**uotient (**RQ**) is the ratio of CO_2 production to O_2 consumption and is highest for carbohydrates (1.0) and lowest for fats (0.7)

HEMODYNAMIC MONITORING

Why are indwelling arterial lines used for blood pressure monitoring in critically ill patients?

Because of the need for frequent measurements, the inaccuracy of frequently repeated cuff measurements, the inaccuracy of cuff measurements in hypotension, and the need for frequent arterial blood sampling/labs

Which pressures/values are obtained from a Swan-Ganz catheter?

CVP, PA pressures, PCWP, CO, PVR, SVR, mixed venous O_2 saturation

Identify the Swan-Ganz waveforms:

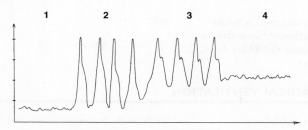

1. CVP/right atrium
2. Right ventricle
3. Pulmonary artery
4. Wedge

What does the abbreviation PCWP stand for?

Pulmonary **C**apillary **W**edge **P**ressure

Give other names for PCWP.

Wedge or wedge pressure, pulmonary artery occlusion pressure (PAOP)

What is it?

Pulmonary capillary pressure after balloon occlusion of the pulmonary artery, which is equal to left atrial pressure because there are no valves in the pulmonary system

Left atrial pressure is essentially equal to left ventricular end diastolic pressure (LVEDP): left heart preload, and, thus, intravascular volume status.

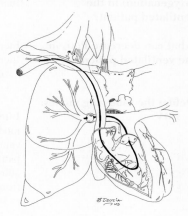

What is the primary use of the PCWP?	As an indirect measure of preload = intravascular volume
Has the usage of a Swan-Ganz catheter been shown to decrease mortality in ICU patients?	NO

MECHANICAL VENTILATION

Define ventilation.	Air through the lungs; monitored by P_{CO_2}
Define oxygenation.	Oxygen delivery to the alveoli; monitored by O_2 sats and P_{O_2}
What can increase ventilation to decrease P_{CO_2}?	Increased respiratory rate (RR), increased tidal volume (minute ventilation)
What is minute ventilation?	Volume of gas ventilated through the lungs (RR × tidal volume)
Define tidal volume.	Volume delivered with each breath; should be 6 to 8 cc/kg on the ventilator
Are ventilation and oxygenation related?	Basically no; you can have an O_2 sat of 100% and a P_{CO_2} of 150; O_2 sats do not tell you anything about the P_{CO_2} (key point!)
What can increase P_{O_2} (oxygenation) in the ventilated patient?	Increased F_{IO_2} Increased PEEP
What can decrease P_{CO_2} in the ventilated patient?	Increased RR Increased tidal volume (i.e., increase minute ventilation)
Define the following modes: **IMV**	**I**ntermittent **M**andatory **V**entilation: mode with intermittent mandatory ventilations at a predetermined rate; patients can also breathe on their own above the mandatory rate **without** help from the ventilator

SIMV	**S**ynchronous **IMV:** mode of IMV that delivers the mandatory breath synchronously with patient's initiated effort; if no breath is initiated, the ventilator delivers the predetermined mandatory breath
A-C	**A**ssist-**C**ontrol ventilation: mode in which the ventilator delivers a breath when the patient initiates a breath, or the ventilator "assists" the patient to breathe; if the patient does not initiate a breath, the ventilator takes "control" and delivers a breath at a predetermined rate In contrast to IMV, all breaths are by the ventilator
CPAP	**C**ontinuous **P**ositive **A**irway **P**ressure: positive pressure delivered **continuously** (during expiration and inspiration) by ventilator, but no volume breaths (patient breathes on own)
Pressure support	Pressure is delivered only **with an initiated breath;** pressure support decreases the work of breathing by overcoming the resistance in the ventilator circuit
APRV	**A**irway **P**ressure **R**elease **V**entilation: high airway pressure intermittently released to a low airway pressure (shorter period of time)
HFV	**H**igh **F**requency **V**entilation: rapid rates of ventilation with small tidal volumes
What are the effects of positive pressure ventilation in a patient with hypovolemia or low lung compliance?	Venous return and cardiac output are decreased
Define PEEP.	**P**ositive **E**nd **E**xpiration **P**ressure: positive pressure maintained at the end of a breath; keeps alveoli open

What is "physiologic PEEP"?

PEEP of 5 cm H_2O; thought to approximate normal pressure in normal nonintubated people caused by the closed glottis

What are the side effects of increasing levels of PEEP?

Barotrauma (injury to airway = pneumothorax), decreased CO from decreased preload

What are the typical initial ventilator settings:
  Mode?

Intermittent mandatory ventilation

  Tidal volume?

6–8 ml/kg

  Ventilator rate?

10 breaths/min

  Fio$_2$?

100% and wean down

  PEEP?

5 cm H_2O
From these parameters, change according to blood-gas analysis

What is a normal I:E (inspiratory to expiratory time)?

1:2

When would you use an inverse I:E ratio (e.g., 2:1, 3:1, etc.)?

To allow for longer inspiration in patients with poor compliance, to allow for "alveolar recruitment"

When would you use a prolonged I:E ratio (e.g., 1:4)?

COPD, to allow time for complete exhalation (prevents "breath stacking")

What clinical situations cause increased airway resistance?

Airway or endotracheal tube obstruction, bronchospasm, ARDS, mucous plug, CHF (pulmonary edema)

What are the presumed advantages of PEEP?

Prevention of alveolar collapse and atelectasis, improved gas exchange, increased pulmonary compliance, decreased shunt fraction

What are the possible disadvantages of PEEP?

Decreased cardiac output, especially in the setting of hypovolemia; decreased gas exchange; ↓ compliance with high levels of PEEP, fluid retention, increased intracranial pressure, barotrauma

What parameters must be evaluated in deciding if a patient is ready to be extubated?	Patient alert and able to protect airway, gas exchange (PaO$_2$ >70, PaCO$_2$ <50), tidal volume (>5 cc/kg), minute ventilation (<10 L/min), negative inspiratory pressure (<−20 cm H$_2$O, or more negative), FiO$_2$ ≤40%, PEEP 5, PH >7.25, RR <35, Tobin index <105
What is the Rapid-Shallow Breathing (a.k.a. Tobin) index?	**R**ate: **T**idal volume ratio; Tobin index <105 is associated with successful extubation (Think: **R**espiratory **T**herapist = **RT** = **R**ate: **T**idal volume)
What is a possible source of fever in a patient with an NG or nasal endotracheal tube?	Sinusitis (diagnosed by sinus films/CT)
What is the 35−45 rule of blood gas values?	Normal values: pH = **7.35−7.45** PCO$_2$ = **35−45**
Which medications can be delivered via an endotracheal tube?	Think "**NAVEL**": **N**arcan **A**tropine **V**asopressin **E**pinephrine **L**idocaine
What conditions should you think of with ↑ peak airway pressure and ↓ urine output?	1. Tension pneumothorax 2. Abdominal compartment syndrome

Chapter 66 — Vascular Surgery

What is atherosclerosis?	Diffuse disease process in arteries; atheromas containing cholesterol and lipid form within the intima and inner media, often accompanied by ulcerations and smooth muscle hyperplasia

What is the common theory of how atherosclerosis is initiated?

Endothelial injury → platelets adhere → growth factors released → smooth muscle hyperplasia/plaque deposition

What are the risk factors for atherosclerosis?

Hypertension, **smoking,** diabetes mellitus, family history, hyper-cholesterolemia, high LDL, obesity, and sedentary lifestyle

What are the common sites of plaque formation in arteries?

Branch points (carotid bifurcation), tethered sites (superficial femoral artery [SFA] in Hunter's canal in the leg)

What must be present for a successful arterial bypass operation?

1. Inflow (e.g., patent aorta)
2. Outflow (e.g., open distal popliteal artery)
3. Run off (e.g., patent trifurcation vessels down to the foot)

What is the major principle of safe vascular surgery?

Get **proximal** and **distal** control of the vessel to be worked on!

What does it mean to "POTTS" a vessel?

Place a vessel loop twice around a vessel so that if you put tension on the vessel loop, it will occlude the vessel

What is the suture needle orientation through graft versus diseased artery in a graft to artery anastomosis?

Needle "in-to-out" of the lumen in diseased artery to help **tack down the plaque** and the needle "out-to-in" on the graft

What are the three layers of an artery?

1. Intima
2. Media
3. Adventitia

Which arteries supply the blood vessel itself?

Vaso vasorum

What is a true aneurysm?

Dilation (>2× nL diameter) of all three layers of a vessel

What is a false aneurysm (a.k.a pseudoaneurysm)?

Dilation of artery not involving all three layers (e.g., hematoma with fibrous covering)

Often connects with vessel lumen and blood swirls inside the false aneurysm

What is "ENDOVASCULAR" repair?	Placement of a catheter in artery and then deployment of a graft intraluminally

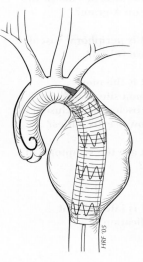

PERIPHERAL VASCULAR DISEASE

Define the arterial anatomy:

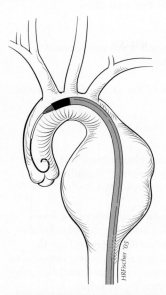

1. Aorta
2. Internal iliac (hypogastric)
3. External iliac
4. Common femoral artery
5. Profundi femoral artery
6. Superficial femoral artery (SFA)
7. Popliteal artery
8. Trifurcation
9. Anterior tibial artery
10. Peroneal artery
11. Posterior tibial artery
12. Dorsalis pedis artery

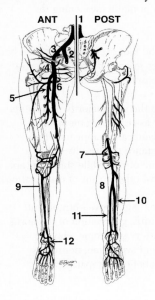

How can you remember the orientation of the lower exterior arteries below the knee on A-gram?	Use the acronym **"LAMP"**: **L**ateral **A**nterior tibial **M**edial **P**osterior tibial
What is peripheral vascular disease (PVD)?	Occlusive atherosclerotic disease in the lower extremities
What is the most common site of arterial atherosclerotic occlusion in the lower extremities?	Occlusion of the SFA in Hunter's canal
What are the symptoms of PVD?	Intermittent claudication, rest pain, erectile dysfunction, sensorimotor impairment, tissue loss
What is intermittent claudication?	Pain, cramping, or both of the lower extremity, usually the calf muscle, after walking a specific distance; then the pain/cramping resolves after stopping for a specific amount of time while standing; this pattern is reproducible
What is rest pain?	Pain in the foot, usually over the distal metatarsals; this pain arises at rest (classically at night, awakening the patient)
What classically resolves rest pain?	Hanging the foot over the side of the bed or standing; gravity affords some extra flow to the ischemic areas
How can vascular causes of claudication be differentiated from nonvascular causes, such as neurogenic claudication or arthritis?	History (in the vast majority of patients) and noninvasive tests; remember, vascular claudication appears after a specific distance and resolves after a specific time of rest while standing (not so with most other forms of claudication)
What is the differential diagnosis of lower extremity claudication?	Neurogenic (e.g., nerve entrapment/discs), arthritis, coarctation of the aorta, popliteal artery syndrome, chronic compartment syndrome, neuromas, anemia, diabetic neuropathy pain

What are the signs of PVD?

Absent pulses, bruits, muscular atrophy, decreased hair growth, thick toenails, tissue necrosis/ulcers/infection

What is the site of a PVD ulcer vs. a venous stasis ulcer?

PVD arterial insufficiency ulcer—usually on the toes/foot
Venous stasis ulcer—medial malleolus (ankle)

What is the ABI?

Ankle to Brachial Index (ABI); simply, the ratio of the systolic blood pressure at the ankle to the systolic blood pressure at the arm (brachial artery) A:B; ankle pressure taken with Doppler; the ABI is noninvasive

What ABIs are associated with normals, claudicators, and rest pain?

Normal ABI— ≥1.0
Claudicator ABI— <0.6
Rest pain ABI— <0.4

Who gets false ABI readings?

Patients with calcified arteries, especially those with diabetes

What are PVRs?

Pulse Volume Recordings; pulse wave forms are recorded from lower extremities representing volume of blood per heart beat at sequential sites down leg
Large wave form means good collateral blood flow
(Noninvasive using pressure cuffs)

Prior to surgery for chronic PVD, what diagnostic test will every patient receive?

A-gram (arteriogram: dye in vessel and x-rays) maps disease and allows for best treatment option (i.e., angioplasty vs. surgical bypass vs. endarterectomy)
Gold standard for diagnosing PVD

What is the bedside management of a patient with PVD?

1. Sheep skin (easy on the heels)
2. Foot cradle (keeps sheets/blankets off the feet)
3. Skin lotion to avoid further cracks in the skin that can go on to form a fissure and then an ulcer

What are the indications for surgical treatment in PVD?

Use the acronym **"STIR"**:
Severe claudication refractory to conservative treatment that affects quality of life/livelihood (e.g., can't work because of the claudication)
Tissue necrosis
Infection
Rest pain

What is the treatment of claudication?

For the vast majority, conservative treatment, including exercise, smoking cessation, treatment of HTN, diet, aspirin, with or without Trental (pentoxifylline)

How can the medical conservative treatment for claudication be remembered?

Use the acronym **"PACE"**:
Pentoxifylline
Aspirin
Cessation of smoking
Exercise

How does aspirin work?

Inhibits platelets (inhibits cyclooxygenase and platelet aggregation)

How does Trental® (pentoxifylline) work?

Results in increased RBC deformity and flexibility (Think: pento**X**ifylline = RBC fle**X**ibility)

What is the risk of limb loss with claudication?

5% limb loss at 5 years (Think: 5 in 5), 10% at 10 years (Think: 10 in 10)

What is the risk of limb loss with rest pain?

>50% of patients will have amputation of the limb at some point

In the patient with PVD, what is the main postoperative concern?

Cardiac status, because most patients with PVD have coronary artery disease; ≈20% have an AAA
MI is the most common cause of postoperative death after a PVD operation

What is Leriche's syndrome?   Buttock **C**laudication, **I**mpotence (erectile
dysfunction), and leg muscle **A**trophy
from occlusive disease of the iliacs/distal
aorta
Think: **"CIA"**:
    Claudication
    Impotence
    Atrophy
    (Think: CIA spy Leriche)

What are the treatment
options for severe PVD?

1. Surgical graft bypass
2. Angioplasty—balloon dilation
3. Endarterectomy—remove diseased
   intima and media
4. Surgical patch angioplasty (place patch
   over stenosis)

What is a FEM-POP bypass?   Bypass SFA occlusion with a graft from the
FEMoral artery to the **POP**liteal artery

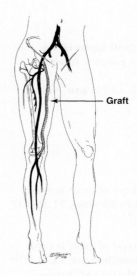

Graft

**What is a FEM-DISTAL
bypass?**

Bypass from the **FEM**oral artery to a
DISTAL artery (peroneal artery, anterior
tibial artery, or posterior tibial artery)

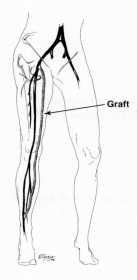

Graft

**What graft material has the
longest patency rate?**

Autologous vein graft

**What is an "in situ" vein
graft?**

Saphenous vein is more or less left in
place, all branches are ligated, and the
vein valves are broken with a small hook
or cut out; a vein can also be used if
reversed so that the valves do not cause a
problem

**What type of graft is used
for above-the-knee FEM-POP
bypass?**

Either vein or Gortex® graft; vein still has
better patency

**What type of graft is used
for below-the-knee FEM-POP
or FEM-DISTAL bypass?**

Must use vein graft; prosthetic grafts
have a prohibitive thrombosis rate

What is DRY gangrene?

Dry necrosis of tissue without signs of
infection ("mummified tissue")

What is WET gangrene?   Moist necrotic tissue with signs of infection

What is blue toe syndrome?   Intermittent painful blue toes (or fingers) due to microemboli from a proximal arterial plaque

LOWER EXTREMITY AMPUTATIONS

What are the indications?   Irreversible tissue ischemia (no hope for revascularization bypass) and necrotic tissue, severe infection, severe pain with no bypassable vessels, or if patient is not interested in a bypass procedure

Identify the level of the following amputations:

1. **A**bove-the-**K**nee **A**mputation (**AKA**)
2. **B**elow-the-**K**nee **A**mputation (**BKA**)
3. Symes amputation
4. Transmetatarsal amputation
5. Toe amputation

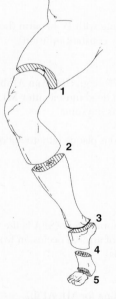

What is a Ray amputation?   Removal of toe and head of metatarsal

ACUTE ARTERIAL OCCLUSION

What is it?	Acute occlusion of an artery, usually by embolization; other causes include acute thrombosis of an atheromatous lesion, vascular trauma
What are the classic signs/symptoms of acute arterial occlusion?	The **"six P's"**: **P**ain **P**aralysis **P**allor **P**aresthesia **P**olar (some say **P**oikilothermia—you pick) **P**ulselessness (You **must** know these!)
What is the classic timing of pain with acute arterial occlusion from an embolus?	Acute onset; the patient can classically tell you exactly when and where it happened
What is the immediate preoperative management?	1. Anticoagulate with IV heparin (bolus followed by constant infusion) 2. A-gram
What are the sources of emboli?	1. Heart—85% (e.g., clot from AFib, clot forming on dead muscle after MI, endocarditis, myxoma) 2. Aneurysms 3. Atheromatous plaque (atheroembolism)
What is the most common cause of embolus from the heart?	AFib
What is the most common site of arterial occlusion by an embolus?	Common femoral artery (SFA is the most common site of arterial occlusion from atherosclerosis)
What diagnostic studies are in order?	1. A-gram 2. ECG (looking for MI, AFib) 3. Echocardiogram ($\pm$) looking for clot, MI, valve vegetation

What is the treatment?

Surgical embolectomy via cutdown and Fogarty balloon (bypass is reserved for embolectomy failure)

What is a Fogarty?

Fogarty balloon catheter—catheter with a balloon tip that can be inflated with saline; used for embolectomy

How is a Fogarty catheter used?

Insinuate the catheter with the balloon deflated past the embolus and then inflate the balloon and pull the catheter out; the balloon brings the embolus with it

How many mm in diameter is a 12 French Fogarty catheter?

Simple: To get mm from French measurements, divide the French number by π, or 3.14; thus, a 12 French catheter is $12/3 = 4$ mm in diameter

What must be looked for postoperatively after reperfusion of a limb?

Compartment syndrome, hyperkalemia, renal failure from myoglobinuria, MI

What is compartment syndrome?

Leg (calf) is separated into compartments by very unyielding fascia; **tissue swelling** from reperfusion can increase the intracompartmental pressure, resulting in decreased capillary flow, ischemia, and myonecrosis; myonecrosis may occur after the intracompartment pressure reaches only 30 mm Hg

What are the signs/ symptoms of compartment syndrome?

Classic signs include pain, especially after passive flexing/extension of the foot, paralysis, paresthesias, and pallor; **pulses are present** in most cases because systolic pressure is much higher than the minimal 30 mm Hg needed for the syndrome!

Can a patient have a pulse and compartment syndrome?

YES!

How is the diagnosis made?

History/suspicion, compartment pressure measurement

What is the treatment of compartment syndrome?	Treatment includes opening compartments via bilateral calf-incision fasciotomies of all four compartments in the calf

ABDOMINAL AORTIC ANEURYSMS

What is it also known as?	AAA, or "triple A"
What is it?	Abnormal dilation of the abdominal aorta (>1.5–$2\times$ normal), forming a true aneurysm

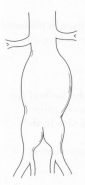

What is the male to female ratio?	$\approx6{:}1$
By far, who is at the highest risk?	White males
What is the common etiology?	Believed to be **atherosclerotic** in 95% of cases; 5% inflammatory
What is the most common site?	Infrarenal (95%)
What is the incidence?	5% of all adults older than 60 years of age
What percentage of patients with AAA have a peripheral arterial aneurysm?	20%

What are the risk factors?

Atherosclerosis, hypertension, smoking, male gender, advanced age, connective tissue disease

What are the symptoms?

Most AAAs are **asymptomatic** and discovered during routine abdominal exam by primary care physicians; in the remainder, symptoms range from vague epigastric discomfort to back and abdominal pain

Classically, what do testicular pain and an AAA signify?

Retroperitoneal rupture with ureteral stretch and referred pain to the testicle

What are the risk factors for rupture?

Increasing aneurysm diameter, COPD, HTN, recent rapid expansion, large diameter, hypertension, symptomatic

What are the signs of rupture?

Classic triad of ruptured AAA:
1. **Abdominal pain**
2. **Pulsatile abdominal mass**
3. **Hypotension**

By how much each year do AAAs grow?

≈3 mm/year on average (larger AAAs grow faster than smaller AAAs)

Why do larger AAAs rupture more often and grow faster than smaller AAAs?

Probably because of Laplace's law (wall tension = pressure × diameter)

What is the risk of rupture per year based on AAA diameter size?

<5 cm = 4%
5–7 cm = 7%
>7 cm = 20%

What are other risks for rupture?

Hypertension, smoking, COPD

Where does the aorta bifurcate?

At the level of the **umbilicus;** therefore, when palpating for an AAA, palpate above the umbilicus and below the xiphoid process

What is the differential diagnosis?

Acute pancreatitis, aortic dissection, mesenteric ischemia, MI, perforated ulcer, diverticulosis, renal colic, etc.

What are the diagnostic tests?

Use U/S to follow AAA clinically; other tests involve contrast CT scan and A-gram; A-gram will assess lumen patency and iliac/renal involvement

What is the limitation of A-gram?

AAAs often have large mural thrombi, which result in a falsely reduced diameter because only the patent lumen is visualized

What are the signs of AAA on AXR?

Calcification in the aneurysm wall, best seen on lateral projection (a.k.a. "eggshell" calcifications)

What are the indications for surgical repair of AAA?

AAA >5.5 cm in diameter, if the patient is not an overwhelming high risk for surgery; also, rupture of the AAA, any size AAA with rapid growth, symptoms/embolization of plaque

What is the treatment?

1. Prosthetic graft placement, with rewrapping of the native aneurysm adventitia around the prosthetic graft after the thrombus is removed; when rupture is strongly suspected, **proceed to immediate laparotomy; there is no time for diagnostic tests!**

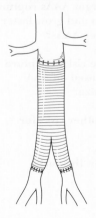

2. Endovascular repair

What is endovascular repair?

Repair of the AAA by femoral catheter placed stents

Why wrap the graft in the native aorta?	To reduce the incidence of enterograft fistula formation
What type of repair should be performed with AAA and iliacs severely occluded or iliac aneurysm(s)?	Aortobi-iliac or aortobifemoral graft replacement (bifurcated graft)
What is the treatment if the patient has abdominal pain, pulsatile abdominal mass, and hypotension?	Take the patient to the **O.R.** for emergent AAA repair
What is the treatment if the patient has known AAA and new onset of abdominal pain or back pain?	CT scan: 1. Leak → straight to OR 2. No leak → repair during next elective slot
What is the mortality rate associated with the following types of AAA treatment: **Elective?**	Good; <4% operative mortality
Ruptured?	≈50% operative mortality
What is the leading cause of postoperative death in a patient undergoing elective AAA treatment?	Myocardial infarction (MI)
What are the other etiologies of AAA?	Inflammatory (connective tissue diseases), mycotic (a misnomer because most result from bacteria, not fungi)
What is the mean normal abdominal aortic diameter?	2 cm
What are the possible operative complications?	MI, atheroembolism, declamping hypotension, acute renal failure (especially if aneurysm involves the renal arteries), ureteral injury, hemorrhage
Why is colonic ischemia a concern in the repair of AAAs?	Often the IMA is sacrificed during surgery; if the collaterals are not adequate, the patient will have colonic ischemia

What are the signs of colonic ischemia?

Heme-positive stool, or bright red blood per rectum (BRBPR), diarrhea, abdominal pain

What is the study of choice to diagnose colonic ischemia?

Colonoscopy

When is colonic ischemia seen postoperatively?

Usually in the first week

What is the treatment of necrotic sigmoid colon from colonic ischemia?

1. Resection of necrotic colon
2. Hartmann's pouch or mucous fistula
3. End colostomy

What is the possible long-term complication that often presents with both upper and lower GI bleeding?

Aortoenteric fistula (fistula between aorta and duodenum)

What are the other possible postoperative complications?

Erectile dysfunction (sympathetic plexus injury), retrograde ejaculation, aortovenous fistula (to IVC), graft infection, **anterior spinal syndrome**

What is anterior spinal syndrome?

Classically:
1. Paraplegia
2. Loss of bladder/bowel control
3. Loss of pain/temperature sensation below level of involvement
4. **Sparing of proprioception**

Which artery is involved in anterior spinal cord syndrome?

Artery of **Adamkiewicz**—supplies the anterior spinal cord

What are the most common bacteria involved in aortic graft infections?

1. *Staphylococcus aureus*
2. *Staphylococcus epidermidis* (usually late)

How is a graft infection with an aortoenteric fistula treated?

Perform an **extra-anatomic bypass** with resection of the graft

What is an extra-anatomic bypass graft?	Axillofemoral bypass graft—**graft not in a normal vascular path;** usually, the graft goes from the axillary artery to the femoral artery and then from one femoral artery to the other (fem-fem bypass)

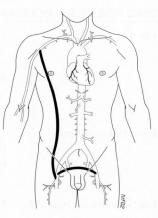

What is an endovascular repair?	Placement of a stent proximal and distal to an AAA through a distant percutaneous access (usually through the groin); less invasive; long-term results pending

CLASSIC INTRAOP QUESTIONS DURING AAA REPAIR

Which vein crosses the neck of the AAA proximally?	Renal vein (left)
What part of the small bowel crosses in front of the AAA?	Duodenum
Which large vein runs to the left of the AAA?	IMV
Which artery comes off the middle of the AAA and runs to the left?	IMA

Which vein runs behind the RIGHT common iliac artery?	**LEFT** common iliac vein
Which renal vein is longer?	Left

MESENTERIC ISCHEMIA

CHRONIC MESENTERIC ISCHEMIA

What is it?	Chronic intestinal ischemia from long-term occlusion of the intestinal arteries; most commonly results from atherosclerosis; usually in two or more arteries because of the extensive collaterals
What are the symptoms?	Weight loss, postprandial abdominal pain, anxiety/fear of food because of postprandial pain, ± heme occult, ± diarrhea/vomiting
What is "intestinal angina"?	Postprandial pain from gut ischemia
What are the signs?	Abdominal bruit is commonly heard
How is the diagnosis made?	A-gram, duplex, MRA
What supplies blood to the gut?	1. Celiac axis vessels 2. SMA 3. IMA
What is the classic finding on A-gram?	Two of the three mesenteric arteries are occluded, and there is atherosclerotic narrowing of the third patent artery
What are the treatment options?	Bypass, endarterectomy, angioplasty, stenting

ACUTE MESENTERIC ISCHEMIA

What is it?	Acute onset of intestinal ischemia
What are the causes?	1. **Emboli** to a mesenteric vessel from the heart 2. **Acute thrombosis** of long-standing atherosclerosis of mesenteric artery

What are the causes of emboli from the heart?	**AFib,** MI, cardiomyopathy, valve disease/endocarditis, mechanical heart valve
What drug has been associated with acute intestinal ischemia?	Digitalis
To which intestinal artery do emboli preferentially go?	Superior Mesenteric Artery (**SMA**)
What are the signs/symptoms of acute mesenteric ischemia?	Severe pain—classically **"pain out of proportion to physical exam,"** no peritoneal signs until necrosis, vomiting/diarrhea/hyperdefecation, ± heme stools
What is the classic triad of acute mesenteric ischemia?	1. Acute onset of pain 2. Vomiting, diarrhea, or both 3. History of AFib or heart disease
What is the gold standard diagnostic test?	Mesenteric A-gram
What is the treatment of a mesenteric embolus?	Perform Fogarty catheter embolectomy, resect obviously necrotic intestine, and leave marginal looking bowel until a "second look" laparotomy is performed 24 to 72 hours postoperatively
What is the treatment of acute thrombosis?	**Papaverine** vasodilator via A-gram catheter until **patient is in the OR;** then, most surgeons would perform a supraceliac aorta graft to the involved intestinal artery or endarterectomy; intestinal resection/second look as needed

MEDIAN ARCUATE LIGAMENT SYNDROME

What is it?	Mesenteric ischemia resulting from narrowing of the celiac axis vessels by extrinsic compression by the median arcuate ligament
What is the median arcuate ligament comprised of?	Diaphragm hiatus fibers

What are the symptoms?	Postprandial pain, weight loss
What are the signs?	Abdominal bruit in almost all patients
How is the diagnosis made?	A-gram
What is the treatment?	Release arcuate ligament surgically

CAROTID VASCULAR DISEASE

ANATOMY

Identify the following structures:

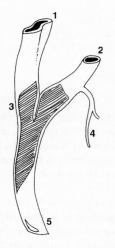

1. Internal carotid artery
2. External carotid artery
3. Carotid "bulb"
4. Superior thyroid artery
5. Common carotid artery
(Shaded area: common site of plaque formation)

What are the signs/ symptoms?	Amaurosis fugax, TIA, RIND, CVA
Define the following terms:	
Amaurosis fugax	Temporary monocular blindness ("curtain coming down"): seen with microemboli to retina; example of TIA
TIA	**T**ransient **I**schemic **A**ttack: focal neurologic deficit with resolution of all symptoms within 24 hours

RIND

Reversible **I**schemic **N**eurologic **D**eficit: transient neurologic impairment (without any lasting sequelae) lasting 24 to 72 hours

CVA

Cerebro**V**ascular **A**ccident (stroke): neurologic deficit with permanent brain damage

What is the risk of a CVA in patients with TIA?

≈10% a year

What is the noninvasive method of evaluating carotid disease?

Carotid ultrasound/Doppler: gives general location and degree of stenosis

What is the gold standard invasive method of evaluating carotid disease?

A-gram

What is the surgical treatment of carotid stenosis?

Carotid **E**nd**A**rterectomy (**CEA**): the removal of the diseased intima and media of the carotid artery, often performed with a shunt in place

What are the indications for CEA in the ASYMPTOMATIC patient?

Carotid artery stenosis >60% (greatest benefit is probably in patients with >80% stenosis)

What are the indications for CEA in the SYMPTOMATIC (CVA, TIA, RIND) patient?

Carotid stenosis >50%

Before performing a CEA in the symptomatic patient, what study other than the A-gram should be performed?

Head CT

In bilateral high-grade carotid stenosis, on which side should the CEA be performed in the asymptomatic, right-handed patient?

Left CEA first, to protect the dominant hemisphere and speech center

What is the dreaded complication after a CEA?

Stroke (CVA)

What are the possible postoperative complications after a CEA?	CVA, MI, hematoma, wound infection, hemorrhage, hypotension/hypertension, thrombosis, vagus nerve injury (change in voice), hypoglossal nerve injury (tongue deviation toward side of injury—"wheel-barrow" effect), intracranial hemorrhage
What is the mortality rate after CEA?	≈1%
What is the perioperative stroke rate after CEA?	Between 1% (asymptomatic patient) and 5% (symptomatic patient)
What is the postoperative medication?	Aspirin (inhibits platelets by inhibiting cyclo-oxygenase)
What is the most common cause of death during the early postoperative period after a CEA?	MI
Define "Hollenhorst plaque"?	Microemboli to retinal arterioles seen as bright defects

CLASSIC CEA INTRAOP QUESTIONS

What thin muscle is cut right under the skin in the neck?	Platysma muscle
What are the extracranial branches of the internal carotid artery?	None
Which vein crosses the carotid bifurcation?	Facial vein
What is the first branch of the external carotid?	Superior thyroidal artery
Which muscle crosses the common carotid proximally?	Omohyoid muscle
Which muscle crosses the carotid artery distally?	Digastric muscle (Think: **D**igastric = **D**istal)

Which nerve crosses approximately 1 cm distal to the carotid bifurcation?

Hypoglossal nerve; cut it and the tongue will deviate toward the side of the injury (the "wheelbarrow effect")

Which nerve crosses the internal carotid near the ear?

Facial nerve (marginal branch)

What is in the carotid sheath?

1. Carotid artery
2. Internal jugular vein
3. **Vagus** nerve (lies posteriorly in 98% of patients and anteriorly in 2%)
4. Deep cervical lymph nodes

SUBCLAVIAN STEAL SYNDROME

What is it?

Arm fatigue and vertebrobasilar insufficiency from obstruction of the left subclavian artery or innominate proximal to the vertebral artery branch point; ipsilateral arm movement causes increased blood flow demand, which is met by retrograde flow from the vertebral artery, thereby "stealing" from the vertebrobasilar arteries

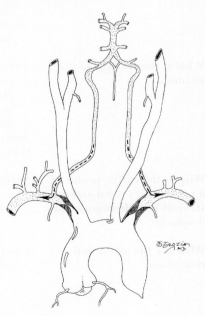

Which artery is most commonly occluded?	Left subclavian
What are the symptoms?	Upper extremity claudication, syncopal attacks, vertigo, confusion, dysarthria, blindness, ataxia
What are the signs?	Upper extremity blood pressure discrepancy, bruit (above the clavicle), vertebrobasilar insufficiency
What is the treatment?	Surgical bypass or endovascular stent

RENAL ARTERY STENOSIS

What is it?	Stenosis of renal artery, resulting in decreased perfusion of the juxtaglomerular apparatus and subsequent activation of the renin-angiotensin-aldosterone system (i.e., hypertension from renal artery stenosis)
What is the incidence?	≈10% to 15% of the U.S. population have HTN; of these, ≈4% have potentially correctable renovascular HTN Also note that 30% of malignant HTN have a renovascular etiology
What is the etiology of the stenosis?	≈66% result from atherosclerosis (men > women), ≈33% result from fibromuscular dysplasia (women > men, average age 40 years, and 50% with bilateral disease) *Note:* Another rare cause is hypoplasia of the renal artery
What is the classic profile of a patient with renal artery stenosis from fibromuscular dysplasia?	Young woman with hypertension
What are the associated risks/clues?	Family history, early onset of HTN, HTN refractory to medical treatment

What are the signs/ symptoms?	Most patients are asymptomatic but may have headache, **diastolic** HTN, flank bruits (present in 50%), and decreased renal function
What are the diagnostic tests?	
A-gram	Maps artery and extent of stenosis (gold standard)
IVP	80% of patients have delayed nephrogram phase (i.e., delayed filling of contrast)
Renal vein renin ratio (RVRR)	If sampling of renal vein renin levels shows ratio between the two kidneys ≥1.5, then diagnostic for a unilateral stenosis
Captopril provocation test	Will show a drop in BP
Are renin levels in serum ALWAYS elevated?	No: Systemic renin levels may also be measured but are only increased in malignant HTN, as the increased intravascular volume dilutes the elevated renin level in most patients
What is the invasive nonsurgical treatment?	Percutaneous **R**enal **T**ransluminal **A**ngioplasty (**PRTA**)/stenting: With FM dysplasia: use PRTA With atherosclerosis: use PRTA/stent
What is the surgical treatment?	Resection, bypass, vein/graft interposition, or endarterectomy
What antihypertensive medication is CONTRAINDICATED in patients with hypertension from renovascular stenosis?	ACE inhibitors (result in renal insufficiency)

SPLENIC ARTERY ANEURYSM

What are the causes?	Women—medial dysplasia Men—atherosclerosis

How is the diagnosis made?	Usually by abdominal pain → U/S or CT scan, in the O.R. after rupture, or incidentally **by eggshell calcifications seen on AXR**
What is the risk factor for rupture?	Pregnancy
What are the indications for splenic artery aneurysm removal?	Pregnancy, >2 cm in diameter, symptoms, and in women of childbearing age
What is the treatment for splenic aneurysm?	Resection or percutaneous catheter embolization in high-risk (e.g., portal hypertension) patients

POPLITEAL ARTERY ANEURYSM

What is it?	Aneurysm of the popliteal artery caused by atherosclerosis and, rarely, bacterial infection
How is the diagnosis made?	Usually by physical exam → A-gram, U/S
Why examine the contralateral popliteal artery?	50% of all patients with a popliteal artery aneurysm have a popliteal artery aneurysm in the contralateral popliteal artery
What are the indications for elective surgical repair of a popliteal aneurysm?	1. ≥2 cm in diameter 2. Intraluminal thrombus 3. Artery deformation
Why examine the rest of the arterial tree (especially the abdominal aorta)?	**75% of all patients with popliteal aneurysms have additional aneurysms elsewhere;** >50% of these are located in the abdominal aorta/iliacs
What size of the following aneurysms are usually considered indications for surgical repair:	
Thoracic aorta?	>6.5 cm
Abdominal aorta?	>5.5 cm

Iliac artery?	>4 cm
Femoral artery?	>2.5 cm
Popliteal artery?	>2 cm

MISCELLANEOUS

Define the following terms:

"Milk leg"

A.k.a. phlegmasia alba dolens (alba = white): often seen in pregnant women with occlusion of iliac vein resulting from extrinsic compression by the uterus (thus, the leg is "white" because of subcutaneous edema)

Phlegmasia cerulea dolens

In comparison, phlegmasia cerulea dolens is secondary to severe venous outflow obstruction and results in a cyanotic leg; the extensive venous thrombosis results in arterial inflow impairment

Raynaud's phenomenon

Vasospasm of digital arteries with color changes of the digits; usually initiated by cold/emotion

White (spasm), then blue (cyanosis), then red (hyperemia)

Takayasu's arteritis

Arteritis of the aorta and aortic branches, resulting in stenosis/occlusion/aneurysms

Seen mostly in women

Buerger's disease

A.k.a. thromboangiitis obliterans: occlusion of the small vessels of the hands and feet; seen in **young men who smoke;** often results in digital gangrene → amputations

What is the treatment for Buerger's disease?

Smoking **cessation,** +/− sympathectomy

What is blue toe syndrome?

Microembolization from proximal atherosclerotic disease of the aorta resulting in blue, painful, ischemic toes

What is a "paradoxical embolus"?

Venous embolus gains access to the left heart after going through an intracardiac defect, most commonly a patent foramen ovale, and then lodges in a peripheral artery

What size iliac aneurysm should be repaired?

>4 cm diameter

What is Behçet's disease?

Genetic disease with aneurysms from loss of vaso vasorum; seen with oral, ocular, and genital ulcers/inflammation (↑ incidence in Japan, Mediterranean)

Chapter 67
Pediatric Surgery

What is the motto of pediatric surgery?	"Children are NOT little adults!"
What is a simple way to distract a pediatric patient when examining the abdomen for tenderness?	Listen to the abdomen with the stethoscope and then push down on the abdomen with the stethoscope to check for tenderness

PEDIATRIC IV FLUIDS AND NUTRITION

What is the estimated blood volume of infants and children?	$\approx 8\%$ of body weight or $\approx$ **80 cc/kg**
What is the maintenance IV fluid for children?	D5 1/4 NS + 20 mEq KCl
Why 1/4 NS?	Children (especially those younger than 4 years of age) cannot concentrate their urine and cannot clear excess sodium
How are maintenance fluid rates calculated in children?	**4, 2, 1 per hour:** **4 cc/kg for the first 10 kg of body weight** **2 cc/kg for the second 10 kg of body weight** **1 cc/kg for every kilogram over the first 20** (e.g., the rate for a child weighing 25 kg is $4 \times 10 = 40$ plus $2 \times 10 = 20$ plus $1 \times 5 = 5$, for an IVF rate of 65 cc/hr)
What is the minimal urine output for children?	From 1 to 2 mL/kg/hr

What is the best way to present urine output measurements on rounds?	Urine output total per shift, THEN cc/kg/hr
What is the major difference between adult and pediatric nutritional needs?	Premature infants/infants/children need more calories and protein/kg/day

What are the caloric requirements by age for the following patients:

Premature infants?	80 Kcal/kg/day and then go up
Children younger than 1 year?	≈100 Kcal/kg/day (90–120)
Children ages 1 to 7?	≈85 Kcal/kg/day (75–90)
Children ages 7 to 12?	≈70 Kcal/kg/day (60–75)
Youths ages 12 to 18	≈40 Kcal/kg/day (30–60)

What are the protein requirements by age for the following patients:

Children younger than 1 year?	3 g/kg/day (2–3.5)
Children ages 1 to 7?	2 g/kg/day (2–2.5)
Children ages 7 to 12?	2 g/kg/day
Youths ages 12 to 18?	1.5 grams/kg/day
How many calories are in breast milk?	20 Kcal/30 cc (same as most formulas)

PEDIATRIC BLOOD VOLUMES

Give blood volume per kilogram:

Newborn infant?	85 cc
Infant 1–3 months of age?	75 cc
Child?	70 cc

FETAL CIRCULATION

What is the number of umbilical veins?	1 (usually)
What is the number of umbilical arteries?	2
Which umbilical vessel carries oxygenated blood?	Umbilical vein
The oxygenated blood travels through the liver to the IVC through which structure?	Ductus venosus
Oxygenated blood passes from the right atrium to the left atrium through which structure?	Foramen ovale
Unsaturated blood goes from the right ventricle to the descending aorta through which structure?	Ductus arteriosum
Define the overall fetal circulation.	

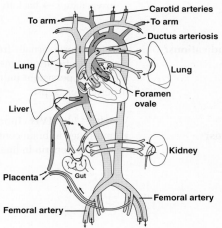

What are the ADULT structures of the following fetal structures:

Ductus venosus?	Ligamentum venosum
Umbilical vein?	Ligamentum teres
Umbilical artery?	Medial umbilical ligament
Ductus arteriosus?	Ligamentum arteriosum
Urachus?	Median umbilical ligament
Tongue remnant of thyroid's descent?	Foramen cecum
Persistent remnant of vitelline duct?	Meckel's diverticulum

ECMO

What is ECMO?　　ExtraCorporeal Membrane Oxygenation: chronic cardiopulmonary bypass—for complete respiratory support

What are the types of ECMO?　　Venovenous: Blood from vein → oxygenated → back to vein
Venoarterial: Blood from vein (IJ) → oxygenated → back to artery (carotid)

What are the indications?　　Severe hypoxia, usually from congenital diaphragmatic hernia, meconium aspiration, persistent pulmonary hypertension, sepsis

What are the contraindications?　　Weight <2 kg, **IVH** (**I**ntra**V**entricular **H**emorrhage in brain contraindicated because of heparin in line)

NECK

What is the major differential diagnosis of a pediatric neck mass?	Thyroglossal duct cyst (midline), branchial cleft cyst (lateral), lymphadenopathy, abscess, cystic hygroma, hemangioma, teratoma/dermoid cyst, thyroid nodule, lymphoma/leukemia (also parathyroid tumors, neuroblastoma, histiocytosis X, rhabdomyosarcoma, salivary gland tumors, neurofibroma)

THYROGLOSSAL DUCT CYST

What is it?	Remnant of the diverticulum formed by migration of thyroid tissue; normal development involves migration of thyroid tissue from the foramen cecum at the base of the tongue through the hyoid bone to its final position around the tracheal cartilage

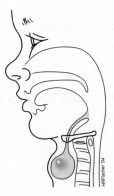

What is the average age at diagnosis?	Usually presents around 5 years of age
How is the diagnosis made?	Ultrasound
What are the complications?	Enlargement, infection, and fistula formation between oropharynx or salivary gland; aberrant thyroid tissue may masquerade as thyroglossal duct cyst, and if it is not cystic, deserves a thyroid scan

What is the anatomic location?	Almost always in the **midline**
How can one remember the position of the thyroglossal duct cyst?	Think: thyro**GLOSSAL** = **TONGUE** midline sticking out

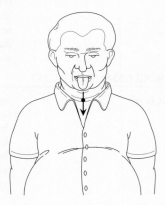

What is the treatment?	Antibiotics if infection is present, then excision, which must include the midportion of the hyoid bone and entire tract to foramen cecum (**Sistrunk** procedure)

BRANCHIAL CLEFT ANOMALIES

What is it?	Remnant of the primitive branchial clefts in which epithelium forms a sinus tract between the pharynx (second cleft), or the external auditory canal (first cleft), and the skin of the anterior neck; if the sinus ends blindly, a cyst may form
What is the common presentation?	Infection because of communication between pharynx and external ear canal
What is the anatomic position?	Second cleft anomaly—**lateral to the midline** along anterior border of the sternocleidomastoid, anywhere from angle of jaw to clavicle First cleft anomaly—less common than second cleft anomalies; tend to be located higher under the mandible

What is the most common cleft remnant?	Second; thus, these are found most often laterally versus thyroglossal cysts, which are found centrally (Think: **S**econd = **S**uperior)
What is the treatment?	Antibiotics if infection is present, then surgical excision of cyst and tract once inflammation is resolved
What is the major anatomic difference between thyroglossal cyst and branchial cleft cyst?	Thyroglossal cyst = **midline** Branchial cleft cyst = **lateral** (Think: br**A**nchial = l**A**teral)

STRIDOR

What is stridor?	Harsh, high-pitched sound heard on breathing caused by obstruction of the trachea or larynx
What are the signs/ symptoms?	Dyspnea, cyanosis, difficulty with feedings
What is the differential diagnosis?	Laryngomalacia—leading cause of stridor in infants; results from inadequate development of supporting laryngeal structures; usually self-limited and treatment is expectant unless respiratory compromise is present Tracheobronchomalacia—similar to laryngomalacia, but involves the entire trachea Vascular rings and slings—abnormal development or placement of thoracic large vessels resulting in obstruction of trachea/bronchus
What are the symptoms of vascular rings?	Stridor, dyspnea on exertion, or dysphagia
How is the diagnosis of vascular rings made?	Barium swallow revealing typical configuration of esophageal compression Echo/arteriogram
What is the treatment of vascular rings?	Surgical division of the ring, if the patient is symptomatic

CYSTIC HYGROMA

What is it?	Congenital abnormality of lymph sac resulting in lymphangioma
What is the anatomic location?	Occurs in sites of primitive lymphatic lakes and can occur virtually anywhere in the body, most commonly in the floor of mouth, under the jaw, or in the neck, axilla, or thorax
What is the treatment?	Early total surgical removal because they tend to enlarge; sclerosis may be needed if the lesion is unresectable
What are the possible complications?	Enlargement in critical regions, such as the floor of the mouth or paratracheal region, may cause airway obstruction; also, they tend to insinuate onto major structures (although not malignant), making excision difficult and hazardous

ASPIRATED FOREIGN BODY (FB)

Which bronchus do FBs go into more commonly (left or right)?	Younger than age 4—50/50 Age 4 and older—most go into right bronchus because it develops into a straight shot (less of an angle)
What is the most commonly aspirated object?	Peanut
What is the associated risk with peanut aspiration?	Lipoid pneumonia
How can an FB result in "air trapping and hyperinflation"?	By forming a "ball valve" (i.e., air in, no air out) as seen on CXR as a hyperinflated lung on expiratory film
How can you tell on A-P CXR if a coin is in the esophagus or the trachea?	Coin in **esophagus** results in the coin lying "en face" with face of the coin viewed as a **round object** because of compression by anterior and posterior structures If coin is in the **trachea,** it is viewed as a **side projection** due to the U-shaped cartilage with membrane posteriorly

What is the treatment of tracheal or esophageal FB?	Remove FB with **rigid** bronchoscope or **rigid** esophagoscope

CHEST

What is the differential diagnosis of a lung mass?	Bronchial adenoma (carcinoid is most common), pulmonary sequestration, pulmonary blastoma, rhabdomyosarcoma, chondroma, hamartoma, leiomyoma, mucus gland adenoma, metastasis
What is the differential diagnosis of mediastinal tumor/mass?	1. Neurogenic tumor (ganglioneuromas, neurofibromas) 2. Teratoma 3. Lymphoma 4. Thymoma (Classic **"four T's"**: **T**eratoma, **T**errible lymphoma, **T**hymoma, **T**hyroid tumor) Rare: pheochromocytoma, hemangioma, rhabdomyosarcoma, osteochondroma

PECTUS DEFORMITY

What heart abnormality is associated with pectus abnormality?	Mitral valve prolapse (many patients receive preoperative echocardiogram)

PECTUS EXCAVATUM

What is it?	Chest wall deformity with sternum caving inward (Think: ex**CAV**atum = **CAVE**)

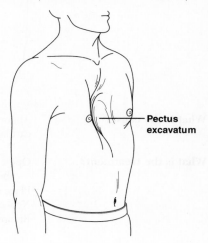

Pectus excavatum

What is the cause?	Abnormal, unequal overgrowth of rib cartilage
What are the signs/ symptoms?	Often asymptomatic; mental distress, dyspnea on exertion, chest pain
What is the treatment?	Open perichondrium, remove abnormal cartilage, place substernal strut; new cartilage grows back in the perichondrium in normal position; remove strut 6 months later
What is the NUSS procedure?	Placement of metal strut to elevate sternum **without** removing cartilage

PECTUS CARINATUM

What is it?	Chest wall deformity with sternum outward (pectus = chest, carinatum = pigeon); much less common than pectus excavatum

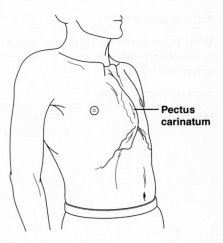

Pectus carinatum

What is the cause?	Abnormal, unequal overgrowth of rib cartilage
What is the treatment?	Open perichondrium and remove abnormal cartilage Place substernal strut New cartilage grows into normal position Remove strut 6 months later

ESOPHAGEAL ATRESIA WITHOUT TRACHEOESOPHAGEAL (TE) FISTULA

What is it?	Blind-ending esophagus from atresia
What are the signs?	Excessive oral secretions and inability to keep food down
How is the diagnosis made?	Inability to pass NG tube; plain x-ray shows tube coiled in upper esophagus and no gas in abdomen
What is the primary treatment?	Suction blind pouch, IVFs, (gastrostomy to drain stomach if prolonged preoperative esophageal stretching is planned)
What is the definitive treatment?	Surgical with 1° anastomosis, often with preoperative stretching of blind pouch (other options include colonic or jejunal interposition graft or gastric tube formation if esophageal gap is long)

ESOPHAGEAL ATRESIA WITH TRACHEOESOPHAGEAL (TE) FISTULA

What is it?	Esophageal atresia occurring with a fistula to the trachea; occurs in >90% of cases of esophageal atresia
What is the incidence?	One in 1500 to 3000 births
Define the following types of fistulas/atresias:	
Type A	Esophageal atresia without TE fistula (8%)

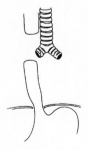

Type B   Proximal esophageal atresia with proximal
                               TE fistula (1%)

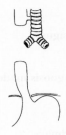

Type C   Proximal esophageal atresia with distal
                               TE fistula (85%); most common type

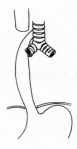

Type D   Proximal esophageal atresia with both
                               proximal and distal TE fistulas (2%)
                               (Think: **D** = **D**ouble connection to
                               trachea)

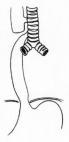

Type E   "H-type" TE fistula without esophageal
                              atresia (4%)

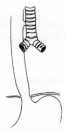

How do you remember   Simple: Most **C**ommon type is type **C**
which type is most common?

What are the symptoms?   Excessive secretions caused by an
                              accumulation of saliva (may not occur
                              with type E)

What are the signs?   Obvious respiratory compromise,
                              aspiration pneumonia, postprandial
                              regurgitation, gastric distention as air
                              enters the stomach directly from the
                              trachea

How is the diagnosis made? Failure to pass an NG tube (although this
                              will not be seen with type E); plain film
                              demonstrates tube coiled in the upper
                              esophagus; "pouchogram" (contrast in
                              esophageal pouch); gas on AXR
                              (tracheoesophageal fistula)

What is the initial   Directed toward minimizing
treatment?   complications from aspiration:
                              1. Suction blind pouch (NPO/TPN)
                              2. Upright position of child
                              3. Prophylactic antibiotics (Amp/gent)

What is the definitive   Surgical correction via a thoracotomy,
treatment?   usually through the right chest with
                              division of fistula and end-to-end
                              esophageal anastomosis, if possible

What can be done to lengthen the proximal esophageal pouch?	Delayed repair: with or without G-tube and daily **stretching** of proximal pouch
Which type should be fixed via a right neck incision?	"H-Type" (type E) is high in the thorax and can most often be approached via a right neck incision
What is the workup of a patient with a TE fistula?	To evaluate the TE fistula and **associated anomalies**: CXR, AXR, U/S of kidneys, cardiac echo (rest of workup directed by physical exam)
What are the associated anomalies?	**VACTERL** cluster (present in about 10% of cases): Vertebral or vascular, Anorectal, Cardiac, TE fistula, Esophageal atresia Radial limb and renal abnormalities, Lumbar and limb Previously known as **VATER**: Vertebral, Anus, TE fistula, Radial
What is the significance of a "gasless" abdomen on AXR?	No air to the stomach and, thus, no tracheoesophageal fistula

CONGENITAL DIAPHRAGMATIC HERNIA

What is it?	Failure of complete formation of the diaphragm, leading to a defect through which abdominal organs are herniated
What is the incidence?	One in 2100 live births; males are more commonly affected
What are the types of hernias?	Bochdalek and Morgagni
What are the associated positions?	Bochdalek—posterolateral with L > R Morgagni—anterior parasternal hernia, relatively uncommon

How to remember the position of the Bochdalek hernia?

Think: **BOCH DA LEK** = **"BACK TO THE LEFT"**

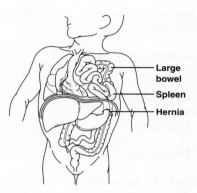

What are the signs?

Respiratory distress, dyspnea, tachypnea, retractions, and cyanosis; bowel sounds in the chest; rarely, maximal heart sounds on the right; ipsilateral chest dullness to percussion

What are the effects on the lungs?

1. Pulmonary hypoplasia
2. Pulmonary hypertension

What inhaled agent is often used?

Inhaled nitric oxide (pulmonary vasodilator), which decreases the shunt and decreases pulmonary hypertension

What is the treatment?

NG tube, ET tube, stabilization, and if patient is stable, surgical repair; if patient is unstable: nitric oxide +/− ECMO then to the O.R. when feasible

PULMONARY SEQUESTRATION

What is it?

Abnormal benign lung tissue with separate blood supply that **DOES NOT** communicate with the normal tracheobronchial airway

Define the following terms:
  Interlobar

Sequestration in the normal lung tissue covered by normal visceral pleura

Extralobar	Sequestration not in the normal lung covered by its own pleura
What are the signs/ symptoms?	Asymptomatic, recurrent pneumonia
How is the diagnosis made?	CXR, chest CT, A-gram, U/S with Doppler flow to ascertain blood supply
What is the treatment of each type:	
Extralobar?	Surgical resection
Intralobar?	Lobectomy
What is the major risk during operation for sequestration?	Anomalous blood supply from below the diaphragm (can be cut and retracted into the abdomen and result in exsanguination!); always document blood supply by A-gram or U/S with Doppler flow

ABDOMEN

What is the differential diagnosis of pediatric upper GI bleeding?	Gastritis, esophagitis, gastric ulcer, duodenal ulcer, esophageal varices, foreign body, epistaxis, coagulopathy, vascular malformation, duplication cyst
What is the differential diagnosis of pediatric lower GI bleeding?	Upper GI bleeding, anal fissures, NEC (premature infants), midgut volvulus (usually children younger than 1 year), strangulated hernia, intussusception, Meckel's diverticulum, infectious diarrhea, polyps, IBD, hemolytic uremic syndrome, Henoch-Schönlein purpura, vascular malformation, coagulopathy
What is the differential diagnosis of neonatal bowel obstruction?	Malrotation with volvulus, intestinal atresia, duodenal web, annular pancreas, imperforate anus, Hirschsprung's disease, NEC, intussusception (rare), Meckel's diverticulum, incarcerated hernia, meconium ileus, meconium plug, maternal narcotic abuse (ileus), maternal hypermagnesemia (ileus), sepsis (ileus)

What is the differential diagnosis of infant constipation?	Hirschsprung's disease, CF (cystic fibrosis), anteriorly displaced anus, polyps

INGUINAL HERNIA

What is the most commonly performed procedure by U.S. pediatric surgeons?	Indirect inguinal hernia repair
What is the most common inguinal hernia in children?	Indirect
What is an indirect inguinal hernia?	Hernia lateral to Hesselbach's triangle into the internal inguinal ring and down the inguinal canal (Think: through the abdominal wall indirectly into the internal ring and out through the external inguinal ring)
What is Hesselbach's triangle?	Triangle formed by: 1. Epigastric vessels 2. Inguinal ligament 3. Lateral border of the rectus sheath
What type of hernia goes through Hesselbach's triangle?	Direct hernia from a weak abdominal floor; rare in children (0.5% of all inguinal hernias)
What is the incidence of indirect inguinal hernia in all children?	≈3%
What is the incidence in premature infants?	Up to 30%
What is the male to female ratio?	6:1
What are the risk factors for an indirect inguinal hernia?	Male gender, ascites, V-P shunt, prematurity, family history, meconium ileus, abdominal wall defect elsewhere, hypo/epispadias, connective tissue disease, bladder exstrophy, undescended testicle, CF

Which side is affected more commonly?	**Right** ($\approx 60\%$)
What percentage are bilateral?	$\approx 15\%$
What percentage have a family history of indirect hernias?	$\approx 10\%$
What are the signs/ symptoms?	Groin bulge, scrotal mass, thickened cord, silk glove sign
What is the silk glove sign?	Hernia sac rolls under the finger like the finger of a silk glove
Why should it be repaired?	Risk of incarcerated/strangulated bowel or ovary; will not go away on its own
How is a pediatric inguinal hernia repaired?	High ligation of hernia sac (no repair of the abdominal wall floor, which is a big difference between the procedure in children vs. adults; high refers to high position on the sac neck next to the peritoneal cavity)
Which infants need overnight apnea monitoring/ observation?	Premature infants; infants younger than 3 months of age
What is the risk of recurrence after high ligation of an indirect pediatric hernia?	$\approx 1\%$
Describe the steps in the repair of an indirect inguinal hernia from skin to skin.	Cut skin, then fat, then Scarpa's fascia, then external oblique fascia through the external inguinal ring; find hernia sac anteriomedially and bluntly separate from the other cord structures; ligate sac high at the neck at the internal inguinal ring; resect sac and allow sac stump to retract into the peritoneal cavity; close external oblique; close Scarpa's fascia; close skin

Define the following terms:

Cryptorchidism

Failure of the testicle to descend into the scrotum

Hydrocele

Fluid-filled sac (i.e., fluid in a patent processus vaginalis or in the tunica vaginalis around the testicle)

Communicating hydrocele

Hydrocele that communicates with the peritoneal cavity and thus fills and drains peritoneal fluid or gets bigger, then smaller

Noncommunicating hydrocele

Hydrocele that does not communicate with the peritoneal cavity; stays about the same size

Can a hernia be ruled out if an inguinal mass transilluminates?

NO; baby bowel is very thin and will often transilluminate

CLASSIC INTRAOPERATIVE QUESTIONS DURING REPAIR OF AN INDIRECT INGUINAL HERNIA

From what abdominal muscle layer is the cremaster muscle derived?

Internal oblique muscle

From what abdominal muscle layer is the inguinal ligament (a.k.a. Poupart's ligament) derived?

External oblique

What nerve travels with the spermatic cord?

Ilioinguinal nerve

Name the 5 structures in the spermatic cord.

1. Cremasteric muscle fibers
2. Vas deferens
3. Testicular artery
4. Testicular pampiniform venous plexus
5. With or without hernia sac

What is the hernia sac made of?

Basically peritoneum or a patent processus vaginalis

What is the name of the fossa between the testicle and epididymis?	Fossa of Geraldi
What attaches the testicle to the scrotum?	Gubernaculum
How can the opposite side be assessed for a hernia intraoperatively?	Many surgeons operatively explore the opposite side when they repair the affected side Laparoscope is placed into the abdomen via the hernia sac and the opposite side internal inguinal ring is examined
Name the remnant of the processus vaginalis around the testicle.	Tunica vaginalis
What is a Littre's inguinal hernia?	Hernia with a Meckel's diverticulum in the hernia sac
What may a yellow/orange tissue that is not fat be on the spermatic cord/testicle?	Adrenal rest
What is the most common organ in an inguinal hernia sac in boys?	Small intestine
What is the most common organ in an inguinal hernia sac in girls?	Ovary/fallopian tube
What lies in the inguinal canal in girls instead of the vas?	Round ligament
Where in the inguinal canal does the hernia sac lie in relation to the other structures?	Anteriomedially
What is a "cord lipoma"?	Preperitoneal fat on the cord structures (pushed in by the hernia sac); not a real lipoma Should be removed surgically, if feasible

Within the spermatic cord, do the vessels or the vas lie medially?

Vas is medial to the testicular vessels

What is a small outpouching of testicular tissue off of the testicle?

Testicular appendage (a.k.a. the appendix testes); should be removed with electrocautery

What is a "blue dot sign"?

Blue dot on the scrotal skin from a twisted testicular appendage

How is a transected vas treated?

Repair with primary anastomosis

How do you treat a transected ilioinguinal nerve?

Should not be repaired; many surgeons ligate it to inhibit neuroma formation

What happens if you cut the ilioinguinal nerve?

Loss of sensation to the medial aspect of the inner thigh and scrotum/labia; loss of cremasteric reflex

UMBILICAL HERNIA

What is it?

Fascial defect at the umbilical ring

What are the risk factors?

1. African American infant
2. Premature infant

What are the indications for surgical repair?

1. >1.5 cm defect
2. Bowel incarceration
3. >4 years of age

GERD

What is it?

GastroEsophageal Reflux Disease

What are the causes?

LES malfunction/malposition, hiatal hernia, gastric outlet obstruction, partial bowel obstruction, common in cerebral palsy

What are the signs/ symptoms?	Spitting up, emesis, URTI, pneumonia, laryngospasm from aspiration of gastric contents into the tracheobronchial tree, failure to thrive
How is the diagnosis made?	24-hour pH probe, bronchoscopy, UGI (manometry, EGD, U/S)
What cytologic aspirate finding on bronchoscopy can diagnose aspiration of gastric contents?	Lipid-laden macrophages (from phagocytosis of fat)
What is the medical/ conservative treatment?	H_2 blockers Small meals/rice cereal Elevation of head
What are the indications for surgery?	"SAFE": **S**tricture **A**spiration, pneumonia/asthma **F**ailure to thrive **E**sophagitis
What is the surgical treatment?	**Nissen** 360° fundoplication, with or without G tube

CONGENITAL PYLORIC STENOSIS

What is it?	Hypertrophy of smooth muscle of pylorus, resulting in obstruction of outflow

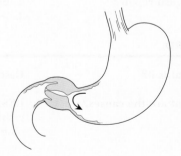

What are the associated risks?	Family history, firstborn males are affected most commonly, decreased incidence in African American population

What is the incidence?

1 in 750 births, M:F ratio = 4:1

What is the average age at onset?

Usually from 2 weeks after birth to about 2 months (**"2 to 2"**)

What are the symptoms?

Increasing frequency of regurgitation, leading to eventual nonbilious projectile vomiting

Why is the vomiting nonbilious?

Obstruction is proximal to the ampulla of Vater

What are the signs?

Abdominal mass or "olive" in epigastric region (85%), hypokalemic hypochloremic metabolic alkalosis, icterus (10%), visible gastric peristalsis, paradoxic aciduria, hematemesis (<10%)

What is the differential diagnosis?

Pylorospasm, milk allergy, increased ICP, hiatal hernia, GERD, adrenal insufficiency, uremia, malrotation, duodenal atresia, annular pancreas, duodenal web

How is the diagnosis made?

Usually by history and physical exam alone
U/S—demonstrates elongated (>15 mm) pyloric channel and thickened muscle wall (>3.5 mm)
If U/S is nondiagnostic, then barium swallow—shows "string sign" or "double railroad track sign"

What is the initial treatment?

Hydration and correction of alkalosis with D10 NS plus 20 mEq of KCl (**Note:** the infant's liver glycogen stores are very small; therefore, use D10; Cl⁻ and hydration will correct the alkalosis)

What is the definitive treatment?

Surgical, via Fredet-Ramstedt pyloromyotomy (division of circular muscle fibers without entering the lumen/mucosa)

What are the postoperative complications?	Unrecognized incision through the duodenal mucosa, bleeding, wound infection, aspiration pneumonia
What is the appropriate postoperative feeding?	Start feeding with Pedialyte® at 6 to 12 hours postoperatively; advance to full-strength formula over 24 hours
Which vein crosses the pylorus?	Vein of Mayo

DUODENAL ATRESIA

What is it?	Complete obstruction or stenosis of duodenum caused by an ischemic insult during development or failure of recanalization
What is the anatomic location?	85% are distal to the ampulla of Vater, 15% are proximal to the ampulla of Vater (these present with nonbilious vomiting)
What are the signs?	Bilious vomiting (if distal to the ampulla), epigastric distention
What is the differential diagnosis?	Malrotation with Ladd's bands, annular pancreas
How is the diagnosis made?	Plain abdominal film revealing "double bubble," with one air bubble in the stomach and the other in the duodenum
What is the treatment?	Duodenoduodenostomy or duodenojejunostomy
What are the associated abnormalities?	50% to 70% have cardiac, renal, or other gastrointestinal defects; 30% have trisomy 21

MECONIUM ILEUS

What is it?	Intestinal obstruction from solid meconium concretions
What is the incidence?	Occurs in ≈15% of infants with CF

What percentage of patients with meconium ileus have CF (cystic fibrosis)?

\>95%

What are the signs/symptoms of meconium ileus?

Bilious vomiting, abdominal distention, failure to pass meconium, Neuhauser's sign, peritoneal calcifications

What is Neuhauser's sign?

A.k.a. "soap bubble" sign: ground glass appearance in the RLQ on AXR from viscous meconium mixing with air

How is the diagnosis made?

Family history of CF, plain abdominal films showing significant dilation of similar-sized bowel loops, but few if any air-fluid levels, BE may demonstrate "microcolon" and inspissated meconium pellets in the terminal ileum

What is the treatment?

70% nonoperative clearance of meconium using gastrografin enema, +/− acetylcysteine, which is hypertonic and therefore draws fluid into lumen, separating meconium pellets from bowel wall (60% success rate)

What is the surgical treatment?

If enema is unsuccessful, then enterotomy with intraoperative catheter irrigation using acetylcysteine (Mucomyst®)

What should you remove during all operative cases?

Appendix

What is the long-term medical treatment?

Pancreatic enzyme replacement

What is cystic fibrosis (CF)?

Inherited disorder of epithelial Cl⁻ transport defect affecting sweat glands, airways, and GI tract (pancreas, intestine); diagnosed by sweat test (elevated levels of NaCl >60 mEq/liter) and genetic testing

What is DIOS?

Distal **I**ntestinal **O**bstruction **S**yndrome: intestinal obstruction in older patients with CF from inspissated luminal contents

MECONIUM PERITONITIS

What is it?	Sign of **intrauterine** bowel perforation; sterile meconium leads to an intense local inflammatory reaction with eventual formation of calcifications
What are the signs?	Calcifications on plain films

MECONIUM PLUG SYNDROME

What is it?	Colonic obstruction from unknown factors that dehydrate meconium, forming a "plug"
What is it also known as?	Neonatal small left colon syndrome
What are the signs/ symptoms?	Abdominal distention and **failure to pass meconium within first 24 hours of life;** plain films demonstrate many loops of distended bowel and air-fluid levels
What is the nonoperative treatment?	Contrast enema is both diagnostic and therapeutic; it demonstrates "microcolon" to the point of dilated colon (usually in transverse colon) and reveals copious intraluminal material
What is the major differential diagnosis?	Hirschsprung's disease
Is meconium plug highly associated with CF?	No; <5% of patients have CF, in contrast to meconium ileus, in which nearly all have CF (95%)

ANORECTAL MALFORMATIONS

What are they?	Malformations of the distal GI tract in the general categories of anal atresia, imperforate anus, and rectal atresia

IMPERFORATE ANUS

What is it?	Congenital absence of normal anus (complete absence or fistula)

Define a "high" imperforate anus.

Rectum patent to level above puborectalis sling

Define "low" imperforate anus.

Rectum patent to below puborectalis sling

Which type is much more common in women?

Low

What are the associated anomalies?

Vertebral abnormalities, **A**nal abnormalities, **C**ardiac, **TE** fistulas, **E**sophageal Atresia, **R**adial/**R**enal abnormalities, **L**umbar abnormalities (**VACTERL**; most commonly TE fistula)

What are the signs/ symptoms?

No anus, fistula to anal skin or bladder, UTI, fistula to vagina or urethra, bowel obstruction, distended abdomen, hyperchloremic acidosis

How is the diagnosis made?

Physical exam, the classic Cross table "invertogram" plain x-ray to see level of rectal gas (not very accurate), perineal ultrasound

What is the treatment of the following conditions:
    Low imperforate anus with anal fistula?

Dilatation of anal fistula and subsequent anoplasty

    High imperforate anus?

Diverting colostomy and mucous fistula; neoanus is usually made at 1 year of age

HIRSCHSPRUNG'S DISEASE

What is it also known as?

Aganglionic megacolon

What is it?

Neurogenic form of intestinal obstruction in which obstruction results from inadequate relaxation and peristalsis; absence of normal ganglion cells of the rectum and colon

What are the associated risks?

Family history; 5% chance of having a second child with the affliction

What is the male to female ratio?	4:1
What is the anatomic location?	Aganglionosis begins at the anorectal line and involves rectosigmoid in 80% of cases (10% have involvement to splenic flexure, and 10% have involvement of entire colon)
What are the signs/ symptoms?	Abdominal distention and bilious vomiting; >95% present with failure to pass meconium in the first 24 hours; may also present later with constipation, diarrhea, and decreased growth
What is the classic history?	Failure to pass meconium in the first 24 hours of life
What is the differential diagnosis?	Meconium plug syndrome, meconium ileus, sepsis with adynamic ileus, colonic neuronal dysplasia, hypothyroidism, maternal narcotic abuse, maternal hypermagnesemia (tocolysis)
What imaging studies should be ordered?	**AXR:** reveals dilated colon **Unprepared barium enema:** reveals constricted aganglionic segment with dilated proximal segment, but this picture may not develop for 3 to 6 weeks; BE will also demonstrate retention of barium for 24 to 48 hours (normal evacuation = 10 to 18 hours)
What is needed for definitive diagnosis?	**Rectal biopsy:** for definitive diagnosis, submucosal suction biopsy is adequate in 90% of cases; otherwise, full-thickness biopsy should be performed to evaluate Auerbach's plexus
What is the "colonic transition zone"?	Transition (taper) from aganglionic small colon into the large dilated normal colon seen on BE
What is the initial treatment?	In neonates, a colostomy proximal to the transition zone prior to correction, to allow for pelvic growth and dilated bowel to return to normal size

What is a "leveling" colostomy?

Colostomy performed for Hirschsprung's disease at the level of normally innervated ganglion cells as ascertained on frozen section intraoperatively

Describe the following procedures:

Swenson

Primary anastomosis between the anal canal and healthy bowel (rectum removed)

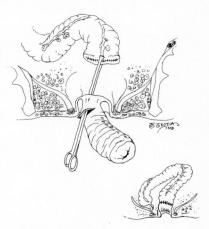

Duhamel

Anterior, aganglionic region of the rectum is preserved and anastomosed to a posterior portion of healthy bowel; a functional rectal pouch is thereby created (Think: **duha** = **dual** barrels side by side)

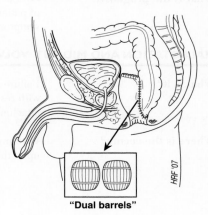

"Dual barrels"

Soave

A.k.a. endorectal pull-through; this procedure involves bringing proximal normal colon through the aganglionic rectum, which has been stripped of its mucosa but otherwise present (Think: **SOAVE** = **SAVE** the rectum, lose the mucosa)

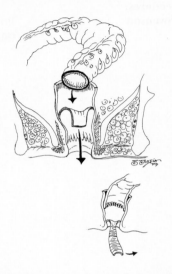

What is the new trend in surgery for Hirschsprung's disease?

No colostomy; remove aganglionic colon (as confirmed on frozen section) and perform pull-through anastomosis at the same time (Boley modification)

What is the prognosis?

Overall survival rate >90%; >96% of patients continent; postoperative symptoms improve with age

MALROTATION AND MIDGUT VOLVULUS

What is it?

Failure of the normal bowel rotation, with resultant abnormal intestinal attachments and anatomic positions

Where is the cecum?

With malrotation, the cecum usually ends up in the RUQ

What are Ladd's bands?

Fibrous bands that extend from the abnormally placed cecum in the RUQ, often crossing over the duodenum and causing obstruction

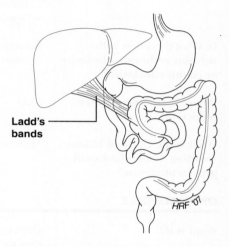

Ladd's bands

HRF '01

What is the usual age at onset?

33% are present by 1 week of age, 75% by 1 month, and 90% by 1 year

What is the usual presentation?

Sudden onset of bilious vomiting (**bilious vomiting in an infant is malrotation until proven otherwise!**)

Why is the vomiting bilious?

"Twist" is distal to the ampulla of Vater

How is the diagnosis made?

Upper GI contrast study showing cutoff in duodenum; BE showing abnormal position of cecum in the upper abdomen

What are the possible complications?

Volvulus with midgut infarction, leading to death or necessitating massive enterectomy (**rapid diagnosis is essential!**)

What is the treatment?

IV antibiotics and fluid resuscitation with LR, followed by emergent laparotomy with Ladd's procedure; second-look laparotomy if bowel is severely ischemic in 24 hours to determine if remaining bowel is viable

What is the Ladd's procedure?	1. **Counterclockwise** reduction of midgut volvulus 2. Splitting of Ladd's bands 3. Division of peritoneal attachments to the cecum, ascending colon 4. Appendectomy
In what direction is the volvulus reduced—clockwise or counterclockwise?	Rotation of the bowel in a counterclockwise direction
Where is the cecum after reduction?	LLQ
What is the cause of bilious vomiting in an infant until proven otherwise?	Malrotation with midgut volvulus

OMPHALOCELE

What is it?	Defect of abdominal wall at umbilical ring; sac **covers** extruded viscera
How is it diagnosed prenatally?	May be seen on **fetal** U/S after 13 weeks' gestation, with elevated maternal AFP
What comprises the "sac"?	Peritoneum and amnion
What organ is often found protruding from an omphalocele, but is almost never found with a gastroschisis?	The liver
What is the incidence?	≈ 1 in 5000 births
How is the diagnosis made?	Prenatal U/S
What are the possible complications?	Malrotation of the gut, anomalies
What is the treatment?	1. NG tube for decompression 2. IV fluids 3. Prophylactic antibiotics 4. Surgical repair of the defect

What is the treatment of a small defect (<2 cm)?

Closure of abdominal wall

What is the treatment of a medium defect (2–10 cm)?

Removal of outer membrane and placement of a silicone patch to form a "silo," temporarily housing abdominal contents; the silo is then slowly decreased in size over 4 to 7 days, as the abdomen accommodates the viscera; then the defect is closed

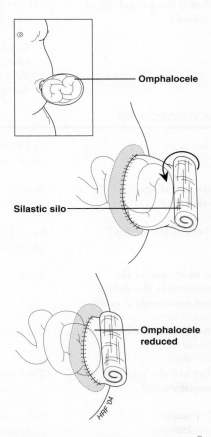

Omphalocele

Silastic silo

Omphalocele reduced

What is the treatment of "giant" defects (>10 cm)?

Skin flaps or treatment with Betadine® spray, mercurochrome, or silver sulfadiazine (Silvadene®) over defect; this allows an eschar to form, which epithelializes over time, allowing opportunity for future repair months to years later

What are the associated abnormalities?	50% of cases occur with abnormalities of the GI tract, cardiovascular system, GU tract, musculoskeletal system, CNS, and chromosomes
Of what "pentalogy" is omphalocele a part?	Pentalogy of Cantrell
What is the pentalogy of Cantrell?	"D COPS": **D**iaphragmatic defect (hernia) **C**ardiac abnormality **O**mphalocele **P**ericardium malformation/absence **S**ternal cleft

GASTROSCHISIS

What is it?	Defect of abdominal wall; sac does not cover extruded viscera
How is it diagnosed prenatally?	Possible at fetal ultrasound after 13 weeks' gestation, elevated maternal AFP
Where is the defect?	Lateral to the umbilicus (Think: g**A**strochisis = l**A**teral)
On what side of the umbilicus is the defect most commonly found?	Right
What is the usual size of the defect?	2 to 4 cm
What are the possible complications?	Thick edematous peritoneum from exposure to amnionic fluid; malrotation of the gut Other complications include hypothermia; hypovolemia from third-spacing; sepsis; and metabolic acidosis from hypovolemia and poor perfusion, NEC, prolonged ileus
How is the diagnosis made?	Prenatal U/S

What is the treatment?	Primary—NG tube decompression, IV fluids (D10 LR), and IV antibiotics
	Definitive—surgical reduction of viscera and abdominal closure; may require staged closure with silo
What is a "silo"?	Silastic silo is a temporary housing for external abdominal contents; silo is slowly tightened over time
What is the prognosis?	>90% survival rate
What are the associated anomalies?	Unlike omphalocele, relatively uncommon except for intestinal atresia, which occurs in 10% to 15% of cases
What are the major differences compared with omphalocele?	No membrane coverings
	Uncommon associated abnormalities
	Lateral to umbilicus—not on umbilicus
How can you remember the position of omphalocele vs. gastroschisis?	Think: **OM**phalocele = **ON** the umbilicus
How do you remember that omphalocele is associated with abnormalities in 50% of cases?	Think: **O**mphalocele = "**O**h no, lots of abnormalities"

POWER REVIEW OF OMPHALOCELE AND GASTROSCHISIS

What are the differences between omphalocele and gastroschisis in terms of the following characteristics:	
Anomalies?	Common in omphalocele (50%), uncommon in gastroschisis
Peritoneal/amnion covering (sac)?	Always with omphalocele—never with gastroschisis
Position of umbilical cord?	On the sac with omphalocele, from skin to the left of the gastroschisis defect

Thick bowel?	Common with gastroschisis, rare with omphalocele (unless sac ruptures)
Protrusion of liver?	Common with omphalocele, almost never with gastroschisis
Large defect?	Omphalocele

APPENDICITIS

What is it?	Obstruction of the appendiceal lumen (fecalith, lymphoid hyperplasia), producing a closed loop with resultant inflammation that can lead to necrosis and perforation
What is its claim to fame?	Most common surgical disease requiring emergency surgery in children
What is the affected age?	Very rare before 3 years of age
What is the usual presentation?	Onset of referred or **periumbilical pain** followed by **anorexia,** nausea, and vomiting (**Note:** Unlike gastroenteritis, **pain precedes vomiting,** then migrates to the **RLQ,** where it intensifies from local peritoneal irritation) If the patient is hungry and can eat, seriously question the diagnosis of appendicitis
How is the diagnosis made?	History and physical exam
What are the signs/ symptoms?	Signs of peritoneal irritation may be present—guarding, muscle spasm, rebound tenderness, obturator and Psoas signs; low-grade fever rising to high grade if perforation occurs
What is the differential diagnosis?	Intussusception, volvulus, Meckel's diverticulum, Crohn's disease, ovarian torsion, cyst, tumor, perforated ulcer, pancreatitis, PID, ruptured ectopic pregnancy, mesenteric lymphadenitis

What is the common bacterial cause of mesenteric lymphadenitis?

Yersinia enterocolitica

What are the associated lab findings with appendicitis?

Increased WBC ($>$10,000 per mm^3 in $>$90% of cases, with a left shift in most)

What is the role of urinalysis?

To evaluate for possible pyelonephritis or renal calculus, but mild hematuria and pyuria are common in appendicitis because of ureteral inflammation

What is the "hamburger" sign?

Ask patients with suspected appendicitis if they would like a hamburger or favorite food; if they can eat, seriously question the diagnosis

What radiographic studies may be performed?

Often none; CXR to rule out RML or RLL pneumonia; abdominal films are usually nonspecific, but calcified fecalith is present in 5% of cases; U/S to evaluate for ovarian/gynecologic pathology

What is the treatment?

Nonperforated—prompt appendectomy and cefoxitin to avoid perforation
Perforated—triple antibiotics, fluid resuscitation, and prompt appendectomy; all pus is drained and cultures obtained, with postoperative antibiotics continued for 5 to 7 days, ± drain

How long should antibiotics be administered if nonperforated?

24 hours

How long if perforated?

Usually 5 to 7 days or until WBCs are normal and patient is afebrile

If a normal appendix is found upon exploration, what must be examined/ ruled out?

Meckel's diverticulum, Crohn's disease, intussusception, gynecologic disease

What is the approximate risk of perforation?	≈25% after 24 hours from onset of symptoms ≈50% by 36 hours ≈75% by 48 hours

INTUSSUSCEPTION

What is it?	Obstruction caused by bowel telescoping into the lumen of adjacent distal bowel; may result when peristalsis carries a "leadpoint" downstream
What is its claim to fame?	Most common cause of small bowel obstruction in toddlers (<2 years old)
What is the usual age at presentation?	Disease of infancy; 60% present from 4 to 12 months of age, 80% by 2 years of age
What is the most common site?	Terminal ileum involving ileocecal valve and extending into ascending colon
What is the most common cause?	Hypertrophic Peyer's patches, which act as a lead point; many patients have prior viral illness
What are the signs/ symptoms?	Alternating lethargy and irritability (colic), bilious vomiting, "currant jelly" stools, RLQ mass on plain abdominal film, empty RLQ on palpation (Dance's sign)
What is the intussuscipiens?	Recipient segment of bowel (Think: **recipiens** = intussus**cipiens**)
What is the intussusceptum?	Leading point or bowel that enters the intussuscipiens
Identify locations 1 and 2 on the following illustration:	1. Intussuscipiens 2. Intussusceptum

How can the spelling of intussusception be remembered?

Imagine a navy ship named The **U.S.S. U.S.—INTUSSUS**CEPTION

What is the treatment?

Air or barium enema; 85% reduce with hydrostatic pressure (i.e., barium = meter elevation air = maximum of 120 mm Hg); if unsuccessful, then laparotomy and reduction by "milking" the ileum from the colon should be performed

What are the causes of intussusception in older patients?

Meckel's diverticulum, polyps, and tumors, all of which act as a lead point

MECKEL'S DIVERTICULUM

What is it?

Remnant of the omphalomesenteric duct/vitelline duct, which connects the yolk sac with the primitive midgut in the embryo

What is the usual location?

Between 45 and 90 cm proximal to the ileocecal valve on the antimesenteric border of the bowel

What is the major differential diagnosis?

Appendicitis

Is it a true diverticulum?

Yes; all layers of the intestine are found in the wall

What is the incidence?

2% of the population at autopsy, but >90% of these are asymptomatic

What is the gender ratio?

2 to 3× more common in males

What is the usual age at onset of symptoms?

Most frequently in the first 2 years of life, but can occur at any age

What are the possible complications?

Intestinal hemorrhage (painless)—50%
Accounts for 50% of all lower GI bleeding in patients younger than 2 years; bleeding results from ectopic gastric mucosa secreting acid → ulcer → bleeding
Intestinal obstruction—25%
Most common complication in adults; includes volvulus and intussusception
Inflammation (± perforation)—20%

What percentage of cases have heterotopic tissue?

>50%; usually gastric mucosa (85%), but duodenal, pancreatic, and colonic mucosa have been described

What is the most common ectopic tissue in a Meckel's diverticulum?

Gastric mucosa

What other pediatric disease entity can also present with GI bleeding secondary to ectopic gastric mucosa?

Enteric duplications

What is the most common cause of lower GI bleeding in children?

Meckel's diverticulum with ectopic gastric mucosa

What is the "rule of 2s"?

2% are symptomatic
Found ≈**2** feet from ileocecal valve
Found in **2%** of the population
Most symptoms occur before age **2**
One of **2** will have ectopic tissue
Most diverticula are about **2** inches long
Male:female ratio = **2**:1

What is a Meckel's scan?

Scan for ectopic gastric mucosa in Meckel's diverticulum; uses **technetium** Tc 99m **pertechnetate** IV, which is preferentially taken up by gastric mucosa

NECROTIZING ENTEROCOLITIS

What is it also known as?	NEC
What is it?	Necrosis of intestinal mucosa, often with bleeding; may progress to transmural intestinal necrosis, shock/sepsis, and death
What are the predisposing conditions?	**PREMATURITY** Stress: shock, hypoxia, RDS, apneic episodes, sepsis, exchange transfusions, PDA and cyanotic heart disease, hyperosmolar feedings, polycythemia, indomethacin
What is the pathophysiologic mechanism?	Probable splanchnic vasoconstriction with decreased perfusion, mucosal injury, and probable bacterial invasion
What is its claim to fame?	Most common cause of emergent laparotomy in the neonate
What are the signs/ symptoms?	Abdominal distention, vomiting, heme positive or gross rectal bleeding, fever or hypothermia, jaundice, abdominal wall erythema (consistent with perforation and abscess formation)
What are the radiographic findings?	Fixed, dilated intestinal loops; pneumatosis intestinalis (air in the bowel wall); free air; and portal vein air (sign of advanced disease)
What are the lab findings?	Low hematocrit, glucose, and platelets
What is the treatment?	Most are managed medically: 1. Cessation of feedings 2. OG tube 3. IV fluids 4. IV antibiotics 5. Ventilator support, as needed
What are the surgical indications?	Free air in abdomen revealing perforation, and positive peritoneal tap revealing transmural bowel necrosis

Operation?	1. Resect
	2. Stoma
What is an option for bowel perforation in <1000 gram NEC patients?	Placement of percutaneous drain (without laparotomy!)
Is portal vein gas or pneumatosis intestinalis alone an indication for operation with NEC?	No
What are the indications for peritoneal tap?	Severe thrombocytopenia, distended abdomen, abdominal wall erythema, unexplained clinical downturn
What are the possible complications?	Bowel necrosis, gram-negative sepsis, DIC, wound infection, cholestasis, short bowel syndrome, strictures, SBO
What is the prognosis?	>80% overall survival rate

BILIARY TRACT

What is "physiologic jaundice"?	Hyperbilirubinemia in the first 2 weeks of life from inadequate conjugation of bilirubin
What enzyme is responsible for conjugation of bilirubin?	Glucuronyl transferase
How is hyperbilirubinemia from "physiologic jaundice" treated?	UV light
What is Gilbert's syndrome?	Partial deficiency of glucuronyl transferase, leading to intermittent asymptomatic jaundice in the second or third decade of life
What is Crigler-Najjar syndrome?	Rare genetic absence of glucuronyl transferase activity, causing unconjugated hyperbilirubinemia, jaundice, and death from kernicterus (usually within the first year)

BILIARY ATRESIA

What is it?	Obliteration of extrahepatic biliary tree
What is the incidence?	One in 16,000 births
What are the signs/ symptoms?	Persistent jaundice (normal physiologic jaundice resolves in <2 weeks), hepatomegaly, splenomegaly, ascites and other signs of portal hypertension, acholic stools, biliuria
What are the lab findings?	Mixed jaundice is always present (i.e., both direct and indirect bilirubin increased), with an elevated serum alkaline phosphatase level
What is the classic "rule of 5s" of indirect bilirubinemia?	Bizarre: with progressive hyperbilirubinemia, jaundice progresses **by levels of 5** from the head to toes: **5** mg/dL = jaundice of head, **10** mg/ dL = jaundice of trunk, **15** mg/dL = jaundice of leg/feet
What is the differential diagnosis?	Neonatal hepatitis (TORCH); biliary hypoplasia
How is the diagnosis made?	1. U/S to rule out choledochal cyst and to examine extrahepatic bile ducts and gallbladder 2. HIDA scan—shows no excretion into the GI tract (with phenobarbital preparation) 3. Operative cholangiogram and liver biopsy
What is the treatment?	Early laparotomy by 2 months of age with a modified form of the Kasai hepatoportoenterostomy
How does a Kasai work?	Anastomosis of the porta hepatis and the small bowel allows drainage of bile via many microscopic bile ducts in the fibrous structure of the porta hepatis

What if the Kasai fails?   Revise or liver transplantation

What are the possible postoperative complications?   Cholangitis (manifested as decreased bile secretion, fever, leukocytosis, and recurrence of jaundice), progressive cirrhosis (manifested as portal hypertension with bleeding varices, ascites, hypoalbuminemia, hypothrombinemia, and fat-soluble vitamin K, A, D, E deficiencies)

What are the associated abnormalities?   Between 25% and 30% have other anomalies, including annular pancreas, duodenal atresia, malrotation, polysplenic syndrome, situs inversus, and preduodenal portal vein; 15% have congenital heart defects

CHOLEDOCHAL CYST

What is it?   Cystic enlargement of bile ducts; most commonly arises in extrahepatic ducts, but can also arise in intrahepatic ducts

What is the usual presentation?   50% present with intermittent jaundice, RUQ mass, and abdominal pain; may also present with pancreatitis

What are the possible complications?   Cholelithiasis, cirrhosis, carcinoma, and portal HTN

What are the anatomic variants:
    I?   Dilation of common hepatic and common bile duct, with cystic duct entering the cyst; most common type (90%)

Type I

II?   Lateral saccular cystic dilation

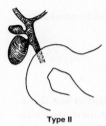

Type II

III?   Choledochocele represented by an
                           intraduodenal cyst

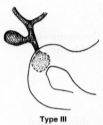

Type III

IV?   Multiple extrahepatic cysts, intrahepatic
                           cysts, or both

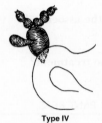

Type IV

V?   Single or multiple intrahepatic cysts

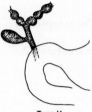

Type V

How is the diagnosis made?	U/S
What is the treatment?	Operative cholangiogram to clarify pathologic process and delineate the pancreatic duct, followed by complete resection of the cyst and a Roux-en-Y hepatojejunostomy
What condition are these patients at increased risk of developing?	**Cholangiocarcinoma** often arises in the cyst; therefore, treat by complete prophylactic resection of the cyst

CHOLELITHIASIS

What is it?	Formation of gallstones
What are the common causes in children?	Etiology differs somewhat from that of adults; the most common cause is cholesterol stones, but there is an increased percentage of pigmented stones from hemolytic disorders
What is the differential diagnosis?	Hereditary spherocytosis, thalassemia, pyruvate kinase deficiency, sickle-cell disease, cystic fibrosis, long-term parenteral nutrition, idiopathic
What are the associated risks?	Use of oral contraceptives, teenage, positive family history
What is the treatment?	Cholecystectomy is recommended for all children with gallstones

ANNULAR PANCREAS

What is an annular pancreas?	Congenital pancreatic abnormality with complete encirclement of the duodenum by the pancreas
What are the symptoms?	Duodenal obstruction
What is the treatment?	Duodenoduodenostomy bypass of obstruction (do not resect the pancreas!)

TUMORS

What is the differential diagnosis of pediatric abdominal mass?	Wilms' tumor, neuroblastoma, hernia, intussusception, malrotation with volvulus, mesenteric cyst, duplication cyst, liver tumor (hepatoblastoma/hemangioma), rhabdomyosarcoma, teratoma

WILMS' TUMOR

What is it?	Embryonal tumor of **renal** origin
What is the incidence?	Very rare: 500 new cases in the United States per year
What is the average age at diagnosis?	Usually between 1 and 5 years of age
What are the symptoms?	Usually asymptomatic except for abdominal mass; 20% of patients present with minimal blunt trauma to mass
What is the classic history?	Found during dressing or bathing
What are the signs?	Abdominal mass (most do not cross the midline); hematuria (10%–15%); HTN in 20% of cases, related to compression of juxtaglomerular apparatus; signs of Beckwith-Wiedemann syndrome
What are the diagnostic radiologic tests?	Abdominal and chest CT
Define the stages:	
Stage I	Limited to kidney and completely resected
Stage II	Extends beyond kidney, but completely resected; capsule invasion and perirenal tissues may be involved
Stage III	Residual nonhematogenous tumor after resection
Stage IV	Hematogenous metastases (lung, distal lymph nodes, and brain)
Stage V	Bilateral renal involvement

What are the best indicators of survival?	Stage and histologic subtype of tumor; 85% of patients have favorable histology (FH); 15% have unfavorable histology (UH); overall survival for FH is 85% for all stages
What is the treatment?	Radical resection of affected kidney with evaluation for staging, followed by chemotherapy (low stages) and radiation (higher stages)
What is the neoadjuvant treatment?	Large tumors may be shrunk with chemotherapy/XRT to allow for surgical resection
What are the associated abnormalities?	**Aniridia,** hemihypertrophy, Beckwith-Wiedemann syndrome, neurofibromatosis, horseshoe kidney
What is the Beckwith-Wiedemann syndrome?	**Syndrome of:** 1. Umbilical defect 2. Macroglossia (big tongue) 3. Gigantism 4. Visceromegaly (big organs) (Think: **W**ilms' = Beckwith-**W**iedemann)

NEUROBLASTOMA

What is it?	Embryonal tumor of neural crest origin
What are the anatomic locations?	**Adrenal medulla**—50% Paraaortic abdominal paraspinal ganglia—25% Posterior mediastinum—20% Neck—3% Pelvis—3%
With which types of tumor does a patient with Horner's syndrome present?	Neck, superior mediastinal tumors
What is the incidence?	One in 7000 to 10,000 live births; most common solid malignant tumor of infancy; most common solid tumor in children outside the CNS
What is the average age at diagnosis?	≈50% are diagnosed by 2 years of age ≈90% are diagnosed by 8 years of age

What are the symptoms?

Vary by tumor location—anemia, failure to thrive, weight loss, and poor nutritional status with advanced disease

What are the signs?

Asymptomatic abdominal mass (palpable in 50% of cases), respiratory distress (mediastinal tumors), Horner's syndrome (upper chest or neck tumors), proptosis (with orbital metastases), subcutaneous tumor nodules, HTN (20%–35%)

LABS?

24-hour urine to measure VMA, HVA, and metanephrines (elevated in >85%); neuron-specific enolase, N-*myc* oncogene, DNA ploidy

What are the diagnostic radiologic tests?

CT scan, MRI, I-MIBG, somatostatin receptor scan

What is the classic abdominal plain x-ray finding?

Calcifications (≈50%)

How do you access bone marrow involvement?

Bone marrow aspirate

What is the difference in position of tumors in neuroblastoma versus Wilms' tumors?

Neuroblastoma may cross the midline, but Wilms' tumors do so only rarely

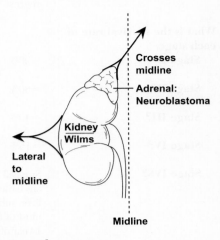

What is the treatment?

Depends on staging

Define the stages:

Stage I	Tumor is confined to organ of origin
Stage II	Tumor extends beyond organ of origin **but not** across the midline
Stage III	Tumor extends **across the midline**
Stage IV	Metastatic disease
Stage IVS	Infants: Localized primary tumor does not cross the midline, but **remote disease** is confined to the liver, subcutaneous/skin, and bone marrow

What is the treatment of each stage:

Stage I?	Surgical resection
Stage II?	Resection and chemotherapy +/− XRT
Stage III?	Resection and chemotherapy/XRT
Stage IV?	Chemotherapy/XRT → resection
Stage IVS?	In the infant with small tumor and asymptomatic = observe as many will regress "spontaneously"

What is the survival rate of each stage:

Stage I?	≈90%
Stage II?	≈80%
Stage III?	≈40%
Stage IV?	≈15%
Stage IVS?	Survival rate is >80%! **Note:** these tumors are basically stage I or II with metastasis to liver, subcutaneous tissue, or bone marrow; most of these patients, if younger than 1 year of age, have a spontaneous cure (Think: Stage IV**S** = **S**pecial condition)

What are the laboratory prognosticators?	Aneuploidy is favorable! The lower the number of N-*myc* oncogene copies, the better the prognosis
Which oncogene is associated with neuroblastoma?	N-*myc* oncogene Think: **N**-*myc* = **N**euroblastoma

RHABDOMYOSARCOMA

What is it?	Highly malignant **striated muscle** sarcoma
What is its claim to fame?	Most common sarcoma in children
What is the age distribution?	Bimodal: 1. 2–5 years 2. 15–19 years
What are the most common sites?	1. Head and neck (40%) 2. GU tract (20%) 3. Extremities (20%)
What are the signs/ symptoms?	Mass
How is the diagnosis made?	Tissue biopsy, CT scan, MRI, bone marrow
What is the treatment: **Resectable?**	Surgical excision, +/− chemotherapy and radiation therapy
Unresectable?	Neoadjuvant chemo/XRT, then surgical excision

HEPATOBLASTOMA

What is it?	Malignant tumor of the liver (derived from embryonic liver cells)
What is the average age at diagnosis?	Presents in the first 3 years of life
What is the male to female ratio?	2:1

How is the diagnosis made?	Physical exam—abdominal distention; **RUQ mass that moves with respiration**
	Elevated serum α-fetoprotein and ferritin (can be used as tumor markers)
	CT scan of abdomen, which often predicts resectability
What percentage will have an elevated α-fetoprotein level?	≈90%
What is the treatment?	Resection by lobectomy or trisegment-ectomy is the treatment of choice (plus postoperative chemotherapy); large tumors may require preoperative chemotherapy and **subsequent** hepatic resection
What is the overall survival rate?	≈50%
What is the major difference in age presentation between hepatoma and hepatoblastoma?	Hepatoblastoma presents at younger than 3 years of age; hepatoma presents at older than 3 years of age and in adolescents

PEDIATRIC TRAUMA

What is the leading cause of death in pediatric patients?	Trauma
How are the vast majority of splenic and liver injuries treated in children?	Observation (i.e., nonoperatively)
What is a common simulator of peritoneal signs in the blunt pediatric trauma victim?	Gastric distention (place an NG tube)
How do you estimate normal systolic blood pressure (SBP) in a child?	80 + 2 × age (e.g., a 5-year-old child should have an SBP of about 90)

What is the 20–20–10 rule for fluid resuscitation of the unstable pediatric trauma patient?

First give a **20**-cc/kg LR bolus followed by a second bolus of **20**-cc/kg LR bolus if needed; if the patient is still unstable after the second LR bolus, then administer a **10**-cc/kg bolus of **blood**

What CT scan findings suggest small bowel injury?

Free fluid with **no** evidence of liver or spleen injury; free air, contrast leak, bowel thickening, mesentery streaking

What is the treatment for duodenal hematoma?

Observation with NGT and TPN

OTHER PEDIATRIC SURGERY QUESTIONS

What is bilious vomiting in an infant?

Malrotation, until proven otherwise! (About 90% of patients with malrotation present before the first year of life)

What does TORCHES stand for?

Nonbacterial fetal and neonatal infections: **TO**xoplasmosis, **R**ubella, **C**ytomegalovirus (CMV), **HE**rpes, **S**yphilis

What is the common pediatric sedative?

Chloral hydrate

What are the contraindications to circumcision?

Hypospadias, etc., because the foreskin might be needed for future repair of the abnormality

When should an umbilical hernia be repaired?

>1.5 cm, after 4 years of age; otherwise observe, because most close spontaneously; repair before school age if it persists

What is the cancer risk in the cryptorchid testicle?

>10× the normal testicular cancer rate

When should orchidopexy be performed?

All patients with undescended testicle undergo orchidopexy after 1 year of age

What are some signs of child abuse?	Cigarette burns, rope burns, scald to posterior thighs and buttocks, multiple fractures/old fractures, genital trauma, delay in accessing health care system
What is the treatment of child abuse?	**Admit the patient** to the hospital
What is Dance's sign?	Empty RLQ in patients with ileocecal intussusception
What is the treatment of hemangioma?	Observation, because most regress spontaneously
What are the indications for operation in hemangiomas?	Severe thrombocytopenia, congestive heart failure, functional impairment (vision, breathing)
What are treatment options for hemangiomas?	Steroids, radiation, surgical resection, angiographic embolization
What is the most common benign liver tumor in children?	Hemangioma
What is Eagle-Barrett's syndrome?	A.k.a. prune belly; congenital inadequate abdominal musculature (very lax and thin)
What is the Pierre-Robin syndrome?	Classic triad: 1. Big, protruding tongue (glossoptosis) 2. Small mandible (micrognathia) 3. Cleft palate
What is the major concern with Pierre-Robin syndrome?	Airway obstruction by the tongue!
What are the most common cancers in children?	1. Leukemia 2. CNS tumors 3. Lymphomas
What is the most common solid neoplasm in infants?	Neuroblastoma
What is the most common solid tumor in children?	CNS tumors

What syndrome must you consider in the patient with abdominal pain, hematuria, history of joint pain, and a purpuric rash?

Henoch-Schönlein syndrome; patient may also have melena (50%) or at least guaiac-positive stools (75%)

What is Apley's law?

The further a chronically recurrent abdominal pain is from the umbilicus, the greater the likelihood of an organic cause for the pain

What is the most common cause of SBO in children?

Hernias

What is a patent urachus?

Persistence of the urachus, a communication between the bladder and umbilicus; presents with urine out of the umbilicus and recurrent UTIs

What is a "Replogle tube"?

10 French sump pump NG tube for babies (originally designed by Dr. Replogle for suction of the esophageal blind pouch of esophageal atresia)

What are "A's and B's"?

Apnea and **B**radycardia episodes in babies

What is the "double bubble" sign on AXR?

Gastric bubble and **duodenal bubble** on AXR; seen with duodenal obstruction (web, annular pancreas, malrotation with volvulus, duodenal atresia, etc.)

What is Poland's syndrome?

Absence of pectoralis major muscle
Absence of pectoralis minor muscle
Often associated with ipsilateral hand malformation
Nipple/breast/right-breast hypoplasia

What is the treatment of ATYPICAL mycobacterial lymph node infection?

Surgical removal of the node

What is the most common cause of rectal bleeding in infants?

Anal fissure

What chromosomal abnormality is associated with duodenal web/atresia/ stenosis?	Trisomy 21
Which foreign body past the pylorus must be surgically removed?	Batteries!

POWER REVIEW

What is the usual age at presentation of the following conditions:

Pyloric stenosis?	2 weeks to 2 months
Intussusception?	4 months to 2 years (>80%)
Wilms' tumor?	1 to 5 years
Malrotation?	Birth to 1 year (>85%)
Neuroblastoma?	≈50% present by 2 years; >80% present by 8 years
Hepatoblastoma?	Younger than 3 years
Appendicitis?	Older than 3 years (but must be considered at *any* age!)

Chapter 68   Plastic Surgery

Define the following terms:

Blepharoplasty	Eyelid surgery—removing excess skin/fat
Face lift	Removal of excess facial skin via hairline/ chin/ear incisions
FTSG	Full Thickness Skin Graft

Langer's lines

Natural skin lines of minimal tension (e.g., lines across the forehead), incisions perpendicular to Langer's lines result in larger scars than incision parallel to the lines

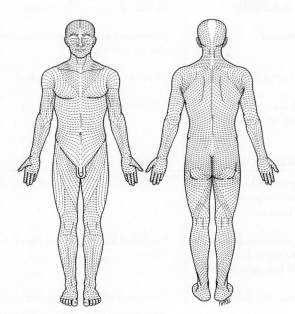

Mammoplasty

Breast surgery (reduction/augmentation)

Polydactyly

Extra fingers

Rhinoplasty

Nose surgery, after trauma or cosmetic

STSG

Split **T**hickness **S**kin **G**raft

Syndactyly

Webbed fingers

WOUND HEALING

What are the phases of wound healing?

Think: "**I**n **E**very **F**resh **C**ut" = **IEFC**:
1. **I**nflammation
2. **E**pithelialization
3. **F**ibroplasia
4. **C**ontraction

**What are the actions of the
following phases:**

Inflammation?

Vasoconstriction followed by vasodilation,
capillary leak

Epithelialization?

Epithelial coverage of wound

Fibroplasia?

Fibroblasts and accumulation of collagen,
elastin, and reticulin

Wound contraction?

Myofibroblasts contract wound

**What is the maximal
contraction of a wound in
mm/day?**

0.75 mm/day

EPITHELIALIZATION

**What degree of bacterial
contamination prevents
epithelialization?**

>100,000 organisms/gm tissue (10^5)

**In which structures does the
epithelium grow from
superficial burns/wounds?**

Epithelial lining of sweat glands and hair
follicles

In full-thickness burns?

From wound margins, grows in <1 cm
from wound edge because no sweat
glands or hair follicles remain; this
epithelium has no underlying dermis

**What malignant ulcer is
associated with a long-
standing scar/burn?**

Marjolin's ulcer (a.k.a. burn scar
carcinoma)

WOUND CONTRACTION

What are myofibroblasts?

Specialized fibroblasts that behave like
smooth muscle cells to pull the wound
edges together following granulation

**Which contracts more: an
STSG or an FTSG?**

STSG contracts up to 41% in surface
area, whereas an FTSG contracts little,
if at all

What is granulation tissue?	Within 4 to 6 days after an open wound, development of capillary beds and fibroblasts provides a healthy base for epithelial growth from wound edges; this tissue also resists bacterial infection
Name the local factors that impair wound healing.	Hematoma, seroma, infection, tight sutures, tight wrap, movement/disturbance of the wound (i.e., poking it with a finger)
What generalized conditions inhibit wound healing?	Anemia Malnutrition Steroids Cancer Radiation Hypoxia Sepsis
What helps wound healing in patients taking steroids?	Vitamin A is thought to counteract the deleterious effect of steroids on wound healing
When does a wound gain more than 90% of its maximal tensile strength?	After ≈6 weeks
Define the following terms: **Laceration**	Jagged wound
Abrasion	Superficial skin removal
Contusion	Bruise without a break in the skin
Hypertrophic scar	Hypertrophic scar **within** original wound margins
Keloid	Proliferative scar tumor progressively enlarging scar **beyond** original wound margins
Why not clean lacerations with Betadine®?	Betadine® is harmful to and inhibits normal healthy tissue
What is the best way to clean out a laceration?	Normal saline irrigation; remember, "The solution to pollution is dilution"

SKIN GRAFTS

What is an STSG?	Split thickness: includes the epidermis and a variable amount of the dermis
How thick is it?	10/1000 to 18/1000 of an inch
What is an FTSG?	Full thickness: includes the entire epidermis and dermis
What are the prerequisites for a skin graft to take?	Bed must be vascularized; a graft to a bone or tendon will not take Bacteria must be <100,000 Shearing motion and fluid beneath the graft must be minimized
What is a better bed for a skin graft: fascia or fat?	Fascia (much better blood supply)
How do you increase surface area of an STSG?	Mesh it (also allows for blood/serum to be removed from underneath the graft)
How does an STSG get nutrition for the first 24 hours?	Imbibition

FLAPS

Where does a random skin flap get its blood supply?	From the dermal-subdermal plexus
Where does an axial skin flap get its blood supply?	It is vascularized by direct cutaneous arteries
Name some axial flaps and their arterial supply.	Forehead flap—superficial temporal artery; often used for intraoral lesions Deltopectoral flap—second, third, and fourth anterior perforators of the internal mammary artery; often used for head and neck wounds Groin flap—superficial circumflex iliac artery; allows coverage of hand and forearm wounds

What is the most common cause of flap loss?

Venous thrombosis

What is a simple advancement flap?

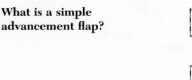

Defect

What is a rotational flap?

Pivot point

Defect

What is a "free flap"?

Flap separated from all vascular supply that requires microvascular anastomosis (microscope)

What is a TRAM flap?

Transverse **R**ectus **A**bdominis **M**yocutaneous flap (see page 410)

What is a "Z-plasty"?

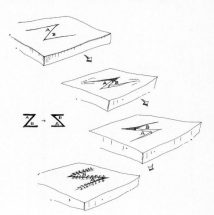

What is a "V-Y advancement flap"?

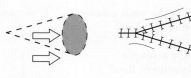

☐ Defect

Chapter 69   **Hand Surgery**

Who operates on hands?	Plastic surgeons **and** orthopaedic surgeons
What are the bones of the hand?	Phalanges (fingers) Metacarpal bones Carpal bones
What is the distal finger joint?	**D**istal **I**nter**P**halangeal (**DIP**) joint
What is the middle finger joint?	**P**roximal **I**nter**P**halangeal (**PIP**) joint
What is the proximal finger joint?	**M**etacarpal **P**halangeal (**MP**) joint
What are the "intrinsic" hand muscles?	Lumbricals, interosseous muscle
What is ADDuction and ABDuction of the fingers?	**ADD**uction is to midline and **ABD**uction is separation from midline

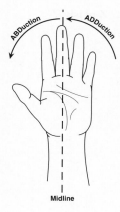

Midline

What are the trauma zones of the hand?

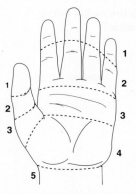

Where is "no man's land"?

Zone extending from the distal palmar crease to just beyond the PIP joint (zone 2)

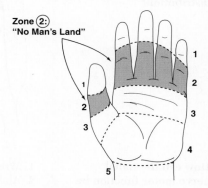

What is the significance of the "no man's land"?

Flexor tendon injuries here have a poor prognosis; a hand expert needs to repair these injuries

SENSORY SUPPLY TO THE HAND

What is the ulnar nerve distribution?

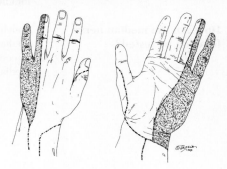

What is the radial nerve distribution?

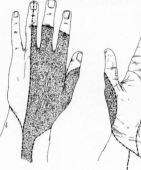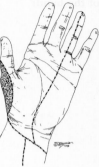

What is the median nerve distribution?

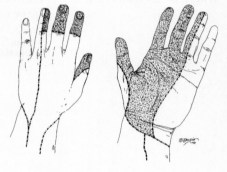

How can the radial nerve motor function be tested?

1. Wrist and MCP extension
2. Abduction and extension of thumb

How can the ulnar nerve motor function be tested?

1. Spread fingers apart against resistance
2. Check ability to cross index and middle fingers

How can the median nerve function be tested?

1. Touch the thumb to the pinky (distal median nerve)
2. Squeeze examiner's finger (proximal median nerve)

How can the flexor digitorum *profundus* (FDP) apparatus be tested?

Check isolated flexion of the finger DIP joint

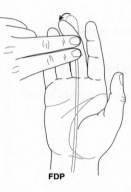

FDP

How can the flexor digitorum *superficialis* (FDS) apparatus be tested?

Check isolated flexion of the finger at the MP joint

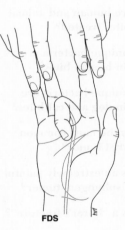

FDS

Where do the digital arteries run?

On medial and lateral sides of the digit

What hand laceration should be left unsutured?

Lacerations from human bites or animal bites

Should a clamp ever be used to stop a laceration bleeder?

No; use pressure and then tourniquet for definitive repair if bleeding does not cease because **nerves run with blood vessels!**

What is a felon?

Infection in **the tip** of the finger pad (Think: felon = fingerprints = infection in pad); treat by incision and drainage

What is a paronychia?

Infection on the **side** of the fingernail (nail fold); treat by incision and drainage

What is tenosynovitis?

Tendon sheath infection

What are Kanavel's signs?

Four signs of tenosynovitis:
1. Affected finger held in flexion
2. Pain over volar aspect of affected finger tendon sheath upon palpation
3. Swelling of affected finger (fusiform)
4. Pain on passive extension of affected finger

Most common bacteria in tenosynovitis and paronychia?

Staphylococcus aureus

How are human and animal hand bites treated?

Débridement/irrigation/administration of antibiotics; **leave wound open**

What unique bacteria are found in human bites?

Eikenella corrodens

What unique bacteria are found in dog and cat bites?

Pasteurella multocida

What is the most common hand/wrist tumor?

Ganglion cyst

What is an extremely painful type of subungual tumor?

Glomus tumor (subungual: under the nail)

What is a "boxer's fracture"?

Fracture of the fourth or fifth metacarpal

What is a "drop finger" injury?

Laceration of extensor tendon over the MP joint

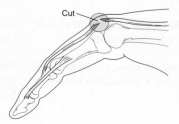

What is the classic deformity resulting from laceration of the extensor tendon over the DIP joint?

Mallet finger

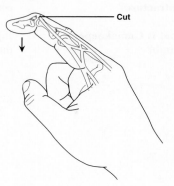

What is the classic deformity resulting from laceration of the extensor tendon over the PIP joint?

Boutonniere deformity

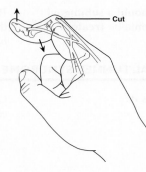

Which fracture causes pain in the "anatomic snuffbox"?

Scaphoid fracture; often not seen on x-ray at presentation, usually seen at a later date (2 weeks) on x-ray
Can result in avascular necrosis
Place in a cast if clinically suspected, **regardless of x-ray findings**

What is the "safe position" of hand splinting?

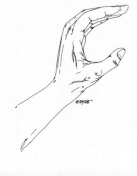

What is Dupuytren's contracture?

Fibrosis of palmar fascia, causing contracture of and inability to extend digits

What is Gamekeeper's thumb?

Injury to the ulnar collateral ligament of the thumb

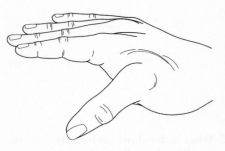

How should a subungual hematoma be treated?

Release pressure by burning a hole in the nail (use hand-held disposable battery-operated coagulation probe)

CARPAL TUNNEL SYNDROME

What is it?

Compression of the median nerve in the carpal tunnel

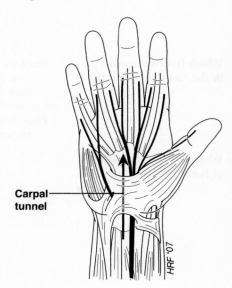

Carpal tunnel

What is the most common cause?	Synovitis
What are other causes?	**"MEDIAN TRAPS":** **M**edian artery (persistent) **E**dema of pregnancy **D**iabetes **I**diopathic **A**cromegaly **N**eoplasm (e.g., ganglioneuroma) **T**hyroid (myxedema) **R**heumatoid arthritis **A**myloid **P**neumatic drill usage **S**LE
What are the symptoms?	Pain and numbness in the median nerve distribution
What are the signs?	Tinel's sign (symptoms with percussion over median nerve), Phalen's test (symptoms with flexion of wrists), thenar atrophy, Wartenberg's sign
What is Wartenberg's sign?	With hand resting on a surface, the fifth digit ("pinky") rests in ABduction compared to the other 4 fingers
What is the workup?	EMG, nerve conduction study
What is initial treatment?	Nonoperative, rest, wrist splint, NSAIDs
What are indications for surgery?	Refractory symptoms, thenar atrophy, thenar weakness
What surgery is performed?	Release transverse carpal ligament

Chapter 70

Otolaryngology: Head and Neck Surgery

Define:

Anosmia	Inability to **smell**
Otorrhea	Fluid discharge from ear
Dysphagia	Difficulty swallowing
Odynophagia	Painful swallowing
Globus	Sensation of a "lump in the throat"
Otalgia	Ear pain (often referred from throat)
Trismus	Difficulty opening mouth

ANATOMY

Define the cranial nerves:

I	Olfactory nerve
II	Optic nerve
III	Oculomotor nerve
IV	Trochlear nerve
V	Trigeminal nerve
VI	Abducens nerve
VII	Facial nerve
VIII	Vestibulocochlear nerve
IX	Glossopharyngeal nerve
X	Vagus nerve

| XI | Accessory nerve |
| XII | Hypoglossal nerve |

Define motor/sensory actions of the following cranial nerves:

I	Smell
II	Sight (**sensory pupil reaction**)
III	Eyeball movement, pupil sphincter, ciliary muscle (**motor pupil reaction**)
IV	Superior oblique muscle movement
V	Motor: chewing (masseter muscle) Sensory: face, teeth, sinuses, cornea
VI	Lateral rectus muscle (lateral gaze)
VII	Motor: facial muscles, lacrimal/ sublingual/submandibular glands Sensory: anterior tongue/soft palate, taste
VIII	Hearing, positioning
IX	Motor: stylopharyngeus, parotid, pharynx Sensory: posterior tongue, pharynx, middle ear

X	Motor: vocal cords, heart, bronchus,
	    GI tract
	Sensory: bronchus, heart, GI tract,
	    larynx, ear

XI	Motor: trapezius muscle, sternocleidomastoid muscle
XII	Motor: tongue, strap muscles (ansa cervicalis branch)

| **What are the three divisions of the trigeminal nerve (cranial nerve V)?** | 1. Ophthalmic
2. Maxillary
3. Mandibular |

What happens when the hypoglossal nerve (cranial nerve XII) is cut?

When the patient sticks out the tongue, it deviates to the same side as the injury (wheelbarrow effect)

Name the duct of the submandibular gland.

Wharton's duct

Name the duct of the parotid gland.

Stensen's duct

What is the source of blood supply to the nose?

1. Internal carotid artery: anterior and posterior ethmoidal arteries via ophthalmic artery
2. External carotid artery: superior labial artery (via facial artery) and sphenopalatine artery (via internal maxillary artery)

Name the three bones that make up the posterior nasal septum.

1. Ethmoid (perpendicular plate)
2. Vomer (Latin for "plow")
3. Palatine (some also include maxillary crest)

Name the seven bones of the bony eyeball orbit.

1. Frontal
2. Zygoma
3. Maxillary
4. Lacrimal
5. Ethmoid
6. Palatine
7. Sphenoid

Name the four strap muscles.

"TOSS":
1. **T**hyrohyoid
2. **O**mohyoid
3. **S**ternothyroid
4. **S**ternohyoid

Which muscle crosses the external and internal carotid arteries?

Digastric muscle

In a neck incision, what is the first muscle incised?

Platysma

Which nerve supplies the strap muscles?

Ansa cervicalis (XII)

What are the anterior and posterior neck triangles?	Two regions of the neck, divided by the sternocleidomastoid muscle

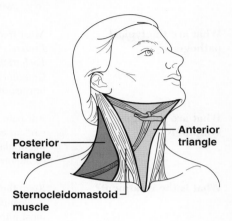

Which nerve runs with the carotid in the carotid sheath?	Vagus
Which nerve crosses the internal carotid artery at approximately 1 to 2 cm above the bifurcation?	Hypoglossal nerve
Name the three auditory ossicle bones.	1. Malleus (hammer) 2. Incus (anvil) 3. Stapes (stirrup)
What comprises the middle ear?	Eustachian tube, ossicle bones, tympanic membrane ("ear drum"), mastoid air cell
What comprises the inner ear?	Cochlea, semicircular canals, internal auditory canal

EAR

OTITIS EXTERNA (SWIMMER'S EAR)

What is it?	Generalized infection involving the external ear canal and often the tympanic membrane

What is the usual cause?	Prolonged water exposure and damaged squamous epithelium of the ear canal (e.g., swimming, hearing aid use)
What are the typical pathogens?	Most frequently *Pseudomonas*, may be *Proteus, Staphylococcus,* occasionally *Escherichia coli,* fungi (*Aspergillus, Candida*), or virus (herpes zoster or herpes simplex)
What are the signs/ symptoms?	Ear pain (otalgia); swelling of external ear, ear canal, or both; erythema; pain on manipulation of the auricle; debris in canal; otorrhea
What is the treatment?	Keep the ear dry; mild infections respond to cleaning and dilute acetic acid drops; most infections require complete removal of all debris and topical antibiotics with or without hydrocortisone (anti-inflammatory)

MALIGNANT OTITIS EXTERNA (MOE)

What is it?	Fulminant **bacterial** otitis externa
Is it malignant cancer?	NO!
Who is affected?	Most common scenario: elderly patient with poorly controlled diabetes (other forms of immunosuppression do not appear to predispose patients to MOE)
What are the causative organisms?	Usually *Pseudomonas aeruginosa*
What is the classic feature?	Nub of granulation tissue on the floor of the external ear canal at the bony–cartilaginous junction
What are the other signs/ symptoms?	Severe ear pain, excessive purulent discharge, and usually **exposed bone**

What are the diagnostic tests?

1. CT scan: shows erosion of bone, inflammation
2. Technetium-99 scan: temporal bone inflammatory process
3. Gallium-tagged white blood cell scan: to follow and document resolution

What are the complications?

Invasion of surrounding structures to produce a cellulitis, osteomyelitis of temporal bone, mastoiditis; later, a facial nerve palsy, meningitis, or brain abscess

What is the treatment?

Control of diabetes, meticulous local care with extensive debridement, hospitalization and IV antibiotics (anti-*Pseudomonas*: usually an aminoglycoside plus a penicillin)

TUMORS OF THE EXTERNAL EAR

What are the most common types?

Squamous cell most common; occasionally, basal cell carcinoma or melanoma

From what location do they usually arise?

Auricle, but occasionally from the external canal

What is the associated risk factor?

Excessive sun exposure

What is the treatment of the following conditions:
  Cancers of the auricle?

Usually wedge excision

  Extension to the canal?

May require excision of the external ear canal or partial temporal bone excision

  Middle ear involvement?

Best treated by en bloc temporal bone resection and lymph node dissection

TYMPANIC MEMBRANE (TM) PERFORATION

What is the etiology?

Usually the result of trauma (direct or indirect) or secondary to middle ear infection; often occurs secondary to slap to the side of the head (compression injury), explosions

What are the symptoms?	Pain, bleeding from the ear, conductive hearing loss, tinnitus
What are the signs?	Clot in the meatus, visible tear in the TM
What is the treatment?	Keep dry; use systemic antibiotics if there is evidence of infection or contamination
What is the prognosis?	Most (90%) heal spontaneously, though larger perforations may require surgery (e.g., fat plug, temporalis fascia tympanoplasty)

CHOLESTEATOMA

What is it?	Epidermal inclusion cyst of the middle ear or mastoid, containing desquamated keratin debris; may be acquired or congenital
What are the causes?	Negative middle ear pressure from eustachian tube dysfunction (primary acquired) or direct growth of epithelium through a TM perforation (secondary acquired)
What other condition is it often associated with?	Chronic middle ear infection
What is the usual history?	Chronic ear infection with chronic, malodorous drainage
What is the appearance?	Grayish-white, shiny keratinous mass behind or involving the TM; often described as a "pearly" lesion
What are the associated problems?	Ossicular erosion, producing conductive hearing loss; also, local invasion resulting in: Vertigo/sensorineural hearing loss Facial paresis/paralysis CNS dysfunction/infection
What is the treatment?	Surgery (tympanoplasty/mastoidectomy) aimed at eradication of disease and reconstruction of the ossicular chain

BULLOUS MYRINGITIS

What is it?	Vesicular infection of the TM and adjacent deep canal
What are the causative agents?	Unknown; viral should be suspected because of frequent association with viral URI (in some instances, *Mycoplasma pneumoniae* has been cultured)
What are the symptoms?	Acute, severe ear pain; low-grade fever; and bloody drainage
What are the findings on otoscopic examination?	Large, reddish blebs on the TM, wall of the meatus, or both
Is hearing affected?	Rarely; occasional reversible sensorineural loss
What is the treatment?	Oral antibiotics (erythromycin if *Mycoplasma* is suspected); topical analgesics may be used, with resolution of symptoms usually occurring in 36 hours

ACUTE SUPPURATIVE OTITIS MEDIA (OM)

What is it?	Bacterial infection of the middle ear, often following a viral URI; may be associated with a middle ear effusion
What is the cause?	Dysfunction of the eustachian tube that allows bacterial entry from nasopharynx; often associated with an occluded eustachian tube, although it is uncertain whether this is a cause or a result of the infection
What are the predisposing factors?	Young age, male gender, bottle feeding, crowded living conditions (e.g., day care), cleft palate, Down's syndrome, cystic fibrosis
What is the etiology?	1. *Streptococcus pneumoniae* (33% of cases) 2. *Haemophilus influenzae* 3. *Moraxella catarrhalis* 4. *Staphylococcus* 5. β-hemolytic strep 6. *Pseudomonas aeruginosa* 7. Viral/no culture

What is the etiology in infants younger than 6 months?	1. *Staphylococcus aureus* 2. *E. coli* 3. *Klebsiella*
What are the symptoms?	Otalgia, fever, decreased hearing, infant pulls on ear, increased irritability; as many as 25% of patients are asymptomatic
What are the signs?	Early, redness of the TM; later, TM bulging with loss of the normal landmarks; finally, impaired TM mobility on pneumatic otoscopy
If pain disappears instantly, what may have happened?	TM perforation!
What are the complications?	TM perforation, acute mastoiditis, meningitis, brain abscess, extradural abscess, labyrinthitis; if recurrent or chronic, OM may have adverse effects on speech and cognitive development as a result of decreased hearing
What is the treatment?	10-day course of antibiotics; amoxicillin is the first-line agent; if the patient is allergic to PCN, trimethoprim-sulfamethoxazole or erythromycin should be administered
What is the usual course?	Symptoms usually resolve in 24 to 36 hours
What are the indications for myringotomy and PE tube placement?	1. Persistent middle ear effusion over 3 months 2. Debilitated or immunocompromised patient 3. More than three episodes over 6 months (especially if bilateral)
What is a PE tube?	**P**neumatic **E**qualization tube (tube placed across tympanic membrane)
What is a Bezold's abscess?	Abscess behind the superior attachment of the sternocleidomastoid muscle resulting from extension of a mastoid infection
What are causes of chronic otitis media?	Mixed, *S. aureus, P. aeruginosa*

What are the signs/symptoms of chronic otitis media?	Otorrhea and hearing loss

OTOSCLEROSIS

What is it?	Genetic disease characterized by abnormal spongy and sclerotic bone formation in the temporal bone around the footplate of the stapes, thus preventing its normal movement
What is the inheritance pattern?	Autosomal dominant with incomplete one-third penetrance
What are the symptoms?	Painless, progressive hearing loss (may be unilateral or bilateral), tinnitus
What is the usual age of onset?	Second through fourth decade
How is the diagnosis made?	Normal TM with conductive hearing loss and no middle-ear effusion (though may be mixed or even sensorineural if bone of cochlea is affected)
What is Schwartze's sign?	Erythema around the stapes from hypervascularity of new bone formation
What is the treatment?	Frequently surgical (stapedectomy with placement of prosthesis), hearing aids, or observation; sodium fluoride may be used if a sensorineural component is present or for preoperative stabilization

MISCELLANEOUS

FACIAL NERVE PARALYSIS

How is the defect localized?	Supranuclear—paralysis of lower face only, forehead muscles are spared because of bilateral corticobulbar supply Intratemporal bone—paralysis of upper and lower face, decreased tearing, altered taste, absent stapedius reflex Distal to stylomastoid foramen—paralysis of facial muscles only

What are the causes?	Bell's palsy
	Trauma
	Cholesteatoma
	Tumor (carcinoma, glomus jugulare)
	Herpes zoster inflammation of geniculate
	    ganglion (Ramsay-Hunt syndrome)
	Peripheral lesions are usually parotid
	    gland tumors

What is the most common cause of bilateral facial nerve palsy?	Lyme disease (*Borrelia burgdorferi*)

BELL'S PALSY

What is it?	Sudden onset, unilateral facial weakness or paralysis in absence of CNS, ear, or cerebellopontine angle disease (i.e., no identifiable cause)
What is the clinical course?	Acute onset, with greatest muscle weakness reached within 3 weeks
What is the incidence?	Most common cause of **unilateral** facial weakness/paralysis
What is the pathogenesis?	Unknown; most widely accepted hypothesis is viral etiology (herpes virus); ischemic and immunologic factors are also implicated
What is the common preceding event?	URI
What are the signs/symptoms?	Pathology is related to swelling of the facial nerve; may present with total facial paralysis, altered lacrimation, increased tearing on affected side, change in taste if region above chorda tympani is affected, dry mouth, and hyperacusis
What is the treatment?	Usually none is required, as most cases resolve spontaneously in 1 month; protect eye with drops and tape closed as needed; most otolaryngologists advocate steroids and acyclovir Surgical decompression of CN VII is indicated if paralysis progresses or tests indicate deterioration

What is the prognosis? Overall, 90% of patients recover completely; if paralysis is incomplete, 95% to 100% will recover without sequelae

SENSORINEURAL HEARING LOSS

What is it? Hearing loss from a lesion occurring in the cochlea or acoustic nerve, rather than the external or middle ear

What are the symptoms? Distortion of hearing, impaired speech discrimination, tinnitus

What are the signs? Air conduction is better than bone conduction (positive Rinne test), Weber lateralizes to the side without the defect; audiogram most commonly shows greatest loss in high-frequency tones

What is the Weber vs. Rinne test? **Weber:** tuning fork on middle of head (lateral louder = either ipsilateral conductive loss or contralateral sensorineural)
Rinne: tuning fork on mastoid and then next to ear (conductive loss louder on mastoid)

What are the causes? Aging (presbycusis)—leading cause
Acoustic injury from sudden or prolonged exposure to loud noises
Perilymph fistula
Congenital (**TORCHES:** maternal **TO**xoplasmosis, **R**ubella, **C**MV, **HE**rpes, and **S**yphilis)
Ménière's disease
Drug/toxin-induced
Acoustic neuroma
Pseudotumor cerebri
CNS disease
Endocrine disorders
Sarcoidosis

What is the most common cause in children? Meningitis (bacterial)

What is the treatment?	Treatment of underlying cause, hearing aids, lip reading, cochlear implant

VERTIGO

What is it?	Sensation of head/body movement, or movement of surroundings (usually rotational)
What is the cause?	Asymmetric neuronal activity between right and left vestibular systems
What is the history of peripheral vertigo?	Severe vertigo, nausea, vomiting, always accompanied by horizontal or rotatory nystagmus (fast component almost always to side opposite disease), other evidence of inner ear disease (tinnitus, hearing loss)
What are the risk factors for peripheral vertigo?	Frequently associated with a previously operated ear, a chronic draining ear, barotrauma, or head trauma
What is the history of central vertigo?	Found in brainstem or cerebellum: insidious onset, less intense and more subtle sensation of vertigo; occasionally, vertical nystagmus
What are the steps in diagnostic evaluation?	Depends on probability of central versus peripheral; careful neurologic and otologic examinations are required May need FTA/VDRL (syphilis), temporal bone scans/CT scan/MRI, ENG, position testing, audiometric testing
What is the most common etiology?	**B**enign **P**aroxysmal **P**ositional **V**ertigo (**BPPV**); history of brief spells of severe vertigo with specific head positions
What is the differential diagnosis?	Central: vertebral basilar insufficiency (often in older patients with DJD of spine), Wallenberg syndrome, MS, epilepsy, migraine Peripheral: BPPV, motion sickness, syphilis, Ménière's disease, vestibular neuronitis, labyrinthitis, acoustic neuroma, syphilis, perilymph fistula

| **What is Tullio's phenomenon?** | Induction of vertigo by loud noises; classically, result of otosyphilis |

MÉNIÈRE'S DISEASE

What is it?	Disorder of the membranous labyrinth, causing fluctuating sensorineural hearing loss, episodic vertigo, nystagmus, tinnitus, and aural fullness, N/V
What is the classic triad?	Hearing loss, **T**innitus, **V**ertigo (**H**, **T**, **V**)
What is the pathophysiology?	Obscure, but most experts believe excessive production/defective resorption of endolymph
What is the medical treatment?	Salt restriction, diuretics (thiazides), antinausea agents; occasionally diazepam is added; 80% of patients respond to medical management, antihistamines
What are the indications for surgery?	Surgery is offered to those who fail medical treatment or who have incapacitating vertigo (60%–80% effective)
What are the surgical options?	1. Shunt from membranous labyrinth to subarachnoid space 2. Vestibular neurectomy 3. Severe cases with hearing loss: labyrinthectomy

GLOMUS TUMORS

What are they?	Benign, slow-growing tumors arising in glomus bodies found in the adventitial layer of blood vessels; often associated with cranial nerves IX and X in the middle ear
What is the usual location?	Middle ear, jugular bulb, course of CN IX to XII
How common are they?	Most common benign tumor of the temporal bone

What is the treatment?	Surgical resection, radiation therapy for poor operative candidates or for recurrences

NOSE AND PARANASAL SINUSES

EPISTAXIS

What is it?	Bleeding from the nose
What are the predisposing factors?	Trauma, "nose picking," sinus infection, allergic or atrophic rhinitis, blood dyscrasias, tumor, environmental extremes (hot, dry climates; winters)
What is the usual cause?	Rupture of superficial mucosal blood vessels (Kiesselbach's plexus if anterior, sphenopalatine artery if posterior)
What is the most common type?	Anterior (90%); usually the result of trauma
Which type is more serious?	Posterior; usually occurs in the elderly or is associated with a systemic disorder (hypertension, tumor, arteriosclerosis)
What is the treatment?	Direct pressure; if this fails, proceed to anterior nasal packing with gauze strips, followed if necessary by posterior packing with Foley catheter or lamb's wool; packs must be removed in <5 days to prevent infectious complications
What is the treatment of last resort?	Ligation or embolization of the sphenopalatine artery (posterior) or ethmoidal artery (anterior)
What infectious disease syndrome is seen with nasal packing?	Toxic shock syndrome: fever, shock, **rash** caused by exotoxin from *Staphylococcus aureus*
What is the treatment of this syndrome?	Supportive with removal of nasal packing, IV hydration, oxygen, and antistaphylococcal antibiotics

ACUTE RHINITIS

What is it?	Inflammation of nasal mucous membrane
What is the most common cause?	URI infection; rhinovirus is the most common agent in adults (other nonallergic causes: nasal deformities and tumors, polyps, atrophy, immune diseases, vasomotor problems)

ALLERGIC RHINITIS

What are the symptoms?	Nasal stuffiness; watery rhinorrhea; paroxysms of morning sneezing; and itching of nose, conjunctiva, or palate
How is the condition characterized?	Early onset (before 20 years of age), familial tendency, other allergic disorders (eczema, asthma), elevated serum IgE, eosinophilia on nasal smear
What are the findings on physical examination?	Pale, boggy, bluish nasal turbinates coated with thin, clear secretions; in children, a transverse nasal crease sometimes results from repeated "allergic salute"
What is the treatment?	Allergen avoidance, antihistamines, decongestants; steroids or sodium cromylate in severe cases; desensitization via allergen immunotherapy is the only "cure"

ACUTE SINUSITIS

What is the typical history?	Previously healthy patient with unrelenting progression of a viral URI or allergic rhinitis beyond the normal 5- to 7-day course
What are the symptoms?	Periorbital pressure/pain, nasal obstruction, nasal/postnasal mucopurulent discharge, fatigue, fever, headache

What are the signs?
Tenderness over affected sinuses, pus in the nasal cavity; may also see reason for obstruction (septal deviation, spur, tight osteomeatal complex); transillumination is unreliable

What is the pathophysiology?
Thought to be secondary to decreased ciliary action of the sinus mucosa and edema causing obstruction of the sinus ostia, lowering intrasinus oxygen tension and predisposing patients to bacterial infection

What are the causative organisms?
Up to 50% of patients have negative cultures and cause is presumably (initially) viral; pneumococcus, *S. aureus*, group A streptococci, and *H. influenzae* are the most common bacteria cultured

What is the treatment?
14-day course of antibiotics (penicillin G, amoxicillin, Ceclor®, and Augmentin® are commonly used), topical and systemic decongestants, and saline nasal irrigation

What is the treatment for fungal sinusitis?
Fungal sinusitis is commonly caused by *Mucor* and seen in immunosuppressed patients; treatment is IV antifungals (e.g., amphotericin or caspofungin) and surgical débridement of all necrotic tissue

CHRONIC SINUSITIS

What is it?
Infection of nasal sinuses lasting longer than 4 weeks, or pattern of recurrent acute sinusitis punctuated by brief asymptomatic periods

What is the pathology?
Permanent mucosal changes secondary to inadequately treated acute sinusitis, consisting of mucosal fibrosis, polypoid growth, and inadequate ciliary action, hyperostosis (increased bone density on CT scan)

What are the symptoms?   Chronic nasal obstruction, postnasal drip, mucopurulent rhinorrhea, low-grade facial and periorbital pressure/pain

What are the causative organisms?   Usually anaerobes (such as *Bacteroides, Veillonella, Rhinobacterium*); also *H. influenzae, Streptococcus viridans, Staphylococcus aureus, Staphylococcus epidermidis*

What is the treatment?   Medical management with decongestants, mucolytics, topical steroids, and antibiotics; if this approach fails, proceed to endoscopic or external surgical intervention

What is FESS?   **F**unctional **E**ndoscopic **S**inus **S**urgery

What are the complications of sinusitis?   Orbital cellulitis (if ethmoid sinusitis), meningitis, epidural or brain abscess (frontal sinus), cavernous sinus thrombosis (ethmoid or sphenoid), osteomyelitis (a.k.a. Pott's puffy tumor if frontal)

CANCER OF THE NASAL CAVITY AND PARANASAL SINUSES

What are the usual locations?   Maxillary sinus (66%)
Nasal cavity
Ethmoid sinus
Rarely in frontal or sphenoid sinuses

What are the associated cell types?   Squamous cell (80%)
Adenocellular (15%)
Uncommon: sarcoma, melanoma

What rare tumor arises from olfactory epithelium?   Esthesioneuroblastoma; usually arises high in the nose (cribriform plate) and is locally invasive

What are the signs/ symptoms?   Early—nasal obstruction, blood-tinged mucus, epistaxis
Late—localized pain, cranial nerve deficits, facial/palate asymmetry, loose teeth

How is the diagnosis made?	CT scan can adequately identify extent of the disease and local invasion; MRI is often also used to evaluate soft-tissue disease
What is the treatment?	Surgery with or without x-ray therapy
What is the prognosis?	5-year survival for T1 or T2 lesions approaches 70%

JUVENILE NASOPHARYNGEAL ANGIOFIBROMA

What is it?	Most commonly encountered vascular mass in the nasal cavity; locally aggressive but nonmetastasizing
What is the usual history?	Adolescent boys who present with nasal obstruction, recurrent massive epistaxis, possibly anosmia
What is the usual location?	Site of origin is the roof of the nasal cavity at the superior margin of sphenopalatine foramen
Into what can the mass transform?	Fibrosarcoma (rare cases reported)
How is the diagnosis made?	Carotid arteriography, CT scan; biopsy is contraindicated secondary to risk of uncontrollable hemorrhage
What are indications for biopsy?	**None!**
What is the treatment?	Surgery via lateral rhinotomy or sublabial maxillotomy with bleeding controlled by internal maxillary artery ligation or preoperative embolization, in the setting of hypotensive anesthesia; preoperative irradiation has also been used to shrink the tumor

ORAL CAVITY AND PHARYNX

PHARYNGOTONSILLITIS

What is the common site of referred throat pain?	EAR
What is it?	Acute or chronic infection of the nasopharynx or oropharynx and/or Waldeyer's ring of lymphoid tissue (consisting of palatine, lingual, and pharyngeal tonsils and the adenoids)
What is the etiology?	Acute attacks can be viral (adenovirus, enterovirus, coxsackievirus, Epstein-Barr virus in infectious mononucleosis) or bacterial (group A β-hemolytic streptococci are the leading bacterial agent); chronic tonsillitis often with mixed population, including streptococci, staphylococci, and *M. catarrhalis*
What are the symptoms?	Acute—Sore throat, fever, local lymphadenopathy, chills, headache, malaise Chronic—Noisy mouth breathing, speech and swallowing difficulties, apnea, halitosis
What are the signs?	Viral—Injected tonsils and pharyngeal mucosa; exudate may occur, but less often than with bacterial tonsillitis Bacterial—Swollen, inflamed tonsils with white-yellow exudate in crypts and on surface; cervical adenopathy
How is the diagnosis made?	CBC, throat culture, Monospot test
What are the possible complications?	Peritonsillar abscess (quinsy), retropharyngeal abscess (causing airway compromise), rheumatic fever, poststreptococcal glomerulonephritis (with β-hemolytic streptococci)

What is the treatment?	Viral—Symptomatic → acetaminophen, warm saline gargles, anesthetic throat spray Bacterial—10 days PCN (erythromycin if PCN-allergic)
What are the indications for tonsillectomy?	Sleep apnea/cor pulmonale secondary to airway obstruction, suspicion of malignancy, hypertrophy causing malocclusion, peritonsillar abscess, recurrent acute or chronic tonsillitis
What are the possible complications?	Acute or delayed hemorrhage

PERITONSILLAR ABSCESS

What is the clinical setting?	Inadequately treated recurrent acute or chronic tonsillitis
What is the associated microbiology?	Mixed aerobes and anaerobes (which may be PCN resistant)
What is the site of formation?	Begins at the superior pole of the tonsil
What are the symptoms?	Severe throat pain, drooling dysphagia, odynophagia, trismus, cervical adenopathy, fever, chills, malaise
What is the classic description of voice?	"Hot-potato voice"
What are the signs?	Bulging, erythematous, edematous tonsillar pillar; swelling of uvula and displacement to contralateral side
What is the treatment?	IV antibiotics and surgical evacuation by incision and drainage; most experts recommend tonsillectomy after resolution of inflammatory changes

LUDWIG ANGINA

What is it?	Infection and inflammation of the floor of the mouth (sublingual and submandibular)

What is the source?	Dental infection
What is the treatment?	Antibiotics, emergency airway, I & D

CANCER OF THE ORAL CAVITY

What is the usual cell type?	Squamous cell (>90% of cases)
What are the most common sites?	**Lip,** tongue, floor of mouth, gingiva, cheek, and palate
What is the etiology?	Linked to smoking, alcohol, and smokeless tobacco products (alcohol and tobacco together greatly increase the risk)
What is the frequency of the following conditions:	
Regional metastasis?	≈30%
Second primary?	≈25%
Nodal metastasis?	Depends on size of tumor and ranges from 10% to 60%, usually to jugular and **jugulodigastric nodes, submandibular nodes**
Distant metastasis?	Infrequent
How is the diagnosis made?	Full history and physical examination, dental assessment, Panorex or bone scan if mandible is thought to be involved, CT scan/MRI for extent of tumor and nodal disease, FNA (often U/S guided)
What is the treatment?	Radiation, surgery, or both for small lesions; localized lesions can usually be treated surgically; larger lesions require combination therapy, possible mandibulectomy and neck dissection

What is the prognosis?

Depends on stage and site:
  Tongue: 20% to 70% survival
  Floor of mouth: 30% to 80% survival
Most common cause of death in
  successfully treated head and neck
  cancer is development of a second
  primary (occurs in 20%–40% of cases)

SALIVARY GLAND TUMORS

What is the frequency of gland involvement?

Parotid gland (80%)
Submandibular gland (15%)
Minor salivary glands (5%)

What is the potential for malignancy?

Greatest in **minor salivary gland** tumors (80% are malignant) and least in parotid gland tumors (80% are benign); **the smaller the gland, the greater the likelihood of malignancy**

How do benign and malignant tumors differ in terms of history and physical examination?

Benign—mobile, nontender, no node
  involvement or facial weakness
Malignant—painful, fixed mass with
  evidence of local metastasis and facial
  paresis/paralysis

What is the diagnostic procedure?

FNA; **never** perform excisional biopsy of a parotid mass; superficial parotidectomy is the procedure of choice for benign lesions of the lateral lobe

What is the treatment?

Involves adequate surgical resection, sparing facial nerve if possible, neck dissection for node-positive necks

What are the indications for postop XRT?

Postoperative radiation therapy if high-grade cancer, recurrent cancer, residual disease, invasion of adjacent structures, any T3 or T4 parotid tumors

What is the most common benign salivary tumor?

Pleomorphic adenoma (benign mixed tumor) 66%
Think: **P**leomorphic = **P**opular

What is the usual location?

Parotid gland

What is the clinical course?	They are well delineated and slow growing
What is the second most common benign salivary gland tumor?	Warthin's tumor (1% of all salivary gland tumors)
What is the usual location?	95% are found in parotid; 3% are bilateral
Describe the lesion.	Slow-growing, cystic mass is usually located in the tail of the superficial portion of the parotid; it rarely becomes malignant
What is the most common malignant salivary tumor?	**Mucoepidermoid carcinoma** (10% of all salivary gland neoplasms) Think: **M**ucoepidermoid = **M**alignant Most common parotid malignancy Second most common submandibular gland malignancy
What is the second most common malignant salivary tumor in adults?	Adenoid cystic carcinoma; most common malignancy in submandibular and minor salivary glands

LARYNX ANATOMY

Define the three parts.	1. Glottis: begins halfway between the true and false cords (in the ventricle) and extends inferiorly 1.0 cm below the edge of the vocal folds 2. Supraglottis: extends from superior glottis to superior border of hyoid and tip of epiglottis 3. Subglottis: extends from lower border of glottis to inferior edge of cricoid cartilage

Innervation?	Vagus nerve: superior laryngeal and recurrent laryngeal nerves; superior laryngeal supplies sensory to supraglottis and motor to inferior constrictor and cricothyroid muscle; recurrent laryngeal supplies sensory to glottis and subglottis and motor to all remaining intrinsic laryngeal muscles

CROUP (LARYNGOTRACHEOBRONCHITIS)

What is it?	Viral infection of the larynx and trachea, generally affecting children (boys > girls)
What is the usual cause?	Parainfluenza virus (Think: crou**P** = **P**arainfluenza)
What age group is affected most?	6 months to 3 years of age
Is the condition considered seasonal?	Yes; outbreaks most often occur in autumn
What are the precipitating events?	Usually preceded by URI
What is the classic symptom?	Barking (seal-like), nonproductive cough
What are the other symptoms?	Respiratory distress, low-grade fever
What are the signs?	Tachypnea, inspiratory retractions, prolonged inspiration, inspiratory stridor, expiratory rhonchi/wheezes
What is the differential diagnosis?	Epiglottitis, bacterial tracheitis, foreign body, diphtheria, retropharyngeal abscess, peritonsillar abscess, asthma
How is the diagnosis made?	A-P neck x-ray shows classic "steeple sign," indicating subglottic narrowing; ABG may show hypoxemia plus hypercapnia

What is the treatment?	**Keep child calm** (agitation only worsens obstruction); cool mist; steroids; aerosolized racemic EPI may be administered to reduce edema/airway obstruction
What are the indications for intubation?	If airway obstruction is severe or child becomes exhausted
What is the usual course?	Resolves in 3 to 4 days
What type of secondary infection occurs?	Secondary bacterial infection (streptococcal, staphylococcal)

EPIGLOTTITIS

What is it?	Severe, rapidly progressive infection of the epiglottis
What is the usual causative agent?	*Haemophilus influenzae* type B
What age group is affected?	Children 2 to 5 years of age
What are the signs/ symptoms?	Sudden onset, high fever (40°C); "hot-potato" voice; dysphagia ($\rightarrow$ drooling); no cough; patient prefers to sit upright, lean forward; patient appears toxic and stridulous
How is the diagnosis made?	Can usually be made clinically and does not involve direct observation of the epiglottis (which may worsen obstruction by causing laryngospasm)
What is the treatment?	Involves immediate airway support in the O.R.: intubation or possibly tracheostomy, medical treatment is comprised of steroids and IV antibiotics *against H. influenzae*

MALIGNANT LESIONS OF THE LARYNX

What is the incidence?	Accounts for $\approx$2% of all malignancies, more often in males
What is the most common site?	Glottis (66%)

What is the second most common type?	Supraglottis (33%)
Which type has the worst prognosis?	Subglottic tumors (infrequent)
What are the risk factors?	Tobacco, alcohol
What is the pathology?	90% are squamous cell carcinoma
What are the symptoms?	Hoarseness, throat pain, dysphagia, odynophagia, neck mass, (referred) ear pain

SUPRAGLOTTIC LESIONS

What is the usual location?	Laryngeal surface of epiglottis
What area is often involved?	Pre-epiglottic space
Extension?	Tend to remain confined to supraglottic region, though may extend to vallecula or base of tongue
What is the associated type of metastasis?	High propensity for nodal metastasis
What is the treatment?	Early stage = XRT Late stage = laryngectomy

GLOTTIC LESIONS

What is the usual location?	Anterior part of true cords
Extension?	May invade thyroid cartilage, cross midline to invade contralateral cord, or invade paraglottic space
What is the associated type of metastasis?	Rare nodal metastasis
What is the treatment?	Early stage = XRT Late stage = laryngectomy

NECK MASS

What is the usual etiology in infants?	Congenital (branchial cleft cysts, thyroglossal duct cysts)
What is the usual etiology in adolescents?	Inflammatory (cervical adenitis is #1), with congenital also possible
What is the usual etiology in adults?	Malignancy (squamous is #1), especially if painless and immobile
What is the "80% rule"?	In general, **80%** of neck masses are **benign** in children; **80%** are **malignant** in adults older than 40 years of age
What are the seven cardinal symptoms of neck masses?	Dysphagia, odynophagia, hoarseness, stridor (signifies upper airway obstruction), globus, speech disorder, referred ear pain (via CN V, IX, or X)
What comprises the workup?	Full head and neck examination, indirect laryngoscopy, CT scan and MRI, FNA for tissue diagnosis; biopsy contraindicated because it may adversely affect survival if malignant
What is the differential diagnosis?	Inflammatory: cervical lymphadenitis, cat-scratch disease, infectious mononucleosis, infection in neck spaces Congenital: thyroglossal duct cyst (midline, elevates with tongue protrusion), branchial cleft cysts (lateral), dermoid cysts (midline submental), hemangioma, cystic hygroma Neoplastic: primary or metastatic
What is the workup of node-positive squamous cell carcinoma and no primary site?	Triple endoscopy (laryngoscopy, esophagoscopy, bronchoscopy) and blind biopsies
What is the treatment?	Surgical excision for congenital or neoplastic; two most important procedures for cancer treatment are radical and modified neck dissection

What is the role of adjuvant treatment in head and neck cancer?	Postoperative chemotherapy/XRT

RADICAL NECK DISSECTION

What is involved?	Classically, removal of **nodes** from clavicle to mandible, sternocleidomastoid muscle, **submandibular gland,** tail of **parotid,** internal **jugular vein, digastric muscles, stylohyoid** and **omohyoid muscles, fascia** within the anterior and posterior triangles, CN XI, and cervical plexus sensory nerves
What are the indications?	1. Clinically positive nodes that likely contain metastatic cancer 2. Clinically negative nodes in neck, but high probability of metastasis from a primary tumor elsewhere 3. Fixed cervical mass that is resectable
What are the contraindications?	1. Distant metastasis 2. Fixation to structure that cannot be removed (e.g., carotid artery) 3. Low neck masses

MODIFIED NECK DISSECTION

What are the types:	
Type I?	Spinal accessory nerve preserved
Type II?	Spinal accessory and internal jugular vein preserved
Type III?	Spinal accessory, IJ, and sternocleidomastoid nerves preserved
What are the advantages?	Increased postoperative function and decreased morbidity (especially if bilateral), most often used in N0 lesions; these modifications are usually intraoperative decisions based on the location and extent of tumor growth

What are the disadvantages?   May result in increased mortality from
                                    local recurrence

FACIAL FRACTURES

MANDIBLE FRACTURES

What are the symptoms?   Gross disfigurement, pain, **malocclusion,
                                    drooling**

What are the signs?   Trismus, fragment mobility and
                                    lacerations of gingiva, hematoma in floor
                                    of mouth

**What are the possible
complications?**   Malunion, nonunion, osteomyelitis, TMJ
                                    ankylosis

What is the treatment?   Open or closed reduction
                                    MMF = **M**axillo**M**andibular **F**ixation
                                    (wire jaw shut)

MIDFACE FRACTURES

How are they evaluated?   Careful physical examination and CT scan

Classification

Le Fort I?   Transverse maxillary fracture above the
                                    dental apices, which also traverses the
                                    pterygoid plate; palate is mobile, but
                                    nasal complex is stable

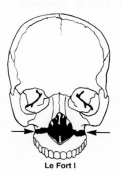

Le Fort I

Le Fort II?

Fracture through the frontal process of the maxilla, through the orbital floor and pterygoid plate; midface is mobile

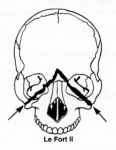

Le Fort II

Le Fort III?

Complete craniofacial separation; differs from II in that it extends through the nasofrontal suture and frontozygomatic sutures

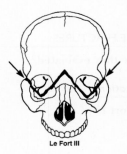

Le Fort III

What is a "tripod" fracture?

Fracture of the zygomatic complex; involves four fractures:
1. Frontozygomatic suture
2. Inferior orbital rim
3. Zygomaticomaxillary suture
4. Zygomaticotemporal suture

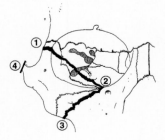

What is a "blowout" fracture? Orbital fracture with "blowout" of supporting bony structural support of orbital floor; patient has enophthalmos (sunken-in eyeball)

What is "entrapment"? Orbital fracture with "entrapment" of periorbital tissues within the fracture opening, including entrapment of extraocular muscles; loss of extraocular muscle mobility (e.g., lateral tracking) and diplopia (double vision)

What is a "step off"? Fracture of the orbit with palpable "step off" of bony orbital rim (inferior or lateral)

Are mandibular fractures usually a single fracture? No; because the mandible forms an anatomic ring, >95% of mandible fractures have more than one fracture site

What is the best x-ray study for mandibular fractures? Panorex

What must be ruled out and treated with a broken nose (nasal fracture)? Septal hematoma; must drain to remove chance of pressure-induced septal necrosis

ENT WARD QUESTIONS

How can otitis externa be distinguished from otitis media on examination? Otitis externa is characterized by severe pain upon manipulation of the auricle

What causes otitis media? Most cases are caused by pneumococci and *H. influenzae*

What causes otitis externa? *Pseudomonas aeruginosa*

What must be considered in unilateral serous otitis? Nasopharyngeal carcinoma

What is the most common cause of facial paralysis? **Bell's palsy,** which has an unidentified etiology

What is the single most important prognostic factor in Bell's palsy?	Whether the affected muscles are completely paralyzed (if not, prognosis is >95% complete recovery)
What is the most common cause of parotid swelling?	Mumps
What is Heerfordt's syndrome?	Sarcoidosis with parotid enlargement, facial nerve paralysis, and uveitis
Which systemic disease causes salivary gland stones?	Gout
What is the most common salivary gland site of stone formation?	Submandibular gland
What is Mikulicz's syndrome?	Any cause of bilateral enlargement of the parotid, lacrimal, and submandibular glands
What are the three major functions of the larynx?	1. Airway protection 2. Airway/respiration 3. Phonation
What is a cricothyroidotomy?	Emergent surgical airway by incising the cricothyroid membrane
Name the four major indications for a tracheostomy.	1. Prolonged mechanical ventilation (usually >2 weeks) 2. Upper airway obstruction 3. Poor life-threatening pulmonary toilet 4. Severe obstructive sleep apnea
What is a ranula?	Sublingual retention cyst arising from sublingual salivary glands
What is Frey's syndrome?	Flushing, pain, and diaphoresis in the auriculotemporal nerve distribution initiated by chewing
What causes Frey's syndrome?	Cutting the auriculotemporal nerve causes abnormal regeneration of the sympathetic/parasympathetic nerves, which, once destined for the parotid gland, find new targets in skin sweat glands; thus, people sweat when eating

What is the classic triad of Ménière's disease?	Hearing loss, tinnitus, vertigo (HTV)
What is the most common posterior fossa tumor and where is it located?	Acoustic neuroma, usually occurring at the cerebellopontine angle
What is the most common site of sinus cancer?	Maxillary sinus
What tumor arises from olfactory epithelium?	Esthesioneuroblastoma
What cell type is most common in head and neck cancer?	Squamous cell
What are the most important predisposing factors to head and neck cancer?	Excessive alcohol use and **tobacco** abuse of any form
What is the most frequent site of salivary gland tumor?	Parotid gland
What is the most common salivary gland neoplasm:	
Benign?	Pleomorphic adenoma
Malignant?	Mucoepidermoid carcinoma
What is the classic feature of croup?	Barking, seal-like cough
What are the classic features of epiglottitis?	"Hot-potato" voice, sitting up, **drooling,** toxic appearance, high fever, **leaning forward**
What comprises the workup of neck mass?	Do **not** biopsy; obtain tissue **via FNA** and complete head and neck examination

What is Ramsay-Hunt syndrome?	Painful facial nerve paralysis from herpes zoster of the ear
What is the most common malignant neck mass in children, adolescents, and young adults?	Lymphoma
What is the most common primary malignant solid tumor of the head and neck in children?	Rhabdomyosarcoma
Throat pain is often referred to what body area?	Ear
What ENT condition is described as "crocodile tears"?	Frey's syndrome!
What is Brown's sign?	Tympanic membrane pulsations that cease with positive pressure (from a "pneumatic" otoscope); seen with middle ear tumor mass

RAPID-FIRE REVIEW OF MOST COMMON CAUSES OF ENT INFECTIONS

Croup?	Parainfluenza virus
Otitis externa?	*Pseudomonas*
Epiglottitis?	*H. influenzae*
Malignant otitis externa?	*Pseudomonas*
Parotitis?	*Staphylococcus*
Acute suppurative otitis media?	*S. pneumoniae* (33%)

Chapter 71

Thoracic Surgery

What does VATS stand for?   Video-Assisted Thoracic Surgery

THORACIC OUTLET SYNDROME (TOS)

What is it?

Compression of the:
Subclavian artery
Subclavian vein or
Brachial plexus at the superior outlet
of the thorax

What are the causes (3)?

1. Various congenital anomalies,
including cervical rib or abnormal
fascial bands to the first rib, or
abnormal anterior scalene muscle
2. Trauma:
Fracture of clavicle or first rib
Dislocation of humeral head
Crush injuries
3. Repetitive motor injuries (baseball
pitchers)

What are the symptoms?

Paresthesias (neck, shoulder, arm, hand);
90% in ulnar nerve distribution
Weakness (neural/arterial)
Coolness of involved extremity (arterial)
Edema, venous distension, discoloration
(venous)

**What are the most common
symptoms with TOS?**

Neurologic

**Which nerve is most often
involved?**

Ulnar nerve

What are the signs?	Paget-von Schroetter syndrome—venous thrombosis leading to edema, arm discoloration, and distension of the superficial veins Weak brachial and radial pulses in the involved arm Hypesthesia/anesthesia Occasionally, atrophy in the distribution of the ulnar nerve Positive Adson maneuver/Tinel's sign Edema

What is the Adson maneuver?	**Evaluates for arterial compromise**
	Patient:
	  1. Extends neck (lifts head)
	  2. Takes a deep breath and holds
	  3. Turns head toward examined side
	Physician:
	  Monitors radial pulse on examined side
	  Test finding is positive if the radial pulse decreases or disappears during maneuver

What is Tinel's test?	Tapping of the supraclavicular fossa producing paresthesias
What is the treatment?	Physical therapy (vast majority of cases) Decompression of the thoracic outlet by resecting the first rib and cervical rib (if present) if physical therapy fails and as a last resort

CHEST WALL TUMORS

BENIGN TUMORS

What are the most common types?	1. Fibrous rib dysplasia (posterolateral rib) 2. Chondroma (at costochondral junction) 3. Osteochondroma (any portion of rib)
What is the treatment?	Wide excision and reconstruction with autologous or prosthetic grafts

MALIGNANT TUMORS

What are the most common types?	1. Fibrosarcoma 2. Chondrosarcoma 3. Osteogenic sarcoma 4. Rhabdomyosarcoma 5. Myeloma 6. Ewing's sarcoma
What is the treatment?	Excision with or without radiation
What is Tietze's syndrome?	Noninfectious costochondral cartilage inflammation

DISEASES OF THE PLEURA

PLEURAL EFFUSION

What is it?	Fluid in the pleural space
What are the causes?	1. Pulmonary infections (pneumonia) 2. Congestive heart failure (CHF) 3. SLE or rheumatoid arthritis 4. Pancreatitis (sympathetic effusion) 5. Trauma 6. Pulmonary embolism 7. Renal disease 8. Cirrhosis 9. Malignancy (mesothelioma, lymphoma, metastasis) 10. Postpericardiotomy syndrome
What are the symptoms?	Dyspnea, pleuritic chest pain
What are the signs?	Decreased breath sounds, dullness to percussion, egophony at the upper limit
What are the properties of a transudate?	Specific gravity <1.016 Protein <3 g/dL Few cells
What are the properties of an exudate?	Specific gravity >1.016 Protein >3 g/dL Many cells

What is the key diagnostic test?	Thoracentesis (needle drainage) with studies including cytology
What is the treatment?	1. Pigtail catheter or thoracostomy (chest tube) 2. Treat underlying condition 3. Consider sclerosis
What is an empyema?	Infected pleural effusion; must be drained, usually with chest tube(s) Decortication may be necessary if the empyema is solid
What is a decortication?	Thoracotomy and removal of an infected fibrous rind from around the lung (think of it as taking off a fibrous "cortex" from the lung)

LUNG ABSCESS

What are the signs/ symptoms?	Fever, sputum, sepsis, fatigue
What are the associated diagnostic studies?	CXR: air-fluid level CT scan to define position and to differentiate from an empyema Bronchoscopy (looking for cancer/culture)
What is the treatment?	Antibiotics and bronchoscopy for culture and toilet, with or without surgery
What are the indications for surgery?	Underlying cancer/tumor Refractory to antibiotics
What are the surgical options?	Lobectomy of lobe with abscess Tube drainage
What is middle lobe syndrome?	Recurrent right middle lobe pneumonia caused most commonly by intermittent extrinsic bronchial obstruction

HEMOPTYSIS

What is it?	Bleeding into the bronchial tree

What are the causes?	1. Bronchitis (50%) 2. Tumor mass (20%) 3. TB (8%) Other causes: bronchiectasis, pulmonary catheters, trauma
Define MASSIVE hemoptysis.	>600 cc/24 hours
What comprises the workup?	CXR Bronchoscopy Bronchial A-gram
What is the treatment if massive?	Bronchoscopy, intubation of unaffected side, Fogarty catheter occlusion of bleeding bronchus, bronchial A-gram with or without embolization, surgical resection of involved lung
What is the treatment of moderate to mild bleeding?	Laser coagulation, +/− epinephrine injection

SPONTANEOUS PNEUMOTHORAX

What is it?	Atraumatic spontaneous development of a pneumothorax
What are the causes?	Idiopathic (primary), bleb disease, emphysema, etc. (secondary)
What body habitus is associated with spontaneous pneumothorax?	Thin and tall
How is the diagnosis made?	CXR
What is the treatment?	Chest tube
What are the options if refractory, recurrent, or bilateral?	Pleurodesis: scar the lung to the parietal pleura with a sclerosant (talc) via chest tube/thoracoscopy, or by thoracotomy and mechanical abrasion
Who might also need a pleurodesis after the first episode?	Those whose lifestyles place them at increased risk for pneumothorax (e.g., pilots, scuba divers)

What is a catamenial pneumothorax?	Pneumothorax due to intrathoracic endometriosis

MESOTHELIOMA

Malignant Mesothelioma

What is it?	Primary pleural neoplasm
What are the two types?	1. Localized 2. Diffuse (highly malignant)
What are the risk factors?	Exposure to asbestos Smoking
What are the symptoms?	Dyspnea and pain = 90% Localized: pleuritic pain, joint pain and swelling, dyspnea Diffuse: chest pain, malaise, weight loss, cough
What are the signs?	Pleural effusion: Localized (10%–15%) Diffuse (>75%)
What are the associated radiographic tests?	X-ray may reveal a peripheral mass, often forming an obtuse angle with the chest wall; **CT scan is also performed**
How is the diagnosis made?	Pleural biopsy, pleural fluid cytology
What is the treatment if localized?	Surgical excision
What is the treatment if diffuse?	Early stages may be resected, followed by radiation; for more advanced stages, radiation, chemotherapy, or both are done
What is the prognosis?	Localized: poor Diffuse: **dismal** (average life span after diagnosis is about 1 year)

Benign Mesothelioma

What is it?	Benign pleural mesothelioma
What pleura is usually involved?	Visceral pleura

What is the gross appearance?	Pedunculated "broccoli or cauliflower" tumor on a stalk coming off of the lung
What is the treatment?	Surgical resection with at least 1 cm clear margin
What is the prognosis?	In contrast to malignant mesothelioma, the benign mesothelioma has an excellent prognosis with cure in the vast majority of cases

DISEASES OF THE LUNGS

BRONCHOGENIC CARCINOMA

What is the annual incidence of lung cancer in the United States?	170,000 new cases/year
What is the number of annual deaths from lung cancer?	150,000; most common cancer death in the United States in men **and** women
What is the #1 risk factor?	Smoking (85%!)
Does asbestos exposure increase the risk in patients who smoke?	Yes
What type of lung cancer arises in nonsmoking?	Adenocarcinoma
Cancer arises more often in which lung?	Right > left; upper lobes > lower lobes
What are the signs/ symptoms?	Change in a chronic cough Hemoptysis, chest pain, dyspnea Pleural effusion (suggests chest wall involvement) Hoarseness (recurrent laryngeal nerve involvement) Superior vena cava syndrome Diaphragmatic paralysis (phrenic nerve involvement) Symptoms of metastasis/paraneoplastic syndrome Finger clubbing

What is Pancoast's tumor?

Tumor at the apex of the lung or superior sulcus that may involve the brachial plexus, sympathetic ganglia, and vertebral bodies, leading to pain, upper extremity weakness, and Horner's syndrome

What is Horner's syndrome?

Injury to the cervical sympathetic chain; Think: **"MAP"**
1. **M**iosis (small pupil)
2. **A**nhydrosis of ipsilateral face
3. **P**tosis

What are the four most common sites of extrathoracic metastases?

1. Bone
2. Liver
3. Adrenals
4. Kidney

What are paraneoplastic syndromes?

Syndromes that are associated with tumors but may affect distant parts of the body; they may be caused by hormones released from endocrinologically active tumors or may be of uncertain etiology

Name five general types of paraneoplastic syndromes.

1. Metabolic: Cushing's, SIADH, hypercalcemia
2. Neuromuscular: Eaton-Lambert, cerebellar ataxia
3. Skeletal: hypertrophic osteoarthropathy
4. Dermatologic: acanthosis nigricans
5. Vascular: thrombophlebitis

What are the associated radiographic tests?

CXR, CT scan, PET scan

How is the tumor diagnosed?

1. Sputum cytology
2. Needle biopsy (CT or fluoro guidance)
3. Bronchoscopy with brushings, biopsies, or both
4. With or without mediastinoscopy, mediastinotomy, scalene node biopsy, or open lung biopsy for definitive diagnosis

For each tumor listed, recall its usual site in the lung and its natural course:

Squamous cell?

66% occur **centrally** in lung hilus; may also be a Pancoast's tumor; slow growth, late metastasis; associated with smoking (Think: **S**quamous = **S**entral)

Adenocarcinoma?

Peripheral, rapid growth with hematogenous/nodal metastasis, associated with lung scarring

Small (oat) cell?

Central, highly malignant, usually not operable

Large cell?

Usually peripheral, very malignant

What are the AJCC stages of carcinoma of the lungs:

Stage Ia?

Tumor <3 cm, no nodes, no metastases

Stage Ib?

Tumor 3–5 cm, no nodes, no metastases

Stage IIa?

1. Tumor <5 cm **and** positive nodes to lung or ipsilateral hilum; **no** metastases, or
2. Tumor 5–7 cm, no nodes, no metastases

Stage IIb?

1. Tumor 5–7 cm and positive nodes in lung or ipsilateral hilum, or
2. Tumor that invades chest wall, diaphragm, mediastinal pleura, phrenic nerve, pericardial sac, or bronchus (not carina) and no nodes, **no** metastases

Stage IIIa?

1. Tumor <7 cm and + nodes in ipsilateral mediastinum or subcarina with **no** metastases
2. Tumor >7 cm or extends into chest wall, parietal pleura, diaphragm, phrenic nerve, or pericardium and + lymph node metastases to ipsilateral, mediastinal, or subcarinal nodes
3. Any size tumor that invades heart, great vessels, trachea, esophagus, carina, or ipsalateral lobe, or + nodes peribronchial and/or ipsilateral hilum, or intrapulmonary nodes

Stage IIIb?

Any tumor, + lymph node metastases to contralateral hilum or mediastinum
Supraclavicular/scalene nodes, NO distant metastases

Stage IV?

Distant metastases

What are the surgical contraindications for NON-small cell carcinoma?

Stage IV, Stage IIIb, poor lung function (FEV$_1$ <0.8L)

What is the treatment by stage for NON-small cell lung carcinoma:

Stage I?

Surgical resection

Stage II?

Surgical resection

Stage IIIa?

Chemotherapy and XRT +/− surgical resection

Stage IIIb?

Chemotherapy and XRT

Stage IV?

Chemotherapy +/− XRT

What is the treatment for isolated brain metastasis?

Surgical resection

What is the approximate prognosis (5-year survival) after treatment of NON-small cell lung carcinoma by stage:	
Stage I?	50%
Stage II?	30%
Stage III?	<10%
Stage IV?	1%
How is small cell carcinoma treated?	Chemotherapy +/− XRT (very small isolated lesions can be surgically resected)
What are the contraindications to surgery for lung cancer?	Think: **"STOP IT"** **S**uperior vena cava syndrome, **S**upraclavicular node metastasis, **S**calene node metastasis **T**racheal carina involvement **O**at cell carcinoma (treat with chemotherapy +/− radiation) **P**ulmonary function tests show FEV$_1$ <0.8L **I**nfarction (myocardial); a.k.a. cardiac cripple **T**umor elsewhere (metastatic disease)
What postoperative FEV$_1$ must you have?	FEV$_1$ >800 cc; thus, a preoperative FEV$_1$ >2L is usually needed for a pneumonectomy If FEV$_1$ is <2L, a ventilation perfusion scan should be performed
What is hypertrophic pulmonary osteoarthropathy?	Periosteal proliferation and new bone formation at the end of long bones and in the bones of the hand (seen in 10% of patients with lung cancer)

SOLITARY PULMONARY NODULES (COIN LESIONS)

What are they?	Peripheral circumscribed pulmonary lesions

What is the differential diagnosis?	Granulomatous disease, benign neoplasms, malignancy
What percentage are malignant?	Overall, 5% to 10% (but >50% are malignant in smokers >50 years)
Is there a gender risk?	Yes; the incidence of coin lesions is 3 to 9× higher and malignancy is nearly twice as common in men as in women
What are the symptoms?	Usually asymptomatic with solitary nodules, but may include coughing, weight loss, chest pain, and hemoptysis
What are the signs?	Physical findings are uncommon; clubbing is rare; hypertrophic osteoarthropathy implies >80% chance of malignancy
How is the diagnosis made?	CXR, chest CT
What is the significance of "popcorn" calcification?	Most likely benign (i.e., hamartoma)
What are the risk factors for malignancy?	1. Size: lesions >1 cm have a significant chance of malignancy, and those >4 cm are very likely to be malignant 2. Indistinct margins (corona radiata) 3. Documented growth on follow-up x-ray (if no change in 2 years, most likely benign) 4. Increasing age
What are the associated lab tests?	1. TB skin tests, etc. 2. Sputum cultures 3. Sputum cytology is diagnostic in 5% to 20% of cases
Which method of tissue diagnosis is used?	Chest CT scan with needle biopsy, bronchoscopy (+/− transtracheal biopsy), excisional biopsy (open or thoracoscopic)

What is the treatment?	Surgical excision is the mainstay of treatment
	Excisional biopsy is therapeutic for benign lesions, solitary metastasis, and for primary cancer in patients who are poor risks for more extensive surgery
	Lobectomy for centrally placed lesions
	Lobectomy with node dissection for primary cancer (if resectable by preop evaluations)
Which solitary nodule can be followed without a tissue diagnosis?	Popcorn calcifications
	Mass unchanged for 2 years on previous CXR
What is the prognosis?	For malignant coin lesions <2 cm, 5-year survival is ≈70%
What if the patient has an SPN and pulmonary hypertrophic osteoarthropathy?	>75% chance of carcinoma
What is hypertrophic pulmonary osteoarthropathy?	Periosteal proliferation and new bone formation at the end of long bones and in bones of the hand
What is its incidence?	≈7% of patients with lung cancer (2%–12%)
What are the signs?	Associated with clubbing of the fingers; diagnosed by x-ray of long bones, revealing periosteal bone hypertrophy

CARCINOID TUMOR

What is it?	**APUD** (**A**mine-**P**recursor **U**ptake and **D**ecarboxylation) cell tumor of the bronchus
What is its natural course in the lung?	Slow growing (but may be malignant)
What are the primary local findings?	Wheezing and atelectasis caused by bronchial obstruction/stenosis

What condition can it be confused with?	Asthma
How is the diagnosis made?	Bronchoscopy reveals round red-yellow-purple mass covered by epithelium that protrudes into bronchial lumen
What is the treatment?	Surgical resection (lobectomy with lymph node dissection) Sleeve resection is also an option for proximal bronchial lesions
What is a sleeve resection?	Resection of a ring segment of bronchus (with tumor inside) and then end-to-end anastomosis of the remaining ends, allowing salvage of lower lobe
What is the prognosis (5-year survival) after complete surgical resection of carcinoid:	
Negative nodes?	>90% alive at 5 years
Positive nodes?	66% alive at 5 years
What is the most common benign lung tumor?	Hamartoma (normal cells in a weird configuration)

PULMONARY SEQUESTRATION

What is it?	Abnormal benign lung tissue with separate blood supply that **DOES NOT** communicate with the normal tracheobronchial airway
Define the following terms:	
Interlobar	Sequestration in normal lung tissue covered by normal visceral pleura
Extralobar	Sequestration not in normal lung covered by its own pleura
What are the signs/symptoms?	Asymptomatic, recurrent pneumonia
How is the diagnosis made?	CXR, chest CT, A-gram, U/S with Doppler flow to ascertain blood supply

What is the treatment in the following cases:

    Extralobar?

Surgical resection

    Intralobar?

Lobectomy

What is the major danger during surgery for sequestration?

Anomalous blood supply from below the diaphragm (these can be cut and retract into the abdomen resulting in exsanguination!)

Always document blood supply by A-gram or U/S with Doppler flow

DISEASES OF THE MEDIASTINUM

MEDIASTINAL ANATOMY

What structures lie in the following locations:

    Superior mediastinum?

Aortic arch, great vessels, upper trachea, esophagus

    Anterior mediastinum?

Thymus, ascending aorta, lymph nodes

    Middle mediastinum?

Heart, lower trachea and bifurcation, lung hila, phrenic nerves, lymph nodes

    Posterior mediastinum?

Esophagus, descending aorta, thoracic duct, vagus and intercostal nerves, sympathetic trunks, azygous and hemizygous veins, lymph nodes

What is the major differential diagnosis for tumors of the mediastinum:

    Anterior mediastinum?

Classic **"four Ts": T**hyroid tumor, **T**hymoma, **T**errible lymphoma, **T**eratoma; also parathyroid tumor, lipoma, vascular aneurysms

    Middle mediastinum?

Lymphadenopathy (e.g., lymphoma, sarcoid), teratoma, fat pad, cysts, hernias, extension of esophageal mass, bronchogenic cancer

Posterior mediastinum? Neurogenic tumors, lymphoma, aortic aneurysm, vertebral lesions, hernias

What is the most common type of tumor arising in the mediastinum? Neurogenic (most commonly in posterior mediastinum)

What is the differential diagnosis for a neurogenic tumor? Schwannoma (a.k.a. neurolemmoma), neurofibroma, neuroblastoma, ganglioneuroma, ganglioneuroblastoma, pheochromocytoma

PRIMARY MEDIASTINAL TUMORS

Thymoma

Where are they found in the mediastinum? Anterior

How is the diagnosis made? CT scan

What is the treatment? All thymomas should be surgically resected via midline sternotomy

What are the indications for *post*op radiation therapy? Invasive malignant tumor

What are the indications for *pre*op chemotherapy? Tumor >6 cm and CT scan with invasion

What percentage of thymomas are malignant? ≈25%

How is a malignant thymoma diagnosed? At surgery with invasion into surrounding structures (not by histology!)

What is myasthenia gravis? Autoimmune disease with antibodies against the muscle acetylcholine receptors

What percentage of patients with myasthenia gravis have a thymoma? ≈15%

What percentage of patients with thymoma have or will have myasthenia gravis? ≈75%!

Teratomas

What are they?	Tumors of branchial cleft cells; the tumors contain ectoderm, endoderm, and mesoderm
What is a dermoid cyst?	Teratoma made up of ectodermal derivatives (e.g., teeth, skin, hair)
Which age group is affected?	Usually adolescents, but can occur at any age
Where in the mediastinum do they occur?	Anterior
What are the characteristic x-ray findings?	Calcifications or teeth; tumors may be cystic
What percentage are malignant?	$\approx 15\%$
What is the treatment of benign dermoid cysts?	Surgical excision
What is the treatment of malignant teratoma?	Preoperative chemotherapy until tumor markers are normal, then surgical resection
Which tumor markers are associated with malignant teratomas?	AFP, CEA

Neurogenic Tumors

What is the incidence?	**Most common** mediastinal tumors in all age groups
Where in the mediastinum do they occur?	Posterior, in the paravertebral gutters
What percentage are malignant?	50% in children 10% in adults

What are the histologic types (5)? (Note cells of origin and whether benign or malignant.)	1. Neurilemmoma or schwannoma (benign)—arise from Schwann cell sheaths of intercostal nerves 2. Neurofibroma (benign)—arise from intercostal nerves; may degenerate into: 3. Neurosarcoma (malignant) 4. Ganglioneuroma (benign)—from sympathetic chain 5. Neuroblastoma (malignant)—also from sympathetic chain

LYMPHOMA

Where in the mediastinum does it occur?	Anywhere, but most often in the anterosuperior mediastinum or hilum in the middle mediastinum
What percentage of lymphomas involve mediastinal nodes?	$\approx 50\%$
What are the symptoms?	Cough, fever, chest pain, weight loss, SVC syndrome, chylothorax
How is the diagnosis made?	1. CXR, CT scan 2. Mediastinoscopy or mediastinotomy with node biopsy
What is the treatment?	Nonsurgical (chemotherapy, radiation, or both)

MEDIASTINITIS

Acute Mediastinitis

What is it?	Acute suppurative mediastinal infection
Name the six etiologies.	1. Esophageal perforation (Boerhaave's syndrome) 2. Postoperative wound infection 3. Head and neck infections 4. Lung or pleural infections 5. Rib or vertebral osteomyelitis 6. Distant infections

What are the clinical features?

Fever, chest pain, dysphagia (especially with esophageal perforation), respiratory distress, leukocytosis

What is the treatment?

1. Wide drainage
2. Treatment of primary cause
3. Antibiotics

Chronic Mediastinitis

What is it?

Mediastinal fibrosis secondary to *chronic* granulomatous infection

What is the most common etiology?

Histoplasma capsulatum

What are the clinical features?

50% are asymptomatic; symptoms are related to compression of adjacent structures: SVC syndrome, bronchial and esophageal strictures, constrictive pericarditis

How is the diagnosis made?

CXR or CT may be helpful, but surgery/ biopsy often makes the diagnosis

What is the treatment?

Antibiotics; surgical removal of the granulomas is rarely helpful

SUPERIOR VENA CAVA SYNDROME

What is it?

Obstruction of the superior vena cava, usually by extrinsic compression

What is the #1 cause?

Malignant tumors cause ≈90% of cases; lung cancer is by far the most common; other tumors include thymoma, lymphoma, and Hodgkin's disease

What are the clinical manifestations?

1. Blue discoloration and puffiness of the face, arms, and shoulders
2. CNS manifestations may include headache, nausea, vomiting, visual distortion, stupor, and convulsions.
3. Cough, hoarseness, and dyspnea

What is the treatment?	1. Diuretics and fluid restriction 2. Prompt radiation therapy +/− chemotherapy for any causative cancer
What is the prognosis?	SVC obstruction itself is fatal in <5% of cases; mean survival time in patients with malignant obstruction is ≈7 months

DISEASES OF THE ESOPHAGUS

ANATOMIC CONSIDERATIONS

What are the primary functions of the Upper and Lower Esophageal Sphincters?	**UES:** swallowing **LES:** prevention of reflux
The esophageal venous plexus drains inferiorly into the gastric veins. Why is this important?	Gastric veins are part of the portal venous system; portal hypertension can thus be referred to the esophageal veins, leading to varices
Identify the esophageal muscle type: Proximal 1/3	Skeletal muscle
Middle 1/3	Smooth muscle > skeletal muscle
Distal 1/3	Smooth muscle
Identify the blood supply to the esophagus: Proximal 1/3	Inferior thyroid, anterior intercostals
Middle 1/3	Esophageal arteries, bronchial arteries
Distal 1/3	Left gastric artery, left inferior phrenic artery
What is the length of the esophagus?	≈25 cm in the adult (40 cm from teeth to LES)
Why is the esophagus notorious for anastomotic leaks?	Esophagus has no serosa (same as the distal rectum)

What nerve runs with the esophagus?	Vagus nerve

ZENKER'S DIVERTICULUM

What is it?	Pharyngoesophageal diverticulum; a false diverticulum containing mucosa and submucosa at the UES at the pharyngoesophageal junction through Killian's triangle

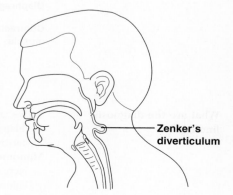

What is the disease's "claim to fame"?	Most common esophageal diverticulum
What are the signs/ symptoms?	Dysphagia, neck mass, halitosis, food regurgitation, heartburn
How is the diagnosis made?	Barium swallow
What is the treatment?	1. Diverticulectomy 2. Cricopharyngeus myotomy, if >2 cm

ACHALASIA

What is it?	1. Failure of the LES to relax during swallowing 2. Loss of esophageal **peristalsis**
What are the proposed etiologies?	1. Neurologic (ganglionic degeneration of Auerbach's plexus, vagus nerve, or both); possibly infectious in nature 2. Chagas' disease in South America

What are the associated long-term conditions?	Esophageal carcinoma secondary to Barrett's esophagus from food stasis
What are the symptoms?	Dysphagia for both solids and liquids, followed by regurgitation; dysphagia for liquids is worse

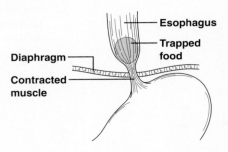

What are the diagnostic findings?	Radiographic contrast studies reveal dilated esophageal body with narrowing inferiorly **Manometry:** motility studies reveal increased pressure in the LES and failure of the LES to relax during swallowing
What are the treatment options?	1. Balloon dilation of the LES 2. Medical treatment of reflux versus Belsey Mark IV 270° fundoplication (do not perform 360° Nissen) 3. Myotomy of the lower esophagus and LES

DIFFUSE ESOPHAGEAL SPASM

What is it?	Strong, nonperistaltic contractions of the esophageal body; sphincter function is usually normal
What is the associated condition?	Gastroesophageal reflux
What are the symptoms?	Spontaneous chest pain that radiates to the back, ears, neck, jaw, or arms

What is the differential diagnosis?	Angina pectoris Psychoneurosis Nutcracker esophagus
What are the associated diagnostic tests?	**Esophageal manometry:** Motility studies reveal repetitive, high-amplitude contractions with normal sphincter response Upper GI may be normal, but 50% show segmented spasms or corkscrew esophagus Endoscopy
What is the classic finding on esophageal contrast study (UGI)?	"Corkscrew esophagus"
What is the treatment?	Medical (antireflux measures, calcium channel blockers, nitrates) Long esophagomyotomy in refractory cases

NUTCRACKER ESOPHAGUS

What is it also known as?	Hypertensive peristalsis
What is it?	Very strong peristaltic waves
What are the symptoms?	Spontaneous chest pain that radiates to the back, ears, neck, jaw, or arms
What is the differential diagnosis?	Angina pectoris Psychoneurosis Diffuse esophageal spasm
What are the associated diagnostic tests?	1. Esophageal manometry: motility studies reveal repetitive, high-amplitude contractions with normal sphincter response 2. Results of UGI may be normal (rule out mass) 3. Endoscopy
What is the treatment?	Medical (antireflux measures, calcium channel blockers, nitrates) Long esophagomyotomy in refractory cases

ESOPHAGEAL REFLUX

What is it?	Reflux of gastric contents into the lower esophagus resulting from the decreased function of the LES
What are the causes?	1. Decreased LES tone 2. Decreased esophageal motility 3. Hiatal hernia 4. Gastric outlet obstruction 5. NGT
Name four associated conditions/factors.	1. Sliding hiatal hernia 2. Tobacco and alcohol 3. Scleroderma 4. Decreased endogenous gastrin production
What are the symptoms?	Substernal pain, heartburn, regurgitation; symptoms are worse when patient is supine and after meals
How is the diagnosis made?	1. pH probe in the lower esophagus reveals acid reflux 2. EGD shows esophagitis 3. Manometry reveals decreased LES pressure 4. Barium swallow
What is the initial treatment?	Medical: H_2-blockers, antacids, metoclopramide, omeprazole Elevation of the head of the bed; small, multiple meals
Which four complications require surgery?	1. Failure of medical therapy 2. Esophageal strictures 3. Progressive pulmonary insufficiency secondary to documented nocturnal aspiration 4. Barrett's esophagus
Describe each of the following types of surgery: **Nissen**	$360°$ fundoplication: wrap fundus of stomach all the way around the esophagus

Belsey Mark IV	270° fundoplication: wrap fundus of stomach, but not all the way around
Hill	Tighten arcuate ligament around esophagus and tack stomach to diaphragm
Lap Nissen	Nissen via laparoscope
Lap Toupet	Lap fundoplication posteriorly with less than 220° to 250° wrap used with decreased esophageal motility; disadvantage is more postoperative reflux
What is Barrett's esophagus?	Replacement of the lower esophageal squamous epithelium with columnar epithelium secondary to reflux
Why is it significant?	This lesion is premalignant
What is the treatment?	People with significant reflux should be followed with regular EGDs with biopsies, H_2-blockers, and antireflux precautions; many experts believe that patients with severe dysplasia should undergo esophagectomy

CAUSTIC ESOPHAGEAL STRICTURES

Which agents may cause strictures if ingested?	Lye, oven cleaners, drain cleaners, batteries, sodium hydroxide tablets (Clinitest)
How is the diagnosis made?	History; EGD is clearly indicated early on to assess the extent of damage (<24 hrs); scope to level of severe injury (deep ulcer) only, water soluble contrast study for deep ulcers to rule out perforation
What is the initial treatment?	1. NPO/IVF/H_2-blocker 2. Do **not** induce emesis 3. Corticosteroids (controversial— probably best for shallow/moderate ulcers), antibiotics (penicillin/ gentamicin) for moderate ulcers 4. Antibiotic for deep ulcers 5. Upper GI at 10 to 14 days

What is the treatment if a stricture develops?	Dilation with Maloney dilator/balloon catheter In severe refractory cases, esophagectomy with colon interposition or gastric pull-up
What is the long-term follow-up?	Because of increased risk of esophageal squamous cancer (especially with ulceration), patients **endoscopies every other year**
What is a Maloney dilator?	Mercury-filled rubber dilator

ESOPHAGEAL CARCINOMA

What are the two main types?	1. Adenocarcinoma at the GE junction 2. Squamous cell carcinoma in most of the esophagus
What is the most common histology?	**Worldwide:** squamous cell carcinoma (95%!) **USA:** adenocarcinoma
What is the age and gender distribution?	Most common in the sixth decade of life; men predominate, especially black men
What are the etiologic factors (5)?	1. Tobacco 2. Alcohol 3. GE reflux 4. Barrett's esophagus 5. Radiation
What are the symptoms?	Dysphagia, weight loss Other symptoms include chest pain, back pain, hoarseness, symptoms of metastasis
What comprises the workup?	1. UGI 2. EGD 3. Transesophageal ultrasound (TEU) 4. CT scan of chest/abdomen
What is the differential diagnosis?	Leiomyoma, metastatic tumor, lymphomas, benign stricture, achalasia, diffuse esophageal spasm, GERD

How is the diagnosis made?

1. Upper GI localizes tumor
2. EGD obtains biopsy and assesses resectability
3. Full metastatic workup (CXR, bone scan, CT scan, LFTs)

Describe the stages of adenocarcinoma esophageal cancer:

    Stage I

Tumor: invades lamina propria, muscularis mucosae, or submucosa
Nodes: negative

    Stage IIa

Tumor: invades muscularis propria (grade 3)
Nodes: negative

    Stage IIb

1. Tumor: invades up to muscularis propria
   Nodes: positive regional nodes
2. Invades adventitia with negative nodes

    Stage III

1. Tumor: invades adventitia
   Nodes: positive regional nodes
2. Tumor: invades adjacent structures

    Stage IV

Distant metastasis

What is the treatment?

Esophagectomy with gastric pull-up or colon interposition

What is an Ivor-Lewis procedure?

Laparotomy and right thoracotomy with gastroesophageal anastomosis in the chest after esophagectomy

Treatment options with metastatic disease (unresectable)?

Chemotherapy and XRT +/− dilation, stent, laser, electrocoagulation, brachytherapy, photodynamic laser therapy

What is a "blunt esophagectomy"?

Esophagectomy with "blunt" transhiatal dissection of esophagus from abdomen and gastroesophageal anastomosis in the neck

What is the operative mortality rate?	≈5%
Has radiation therapy and/or chemotherapy been shown to decrease mortality?	No
What is the postop complication rate?	≈33%!
What is the prognosis (5-year survival) by stage:	
I?	66%
II?	25%
III?	10%
IV?	Basically 0%

Chapter 72   Cardiovascular Surgery

What do the following abbreviations stand for:	
AI?	**A**ortic **I**nsufficiency/regurgitation
AS?	**A**ortic **S**tenosis
ASD?	**A**trial **S**eptal **D**efect
CABG?	**C**oronary **A**rtery **B**ypass **G**rafting
CAD?	**C**oronary **A**rtery **D**isease
CPB?	**C**ardio**P**ulmonary **B**ypass
IABP?	**I**ntra**A**ortic **B**alloon **P**ump
LAD?	**L**eft **A**nterior **D**escending coronary artery

IMA?	**I**nternal **M**ammary **A**rtery
MR?	**M**itral **R**egurgitation
PTCA?	**P**ercutaneous **T**ransluminal **C**oronary **A**ngioplasty (balloon angioplasty)
VAD?	**V**entricular **A**ssist **D**evice
VSD?	**V**entricular **S**eptal **D**efect

Define the following terms:

Stroke volume (SV)	mL of blood pumped per heartbeat (SV = CO/HR)
Cardiac output (CO)	Amount of blood pumped by the heart each minute: heart rate × SV
Cardiac Index (CI)	CO/BSA (body surface area)
Ejection fraction	Percentage of blood pumped out of the left ventricle: SV ÷ end diastolic volume (nl 55%–70%)
Compliance	Change in volume/change in pressure
SVR	**S**ystemic **V**ascular **R**esistance = $\dfrac{\text{MAP} - \text{CVP}}{\text{CO} \times 80}$
Preload	Left ventricular end diastolic pressure or volume
Afterload	Arterial resistance the heart pumps against
PVR	**P**ulmonary **V**ascular **R**esistance = $PA_{(mean)}$ − PCWP/CO × 80
MAP	**M**ean **A**rterial **P**ressure = diastolic BP + 1/3 (systolic BP − diastolic BP)
What is a normal CO?	4 to 8 L/minute
What is a normal CI?	2.5 to 4 L/minute

What are the ways to increase CO?	Remember **"MR. PAIR"**:
	1. **M**echanical assistance (IABP, VAD)
	2. **R**ate—Increase heart rate
	3. **P**reload—Increase preload
	4. **A**fterload—Decrease afterload
	5. **I**notropes—Increase contractility
	6. **R**hythm—Normal sinus

When does most of the coronary blood flow take place?	During diastole (66%)

Name the three major coronary arteries.	1. Left **A**nterior **D**escending (**LAD**)
	2. Circumflex
	3. Right coronary

What are the three main "cardiac electrolytes"?	1. Calcium (inotropic)
	2. Potassium (dysrhythmias)
	3. Magnesium (dysrhythmias)

ACQUIRED HEART DISEASE

CORONARY ARTERY DISEASE (CAD)

What is it?	Atherosclerotic occlusive lesions of the coronary arteries; segmental nature makes CABG possible

What is the incidence?	CAD is the #1 killer in the Western world; >50% of cases are triple vessel diseases involving the LAD, circumflex, and right coronary arteries

What are the symptoms?	If ischemia occurs (low flow, vasospasm, thrombus formation, plaque rupture, or a combination), patient may experience chest pain, crushing, substernal shortness of breath, nausea/upper abdominal pain, sudden death, or may be asymptomatic with fatigue

Who classically gets "silent" MIs?	Patients with diabetes (autonomic dysfunction)

What are the risk factors?

HTN
Smoking
High cholesterol/lipids (>240)
Obesity
Diabetes mellitus
Family history

Which diagnostic tests should be performed?

Exercise stress testing (± thallium)
Echocardiography
Localize dyskinetic wall segments
Valvular dysfunction
Estimate ejection fraction
Cardiac catheterization with coronary
    angiography and left ventriculography
    (the definitive test)

What is the treatment?

Medical therapy (β-blockers, aspirin,
nitrates, HTN medications), angioplasty
(PTCA), +/− stents, surgical therapy: CABG

CABG

What is it?

Coronary Artery Bypass Grafting

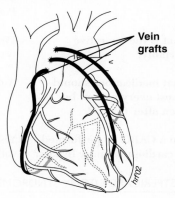

Vein grafts

What are the indications?

Left main disease
≥2-vessel disease (especially diabetics)
Unstable or disabling angina unresponsive
    to medical therapy/PTCA
Postinfarct angina
Coronary artery rupture, dissection,
    thrombosis after PTCA

CABG vs. PTCA +/− stents? CABG = Survival improvement for diabetics and ≥2-vessel disease, ↑ short-term morbidity
PTCA = ↓ short-term morbidity, ↓ cost, ↓ hospital stay, ↑ reintervention, ↑ postprocedure angina

What procedures are most often used in the treatment? Coronary arteries grafted (usually 3–6): internal mammary pedicle graft and saphenous vein free graft are most often used (IMA 95% 10-year patency vs. 50% with saphenous)

What other vessels are occasionally used for grafting? Radial artery, inferior epigastric vein

What are the possible complications? Hemorrhage
Tamponade
MI, dysrhythmias
Infection
Graft thrombosis
Sternal dehiscence
Postpericardiotomy syndrome, stroke

What is the operative mortality? 1% to 3% for elective CABG (vs. 5%–10% for acute MI)

What medications should almost every patient be given after CABG? Aspirin, β-blocker

Can a CABG be performed off cardiopulmonary bypass? Yes, today they are performed with or without bypass

POSTPERICARDIOTOMY SYNDROME

What is it? Pericarditis after pericardiotomy (unknown etiology), occurs weeks to 3 months postoperatively

What are the signs/symptoms? Fever
Chest pain, atrial fibrillation
Malaise
Pericardial friction rub
Pericardial effusion/pleural effusion

What is the treatment?	NSAIDs, +/− steroids
What is pericarditis after an MI called?	Dressler's syndrome

CARDIOPULMONARY BYPASS (CPB)

What is it?	Pump and oxygenation apparatus remove blood from SVC and IVC and return it to the aorta, bypassing the heart and lungs and allowing cardiac arrest for open-heart procedures, heart transplant, lung transplant, or heart-lung transplant as well as procedures on the proximal great vessels

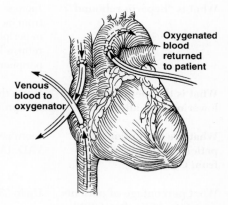

Oxygenated blood returned to patient

Venous blood to oxygenator

Is anticoagulation necessary?	Yes, just before and during the procedure, with heparin
How is anticoagulation reversed?	Protamine
What are the ways to manipulate cardiac output after CPB?	Rate, rhythm, afterload, preload, inotropes, mechanical (IABP and VAD)
What mechanical problems can decrease CO after CPB?	Cardiac tamponade, pneumothorax
What is "tamponade physiology"?	↓ Cardiac output, ↑ heart rate, hypotension, ↑ **CVP = ↑ wedge pressure**

What are the possible complications?

Trauma to formed blood elements (especially thrombocytopenia and platelet dysfunction)
Pancreatitis (low flow)
Heparin rebound
CVA
Failure to wean from bypass
Technical complications (operative technique)
MI

What are the options for treating postop CABG mediastinal bleeding?

Protamine, ↑ PEEP, FFP, platelets, aminocaproic acid

What is "heparin rebound"?

Increased anticoagulation after CPB from increased heparin levels, as increase in peripheral blood flow after CPB returns heparin residual that was in the peripheral tissues

What is the method of lowering SVR after CPB?

Warm the patient; administer sodium nitroprusside (SNP) and dobutamine

What are the options if a patient cannot be weaned from CPB?

Inotropes (e.g., epinephrine)
VAD, IABP

What percentage of patients goes into AFib after CPB?

Up to 33%

What is the workup of a postoperative patient with AFib?

Rule out PTX (ABG, CT scan), acidosis (ABG), electrolyte abnormality (LABS), and ischemia (EKG), CXR

What is a MIDCAB?

Minimally **I**nvasive **D**irect **C**oronary **A**rtery **B**ypass—LIMA to LAD bypass without CPB and through a small thoracotomy

What is TMR?

Trans**M**yocardial laser **R**evascularization: laser through groin catheter makes small holes (intramyocardial sinusoids) in cardiac muscle to allow blood to nourish the muscle

What is OPCAB?	**O**ff **P**ump **C**oronary **A**rtery **B**ypass—median sternotomy but no bypass pump

AORTIC STENOSIS (AS)

What is it?	Destruction and calcification of valve leaflets, resulting in obstruction of left ventricular outflow
What are the causes?	Calcification of bicuspid aortic valve Rheumatic fever Acquired calcific AS (7th to 8th decades)
What are the symptoms?	Angina (5 years life expectancy if left untreated) Syncope (3 years life expectancy if left untreated) CHF (2 years life expectancy if left untreated) Often asymptomatic until late
What is the memory aid for the aortic stenosis complications?	**A**ortic **S**tenosis **C**omplications = **A**ngina **S**yncope **C**HF—5,3,2
What are the signs?	Murmur: crescendo-decrescendo systolic second right intercostal space with radiation to the carotids Left ventricular heave or lift from left ventricular hypertrophy
What tests should be performed?	CXR, ECG, echocardiography Cardiac catheterization—needed to plan operation
What is the surgical treatment?	Valve replacement with tissue or mechanical prosthesis
What are the indications for surgical repair?	If patient is symptomatic or valve cross-sectional area is <0.75 cm^2 (normal 2.5 to 3.5 cm^2) and/or gradient >50 mm Hg
What are the pros/cons of mechanical valve?	Mechanical valve is more durable, but requires lifetime anticoagulation

What is the treatment option in poor surgical candidates?	Balloon aortic "valvuloplasty" (percutaneous)
Why is a loud murmur often a good sign?	Implies a high gradient, which indicates preserved LV function
Why might an AS murmur diminish over time?	It may imply a decreasing gradient from a decline in LV function

AORTIC INSUFFICIENCY (AI)

What is it?	Incompetency of the aortic valve (regurgitant flow)
What are the causes?	Bacterial endocarditis (*Staphylococcus aureus, Streptococcus viridans*) Rheumatic fever (rare) Annular ectasia from collagen vascular disease (especially Marfan's syndrome)
What are the predisposing conditions?	Bicuspid aortic valve, connective tissue disease
What are the symptoms?	Palpitations from dysrhythmias and dilated left ventricle Dyspnea/orthopnea from left ventricular failure Excess fatigue Angina from ↓ diastolic BP and coronary flow (***Note:*** Most coronary blood flow occurs during diastole and aorta rebound) Musset sign (bobble-head)
What are the signs?	↑ diastolic BP Murmur: blowing, decrescendo diastolic at left sternal border Austin-Flint murmur: reverberation of regurgitant flow Increased pulse pressure: "pistol shots," "water-hammer" pulse palpated over peripheral arteries Quincke sign (capillary pulsations of uvula)

Which diagnostic tests should be performed?	1. CXR: increasing heart size can be used to follow progression 2. Echocardiogram 3. Catheterization (definitive) 4. TEE
What is the treatment?	Aortic valve replacement
What are the indications for surgical treatment?	Symptomatic patients (CHF, PND, etc.), left ventricle dilatation, decreasing LV function, decreasing EF, acute AI onset
What is the prognosis?	Surgery gives symptomatic improvement and may improve longevity; low operative risk

MITRAL STENOSIS (MS)

What is it?	Calcific degeneration and narrowing of the mitral valve resulting from rheumatic fever in most cases
What are the symptoms?	1. Dyspnea from increased left atrial pressure, causing pulmonary edema (i.e., CHF) 2. Hemoptysis (rarely life-threatening) 3. Hoarseness from dilated left atrium impinging on the recurrent laryngeal nerve 4. Palpations (AFib)
What are the signs?	Murmur: crescendo diastolic rumble at apex Irregular pulse from AFib caused by dilated left atrium Stroke caused by systemic emboli from left atrium (AFib and obstructed valve allow blood to pool in the left atrium and can lead to thrombus formation)
Which diagnostic tests should be performed?	Echocardiogram Catheterization
What are the indications for intervention?	1. Symptoms (severe) 2. Pulmonary HTN and mitral valve area <1 cm^2/m^2 3. Recurrent thromboembolism

What are the treatment options?	1. Open commissurotomy (open heart operation) 2. Balloon valvuloplasty: percutaneous 3. Valve replacement
What is the medical treatment for mild symptomatic patients?	Diuretics
What is the prognosis?	>80% of patients are well at 10 years with successful operation

MITRAL REGURGITATION (MR)

What is it?	Incompetence of the mitral valve
What are the causes?	Severe mitral valve prolapse (some prolapse is found in 5% of the population, with women ≥ men) Rheumatic fever Post-MI from papillary muscle dysfunction/rupture Ruptured chordae
What are the most common causes?	Rheumatic fever (#1 worldwide), ruptured chordae/papillary muscle dysfunction
What are the symptoms?	Often insidious and late: dyspnea, palpitations, fatigue
What are the signs?	Murmur: holosystolic, apical radiating to the axilla
What are the indications for treatment?	1. Symptoms 2. LV >45 mm end-systolic dimension (left ventricular dilation)
What is the treatment?	1. Valve replacement 2. Annuloplasty: suture a prosthetic ring to the dilated valve annulus

ARTIFICIAL VALVE PLACEMENT

What is it?	Replacement of damaged valves with tissue or mechanical prosthesis
What are the types of artificial valves?	Tissue and mechanical
What are the pros and cons: **Tissue?**	NO anticoagulation but shorter duration (20%–40% need replacement in 10 years); good for elderly
Mechanical?	Last longer (>15 years) but require ANTICOAGULATION
Contraindications for tissue valve?	Dialysis (calcify), youth
Contraindications for mechanical valve?	Pregnancy (or going to be pregnant due to anticoagulation), bleeding risk (alcoholic, PUD)
What is the operative mortality?	From 1% to 5% in most series
What must patients with an artificial valve receive before dental procedures?	Antibiotics
Define the Ross procedure.	Aortic valve replacement with a pulmonary **auto**graft (i.e., patient's own valve!)

INFECTIOUS ENDOCARDITIS

What is it?	Microbial infection of heart valves
What are the predisposing conditions?	Preexisting valvular lesion, procedures that lead to bacteremia, IV drug use
What are the common causative agents?	*S. viridans:* associated with abnormal valves *S. aureus:* associated with IV drug use *S. epidermidis:* associated with prosthetic valves

What are the signs/ symptoms?	Murmur (new or changing) Petechiae Splinter hemorrhage (fingernails) Roth spots (on retina) Osler nodes (raised, **painful** on soles and palms; **O**sler = **O**uch!) Janeway lesions (similar to Osler nodes, but flat and **painless**) (Jane**WAY** = pain a**WAY**)
Which diagnostic tests should be performed?	Echocardiogram, TEE Serial blood cultures (definitive)
What is the treatment?	Prolonged IV therapy with bactericidal antibiotics, to which infecting organisms are sensitive
What is the prognosis?	Infection can progress, requiring valve replacement

CONGENITAL HEART DISEASE

VENTRICULAR SEPTAL DEFECT (VSD)

What is its claim to fame?	Most common congenital heart defect
What is it?	Failure of ventricular septum to completely close; **80% of cases involve the membranous portion of the septum,** resulting in left-to-right shunt, increased pulmonary blood flow, and CHF if pulmonary to systemic flow is >2:1
What is pulmonary vascular obstructive disease?	Pulmonary artery hyperplasia from increased pulmonary pressure caused by a left to right shunt (e.g., VSD)
What is Eisenmenger's syndrome?	Irreversible pulmonary HTN from chronic changes in pulmonary arterioles and increased right heart pressures; cyanosis develops when the shunt reverses (becomes right to left across the VSD)
What is the treatment of Eisenmenger's syndrome?	Only option is heart-lung transplant; otherwise, the disease is untreatable

What is the incidence of VSD?	30% of heart defects (most common defect)

PATENT DUCTUS ARTERIOSUS (PDA)

What is it?	Physiologic right-to-left shunt in fetal circulation connecting the pulmonary artery to the aorta bypassing fetal lungs; often, this shunt persists in the neonate
What are the factors preventing closure?	Hypoxia, increased prostaglandins, prematurity
What are the symptoms?	Often asymptomatic Poor feeding Respiratory distress CHF with respiratory infections
What are the signs?	Acyanotic, unless other cardiac lesions are present; continuous "machinery" murmur
Which diagnostic tests should be performed?	Physical examination Echocardiogram (to rule out associated defects) Catheter (seldom required)
What is the medical treatment?	Indomethacin is an NSAID: prostaglandin (PG) inhibitor (PG keeps PDA open)
What is the surgical treatment?	Surgical ligation or cardiac catheterization closure at 6 months to 2 years of age

TETRALOGY OF FALLOT (TOF)

What is it?	Misalignment of the infundibular septum in early development, leading to the characteristic tetrad: 1. Pulmonary stenosis/obstruction of right ventricular outflow 2. Overriding aorta 3. Right ventricular hypertrophy 4. VSD

What are the symptoms?	Hypoxic spells (squatting behavior increases SVR and increases pulmonary blood flow)
What are the signs?	Cyanosis Clubbing Murmur: SEM at left third intercostal space
Which diagnostic tests should be performed?	CXR: small, "boot-shaped" heart and decreased pulmonary blood flow Echocardiography
What is the prognosis?	95% survival at specialized centers

IHSS

What is IHSS?	**I**diopathic **H**ypertrophic **S**ubaortic **S**tenosis
What is it?	Aortic outflow obstruction from septal tissue
What is the usual presentation?	Similar to aortic stenosis

COARCTATION OF THE AORTA

What is it?	Narrowing of the thoracic aorta, with or without intraluminal "shelf" (infolding of the media); usually found near ductus/ligamentum arteriosum
What are the three types?	1. Preductal (fatal in infancy if untreated) 2. Juxtaductal 3. Postductal
What percentage are associated with other cardiac defects?	60% (bicuspid aortic valve is most common)
What is the major route of collateral circulation?	Subclavian artery to the IMA to the intercostals to the descending aorta
What are the risk factors?	Turner's syndrome, male > female

What are the symptoms?	Headache Epistaxis Lower extremity fatigue → claudication

What are the signs?	Pulses: decreased lower extremity pulses
	Murmurs:
	    1. Systolic—from turbulence across coarctation, often radiating to infrascapular region
	    2. Continuous—from dilated collaterals

Which diagnostic tests should be performed?	CXR: "3" sign is aortic knob, coarctation, and dilated poststenotic aorta; rib notching is bony erosion from dilated intercostal collaterals Echocardiogram Cardiac catheterization if cardiac defects

What is the treatment?	Surgery:
	    Resection with end-to-end anastomosis
	    Subclavian artery flap
	    Patch graft (rare)
	    Interposition graft
	    Endovascular repair an option in adults

What are the indications for surgery?	Symptomatic patient Asymptomatic patient >3 to 4 years
What are the possible postoperative complications?	Paraplegia "Paradoxic" HTN Mesenteric necrotizing panarteritis (GI bleeding), Horner's syndrome, injury to recurrent laryngeal nerve
What are the long-term concerns?	Aortic dissection, HTN

TRANSPOSITION OF THE GREAT VESSELS

What is it?	Aorta originates from the right ventricle and the pulmonary artery from the left ventricle; fatal without PDA, ASD, or VSD—to allow communication between the left and right circulations

What is the incidence?	From 5% to 8% of defects
What are the signs/ symptoms?	Most common lesion that presents with cyanosis and CHF in neonatal period (>90% by day 1)
Which diagnostic tests should be performed?	CXR: "egg-shaped" heart contour Catheterization (definitive)
What is the treatment?	Arterial switch operation—aorta and pulmonary artery are moved to the correct ventricle and the coronaries are reimplanted

EBSTEIN'S ANOMALY

What is it?	Tricuspid valve is placed abnormally low in the right ventricle, forming a large right atrium and a small right ventricle, leading to tricuspid regurgitation and decreased right ventricular output
What are the signs/symptoms?	Cyanosis
What are the risk factors?	400× the risk if the mother has taken lithium

VASCULAR RINGS

What are they?	Many types; represent an anomalous development of the aorta/pulmonary artery from the embryonic aortic arch that surrounds and obstructs the trachea/esophagus
How are they diagnosed?	Barium swallow, MRI
What are the signs/ symptoms?	Most prominent is stridor from tracheal compression

CYANOTIC HEART DISEASE

What are the causes?	Five "Ts" of cyanotic heart disease: Tetralogy of Fallot Truncus arteriosus Totally anomalous pulmonary venous return (TAPVR) Tricuspid atresia Transposition of the great vessels

CARDIAC TUMORS

What is the most common benign lesion?	Myxoma in adults
What is the most common location?	Left atrium with pedunculated morphology
What are the signs/ symptoms?	Dyspnea, emboli
What is the most common malignant tumor in children?	Rhabdomyosarcoma

DISEASES OF THE GREAT VESSELS

THORACIC AORTIC ANEURYSM

What is the cause?	Vast majority result from atherosclerosis, connective tissue disease
What is the major differential diagnosis?	Aortic dissection
What percentage of patients have aneurysms of the aorta at a different site?	≈33%! (Rule out AAA)
What are the signs/ symptoms?	Most are asymptomatic Chest pain, stridor, hemoptysis (rare), recurrent laryngeal nerve compression
How is it most commonly discovered?	Routine CXR
Which diagnostic tests should be performed?	CXR, CT scan, MRI, aortography
What are the indications for treatment?	>6 cm in diameter Symptoms Rapid increase in diameter Rupture

What is the treatment?	Replace with graft, open or endovascular stent
What are the dreaded complications after treatment of a thoracic aortic aneurysm?	Paraplegia (up to 20%) Anterior spinal syndrome
What is anterior spinal syndrome?	Syndrome characterized by: Paraplegia Incontinence (bowel/bladder) Pain and temperature sensation loss
What is the cause?	Occlusion of the great radicular artery of **Adamkiewicz, w**hich is one of the intercostal/lumbar arteries from T8 to L4

AORTIC DISSECTION

What is it?	Separation of the walls of the aorta from an intimal tear and disease of the tunica media; a false lumen is formed and a "reentry" tear may occur, resulting in "double-barrel" aorta
What are the aortic dissection classifications?	DeBakey classification Stanford classification
Define the DeBakey classifications: **DeBakey type I**	Involves ascending **and** descending aorta

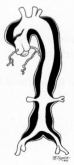

DeBakey type II   Involves ascending aorta only

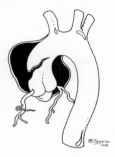

DeBakey type III   Involves descending aorta only

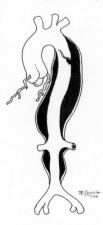

**Define the Stanford
classifications:**

Type A   Ascending aorta (requires surgery)
                              ± Descending aorta (includes DeBakey
                              types I and II)

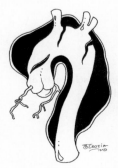

Type B

Descending aorta only (nonoperative, except for complications) (same as DeBakey type III)

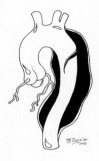

What is the etiology?

HTN (most common)
Marfan's syndrome
Bicuspid aortic valve
Coarctation of the aorta
Cystic medial necrosis
Proximal aortic aneurysm

What are the signs/ symptoms?

Abrupt onset of severe chest pain, most often radiating/"tearing" to the back; onset is typically more abrupt than that of MI; the pain can migrate as the dissection progresses; patient describes a **"tearing pain"**

Note three other sequelae.

1. Cardiac tamponade; Beck's triad—distant heart sounds, ↑ CVP with JVD, ↓ BP
2. Aortic insufficiency—diastolic murmur
3. Aortic arterial branch occlusion/ shearing, leading to ischemia in the involved circulation (i.e., unequal pulses, CVA, paraplegia, renal insufficiency, bowel ischemia, claudication)

Which diagnostic tests are indicated?

CXR:
1. Widened mediastinum
2. Pleural effusion
TEE
CTA (CT angiography)
Aortography (definitive gold standard but time-consuming!)

What is the treatment of the various types:

Types I and II (Stanford type A)?

Surgical because of risk of:
1. Aortic insufficiency
2. Compromise of cerebral and coronary circulation
3. Tamponade
4. Rupture

Type III (Stanford type B)?

Medical (control BP), unless complicated by rupture or significant occlusions

Describe the surgery for an aortic dissection (Type I, II, Stanford A).

Open the aorta at the proximal extent of dissection, and then sew—graft to— intimal flap and adventitia circumferentially (endovascular an option)

What is the preoperative treatment?

Control BP with sodium nitroprusside and β-blockers (e.g., esmolol); β-blockers decrease shear stress

What is the postoperative treatment?

Lifetime control of BP and monitoring of aortic size

What is the possible cause of MI in a patient with aortic dissection?

Dissection involves the coronary arteries or underlying LAD

What is a dissecting aortic aneurysm?

Misnomer! Not an aneurysm!

What are the EKG signs of the following disorders:

Atrial fibrillation?

Irregularly irregular

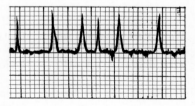

PVC?

Premature Ventricular Complex:
Wide QRS

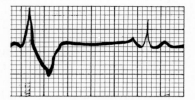

Ventricular aneurysm?

ST elevation

Ischemia?

ST elevation/ST depression/flipped
T waves

Infarction?

Q waves

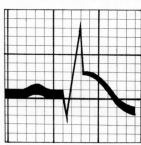

Pericarditis?

ST elevation throughout leads

RBBB?

Right **B**undle **B**ranch **B**lock: wide QRS
and "rabbit ears" or R-R in V1 or V2

LBBB?

Left **B**undle **B**ranch **B**lock: wide QRS
and "rabbit ears" or R-R in V5 or V6

Wolff-Parkinson-White?

Delta wave = slurred upswing on QRS

First degree A-V block?

Prolonged P-R interval (0.2 second)

Second degree A-V block?

Dropped QRS; not all P waves transmit
to produce ventricular contraction

**Wenckebach
phenomenon?**

Second-degree block with progressive
delay in P-R interval prior to dropped beat

Third-degree A-V block?	Complete A-V dissociation; random P wave and QRS

MISCELLANEOUS

What is Mondor's disease?	Thrombophlebitis of the thoracoepigastric veins
What is a VAD?	**V**entricular **A**ssist **D**evice
How does an IABP work?	**I**ntra**A**ortic **B**alloon **P**ump has a balloon tip resting in the aorta Balloon inflates in diastole, increasing diastolic BP and coronary blood flow; in systole the balloon deflates, creating a negative pressure, lowering afterload, and increasing systolic BP
What electrolyte must be monitored during diuresis after CPB?	K^+
How is extent/progress of postbypass diuresis followed?	I's and O's, CXR, JVD, edema, daily weight
What is an Austin Flint murmur?	Diastolic murmur of AI secondary to regurgitant turbulent flow
Where is the least oxygenated blood in the body?	Coronary sinus
What is the most common cause of a cardiac tumor?	Metastasis

Chapter 73 — Transplant Surgery

Define the following terms: **Autograft**	Same individual is both donor and recipient
Isograft	Donor and recipient are genetically identical (identical twins)

Allograft	Donor and recipient are genetically dissimilar, but of the same species
Xenograft	Donor and recipient belong to different species
Orthotopic	Donor organ is placed in normal anatomic position (liver, heart)
Heterotopic	Donor organ is placed in a different site than the normal anatomic position (kidney, pancreas)
Paratopic	Donor organ is placed close to original organ
Chimerism	Sharing cells between the graft and donor

BASIC IMMUNOLOGY

What are histocompatibility antigens?	Distinct (genetically inherited) cell surface proteins of the human leukocyte antigen system (HLA)
Why are they important?	They are targets (class I antigens) and initiators (class II antigens) of immune response to donor tissue (i.e., distinguishing self from nonself)
Which cells have class I antigens?	All nucleated cells (Think: class **1** = **ALL** cells and thus "**ONE** for **ALL**")
Which cells have class II antigens?	Macrophages, monocytes, B cells, activated T cells, endothelial cells
What are the gene products of MHC called in humans?	**HLA** (**H**uman **L**eukocyte **A**ntigen)
What is the location of the MHC complex?	Short arm of chromosome 6
What is a haplotype?	Combination of HLA genes on a chromosome inherited from one parent; therefore, two siblings have a 25% chance of being "haploidentical"

Does HLA matching matter in organ transplantation?	With recent improvements in immunosuppression (i.e., cyclosporine), the effect is largely obscured, but it still does matter; the most important ones to match in order to improve renal allograft survival are HAL-B and HLA-DR

CELLS

T CELLS

What is the source?	Thymus
What is the function?	Cell-mediated immunity/rejection
What are the types?	Th (CD4): helper T—help B cells become plasma cells Ts (CD8): suppressor T—regulate immune response Tc (CD8): cytotoxic T—kill cell by direct contact

B CELLS

What is the function?	Humoral immunity
What is the cell type that produces antibodies?	B cells differentiate into plasma cells

MACROPHAGE

What is it?	Monocyte in parenchymal tissue
What is its function?	Processes foreign protein and presents it to lymphocytes
What is it also known as?	Antigen-**P**resenting **C**ell (**APC**)
Briefly describe the events leading to antibody production.	1. Macrophage engulfs antigen and presents it to Th cells; the macrophage produces IL-1 2. Th cells then produce IL-2, and the Th cells proliferate 3. Th cells then activate (via IL-4) B cells that differentiate into plasma cells, which produce antibodies against the antigen presented

IMMUNOSUPPRESSION

Who needs to be immunosuppressed?	All recipients (except autograft or isograft)
What are the major drugs used for immunosuppression?	Triple therapy: corticosteroids, azathioprine, cyclosporine/tacrolimus
What are the other drugs?	OKT3, ATGAM, mycophenolate
What is the advantage of "triple therapy"?	Employs three immunosuppressive drugs; therefore, a lower dose of each can be used, decreasing the toxic side effects of each
What is "induction therapy"?	High doses of immunosuppressive drugs to "induce" immunosuppression

CORTICOSTEROIDS

Which is most commonly used in transplants?	Prednisone
How does it function?	Primarily blocks production of IL-1 by macrophage and stabilizes lysosomal membrane of macrophage
What is the associated toxicity?	"Cushingoid," alopecia, striae, HTN, diabetes, pancreatitis, ulcer disease, osteomalacia, aseptic necrosis (especially of the femoral head)
What is the relative potency of the following corticosteroids:	
Cortisol?	1
Prednisone?	4
Methylprednisolone?	5
Dexamethasone?	25

AZATHIOPRINE (AZA [IMURAN®])

How does it function?	Prodrug that is cleaved into mercaptopurine; inhibits synthesis of DNA and RNA, leading to decreased cellular (T/B cells) production

What is the associated toxicity?	Toxic to bone marrow (leukopenia + thrombocytopenia), hepatotoxic, associated with pancreatitis
When should a lower dose of AZA be administered?	When WBC is <4
What is the associated drug interaction?	Decrease dose if patient is also on allopurinol, because allopurinol inhibits the enzyme xanthine oxidase, which is necessary for the breakdown of azathioprine

CYCLOSPORINE (CSA)

What is its function?	"Calcineurin inhibitor" inhibits production of IL-2 by Th cells
What is the associated toxicity?	Toxicity for cyclosporine includes the 11 "**H**'s" and three "**N**'s": **H**epatitis, **H**ypertrichosis, gingival **H**yperplasia, **H**yperlipidemia (worse than FK), **H**yperglycemia, **H**ypertension (worse than FK), **H**emolytic uremic syndrome, **H**yperkalemia, **H**ypercalcemia, **H**ypomagnesemia, **H**yperuricemia, **N**ephrotoxicity, **N**eurotoxicity (headache, tremor), **N**eoplasia (lymphoma, KS, squamous cell skin cancers)
What drugs increase CSA levels?	Diltiazem Ketoconazole Erythromycin, fluconazole, **ranitidine**
What drugs decrease CSA levels?	By inducing the p450 system: dilantin, Tegretol®, rifampin, isoniazid, barbiturates
What are the drugs of choice for HTN from CSA?	Clonidine, calcium channel blockers

ATGAM/ANTITHYMOCYTE GLOBULIN

How does it function?	Antibody against thymocytes, lymphocytes (polyclonal)
When is it typically used?	For induction

What is the associated toxicity?	Thrombocytopenia, leukopenia, serum sickness, rigors, fever, anaphylaxis, increased risk of viral infection, arthralgia

OKT3

How does it work?	MONOclonal antibody that binds CD3 receptor (on T cells)
What is a major problem with multiple doses?	Blocking antibodies develop, and OKT3 is less effective each time it is used
What are basiliximab and daclizumab?	Anti-CD25 monoclonal antibodies

TACROLIMUS

What is tacrolimus also known as?	Prograf®(FK506)
How does it work?	Similar to CSA—"calcineurin inhibitor," blocks IL-2 receptor expression, inhibits T cells
What is its potency compared to CSA?	100× more potent than CSA
What are its side effects?	Nephrotoxicity and CNS toxicity (tremor, seizure, parasthesia, coma), hyperkalemia, alopecia, diabetes

SIROLIMUS

What is sirolimus also known as?	Rapamycin, Rapamune®
How does it work?	Like CSA and tacrolimus, it does not bind to and inhibit calcineurin; rather, it blocks T-cell signaling
Toxicity?	Hypertriglyceridemia, thrombocytopenia, wound/healing problems, anemia, oral ulcers

MYCOPHENOLATE MOFETIL (MMF)

What is MMF also known as?	CellCept®

How does it work?
Inhibitor of inosine monophosphate dehydrogenase required for de novo purine synthesis which expanding T and B cells depend on; also inhibits adhesion molecule and antibody production

OVERVIEW OF IMMUNOSUPPRESSION MECHANISMS

What drug acts at the following sites:

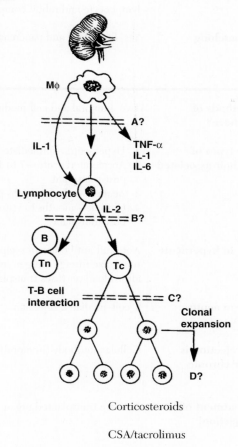

A?	Corticosteroids
B?	CSA/tacrolimus
C?	AZA/MMF
D?	OKT3/ATGAM

MATCHING OF DONOR AND RECIPIENT

How is ABO crossmatching performed?	Same procedure as in blood typing
What is the purpose of lymphocytotoxic cross-matching?	Tests for HLA antibodies in serum; most important in kidney and pancreas transplants
How is the test performed?	Mix recipient serum with donor lymphocyte and rabbit complement
Is HLA crossmatching important?	Yes, for kidney and pancreas transplants

REJECTION

How many methods of rejection are there?	Two: humoral and cell-mediated
Name the four types of rejection and their associated time courses.	1. Hyperacute—immediate in O.R. 2. Accelerated acute—7 to 10 days post-transplant 3. Acute—weeks to months post-transplant 4. Chronic—months to years post-transplant
What happens in hyperacute rejection?	Antigraft antibodies in recipient recognize foreign antigen immediately after blood perfuses transplanted organ
What happens in acute rejection?	T cell–mediated rejection
What type of rejection is responsible for chronic rejection?	Cellular, antibody (humoral), or both
What is the treatment of hyperacute rejection?	Remove transplanted organ

What is the treatment of acute rejection?	High-dose steroids/OKT3
What is the treatment of chronic rejection?	Not much (irreversible) or retransplant

ORGAN PRESERVATION

What is the optimal storage temperature of an organ?	4°C—keep on ice in a cooler
Why should it be kept cold?	Cold decreases the rate of chemical reactions; decreased energy use minimizes effects of hypoxia and ischemia
What is U-W solution?	University of Wisconsin solution; used to perfuse an organ prior to removal from the donor
What is in it?	Potassium phosphate, buffers, starch, steroids, insulin, electrolytes, adenosine
Why should it be used?	Lengthens organ preservation time

MAXIMUM TIME BETWEEN HARVEST AND TRANSPLANT OF ORGAN

Heart?	6 hours
Lungs?	6 hours
Pancreas?	24 hours
Liver?	24 hours
Kidney?	Up to 72 hours

KIDNEY TRANSPLANT

In what year was the first transplant performed in man?	1954
By whom?	Joseph E. Murray—1990 Nobel Prize winner in Medicine

What are the indications for kidney transplant?

Irreversible renal failure from:
1. Glomerulonephritis (leading cause)
2. Pyelonephritis
3. Polycystic kidney disease
4. Malignant HTN
5. Reflux pyelonephritis
6. Goodpasture's syndrome (antibasement membrane)
7. Congenital renal hyperplasia
8. Fabry's disease
9. Alport's syndrome
10. Renal cortical necrosis
11. Damage caused by type 1 diabetes mellitus

Define renal failure.

GFR <20% to 25% of normal; as GFR drops to 5% to 10% of normal, uremic symptoms begin (e.g., lethargy, seizures, neuropathy, electrolyte disorders)

What is the most common cause for kidney transplant?

Diabetes (25%)

STATISTICS

What are the sources of donor kidneys?

Deceased donor (70%)
Living related donor (LRD; 30%)

What survival rate is associated with deceased donor source?

90% at 1 year if HLA matched; 80% at 1 year if not HLA matched; 75% graft survival at 3 years

What survival rate is associated with LRD?

95% patient survival at 1 year; 75% to 85% graft survival at 3 years

What are the tests for compatibility?

ABO, HLA typing

If a choice of left or right donor kidney is available, which is preferred?

Left—longer renal vein allows for easier anastomosis

Should the placement of the kidney be hetero- or orthotopic?

Heterotopic—retroperitoneal in the RLQ or LLQ above the inguinal ligament

Why?

Preserves native kidneys, allows easy access to iliac vessels, places ureter close to the bladder, easy to biopsy kidney

Define anastomoses of a heterotopic kidney transplant.

1. Renal artery to iliac artery
2. Renal vein to iliac vein
3. Ureter to bladder

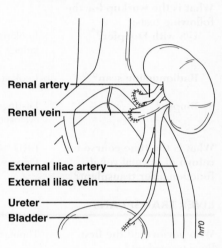

Renal artery

Renal vein

External iliac artery
External iliac vein

Ureter
Bladder

What is the correct placement of the ureter?

Submucosally through the bladder wall—decreases reflux

What is the differential diagnosis of post–renal transplant fluid collection?

"HAUL":
  Hematoma
  Abscess
  Urinoma
  Lymphocele

Why keep native kidneys?

Increased morbidity if they are removed

What is the indication for removal of native kidneys?

Uncontrollable HTN, ongoing renal sepsis

REJECTION

What is the red flag that indicates rejection?

↑ creatinine

What is the differential diagnosis of increased creatinine?

(Remember: "**-TION**") obstruc**TION**, dehydra**TION**, infec**TION**, intoxica**TION** (CSA); plus lymphocele, ATN

What are the signs/ symptoms?

Fever, malaise, HTN, ipsilateral leg edema, pain at transplant site, oliguria

What is the workup for the following tests:
    U/S with Doppler?

Look for fluid collection around the kidney, hydronephrosis, flow in vessels

    Radionuclide scan?

Look at flow and function

    Biopsy?

Distinguish between rejection and cyclosporine toxicity

What is the time course for return of normal renal function after transplant?

LRD—3 to 5 days
Deceased donor—7 to 15 days

LIVER TRANSPLANT

Who performed the first liver transplant?

Thomas Starzl (1963)

What are the indications?

Liver failure from:
  1. Cirrhosis (leading indication in adults)
  2. Budd-Chiari
  3. Biliary atresia (leading indication in children)
  4. Neonatal hepatitis
  5. Chronic active hepatitis
  6. Fulminant hepatitis with drug toxicity—acetaminophen
  7. Sclerosing cholangitis
  8. Caroli's disease
  9. Subacute hepatic necrosis
  10. Congenital hepatic fibrosis
  11. Inborn errors of metabolism
  12. Fibrolamellar hepatocellular carcinoma

What is the MELD score?

"**M**odel for **E**nd Stage **L**iver **D**isease" is the formula currently used to assign points for prioritizing position on the waiting list for deceased donor liver transplant; based on INR, bilirubin, and creatinine with extra points given for the presence of liver cancer

What is the test for compatibility?

ABO typing

What is the placement?

Orthotopic

What are the options for biliary drainage?

1. Donor common bile to recipient common bile duct end to end
2. Roux-en-Y choledochojejunostomy

What is the "piggyback technique"?

Recipient vena cava is left in place; the donor infrahepatic IVC is oversewn; the donor superior IVC is anastomosed onto a cuff made from the recipient hepatic veins (allows for greater hemodynamic stability of the recipient during OLT)

How does Living Donor Liver Transplantation (LDLT) work?

Adult donates a left lateral segment to a child or an adult donates a right lobe to another adult

What is a split liver transplant?

Deceased donor liver is harvested and divided into two "halves" for two recipients

What is chronic liver rejection called?

"Vanishing bile duct syndrome"

REJECTION

What are the red flags indicating rejection?

Decreased bile drainage, increased serum bilirubin, increased LFTs

What is the site of rejection?

Rejection involves the biliary epithelium first, and later, the vascular endothelium

What is the workup with the following tests:

U/S with Doppler?	Look at flow in portal vein, hepatic artery; rule out thrombosis, leaky anastomosis, infection (abscess)
Cholangiogram?	Look at bile ducts (easy to do; patients usually have a T-tube if they have primary biliary anastomosis)
Biopsy?	Especially important 3 to 6 weeks postoperatively, when CMV is of greatest concern

Does hepatorenal syndrome renal function improve after liver transplant?

Yes

SURVIVAL STATISTICS

What is the 1-year survival rate?

≈80% to 85%

What percentage of patients requires retransplant?

≈20%

Why?

Usually primary graft dysfunction, rejection, infection, vascular thrombosis, or recurrence of primary disease

PANCREAS TRANSPLANT

Who performed the first pancreas transplant?

Richard C. Lillehei and William D. Kelly (1966)

What are the indications?

Type I (juvenile) diabetes mellitus associated with severe complications (renal failure, blindness, neuropathy) or very poor glucose control

What are the tests for compatibility?

ABO, DR matching (class II)

What is the placement?

Heterotopic, in iliac fossa or paratopic

Where is anastomosis of the exocrine duct in heterotopic placement?

To the bladder

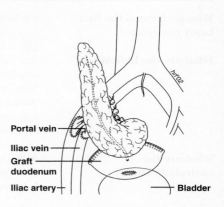

Portal vein
Iliac vein
Graft duodenum
Iliac artery
Bladder

Why?

Measures the amount of amylase in urine, gives an indication of pancreatic function (i.e., high urine amylase indicates good pancreatic function)

What is the associated electrolyte complication?

Loss of bicarbonate

Where is anastomosis of the exocrine duct in paratopic placement?

To the jejunum

Why?

It is close by and physiologic

What is the advantage of paratopic placement?

Endocrine function drains to the portal vein directly to the liver, and pancreatic contents stay within the GI tract (no need to replace bicarbonate)

What are the red flags indicating rejection?

Hyperamylasemia, hyperglycemia, hypoamylasuria, graft tenderness

Why should the kidney and pancreas be transplanted together?

Kidney function is a better indicator of rejection; also better survival of graft is associated with kidney-pancreas transplant than pancreas alone

Why is hyperglycemia not a good indicator for rejection surveillance?

Hyperglycemia appears relatively late with pancreatic rejection

HEART TRANSPLANT

Who performed the first heart transplant?	Christiaan Barnard (1967)
What are the indications?	Age birth to 65 years with terminal acquired heart disease—class IV of New York Heart Association classification (inability to do any physical activity without discomfort = 10% chance of surviving 6 months)
What are the contraindications?	Active infection Poor pulmonary function Increased pulmonary artery resistance
What are the tests for compatibility?	ABO, size
What is the placement?	Orthotopic anastomosis of atria, aorta, pulmonary artery
What is sewn together in a heart transplant?	Donor heart atriums, pulmonary artery, and aorta are sewn to the recipient heart atriums, pulmonary artery, and aorta

What are the red flags of rejection?	Fever, hypotension or hypertension, increased T4/T8 ratio
What is coronary artery vasculopathy?	Small vessel occlusion from chronic rejection—often requires retransplant

What are the tests for rejection?	Endomyocardial biopsy—much more important than clinical signs/symptoms; patient undergoes routine biopsy
What are survival statistics for:	
1 year?	85%
5 years?	65%

INTESTINAL TRANSPLANTATION

What is it?	Transplantation of the small bowel
What types of donors are there?	Living donor, deceased donor
Anastomosis:	
Living donor?	Ileocolic artery and vein
Deceased donor?	SMA, SMV
What are indications?	Short gut syndrome, motility disorders, and inability to sustain TPN (liver failure, lack of venous access, etc.)
What is a common postoperative problem other than rejection?	**GVHD** (**G**raft-**V**ersus-**H**ost **D**isease) from large lymphoid tissue in transplanted intestines
CMV status of donor?	Must be CMV negative if recipient is CMV negative
What is the most common cause of death postoperatively?	**Sepsis**
How is rejection surveillance conducted?	Endoscopic biopsies
What is the clinical clue to rejection?	Watery diarrhea

LUNG TRANSPLANT

Who performed the first lung transplant?	James Hardy (1963)

What are the indications?	Generally, a disease that substantially limits activities of daily living and is likely to result in death within 12 to 18 months:
	    Pulmonary fibrosis
	    COPD
	    Eosinophilic granuloma
	    Primary pulmonary HTN
	    Eisenmenger's syndrome
	    Cystic fibrosis

What are the contraindications?	Current smoking Active infection
What tests comprise the pretransplant assessment of the recipient?	1. Pulmonary—PFTs, V/Q scan 2. Cardiac—Echo, cath, angiogram 3. Exercise tolerance test
What are the donor requirements?	1. 55 years of age or younger 2. Clear chest film 3. PA oxygen tension of 300 on 100% oxygen and 5 cm PEEP 4. No purulent secretions on bronchoscopy
What are necessary anastomoses?	Bronchi, PA, pulmonary veins (Bronchial artery is not necessary)
What are the postop complications?	Bronchial necrosis/stricture, reperfusion, pulmonary edema, rejection
What are the red flags of rejection (4)?	1. Decreased arterial O_2 tension 2. Fever 3. Increased fatigability 4. Infiltrate on x-ray
What is chronic lung rejection called?	**O**bliterative **B**ronchiolitis (**OB**)

What are the survival rates:
    1 year?   80%

    3 yrs?   70%

TRANSPLANT COMPLICATIONS

What are four major complications?

1. Infection
2. Rejection
3. Post-transplant lymphoproliferative disease
4. Complications of steroids

INFECTION

What are the usual agents?	DNA viruses, especially CMV, HSV, VZV
When should CMV infection be suspected?	>21 days post-transplant
What is the time of peak incidence of CMV infections?	4 to 6 weeks post-transplant
What are the signs/ symptoms of CMV?	Fever, neutropenia, signs of rejection of transplant; also can present as viral pneumonitis, hepatitis, colitis
How is CMV diagnosed?	Biopsy of transplant to differentiate rejection, cultures of blood, urine
What is the treatment of CMV?	Ganciclovir, with or without immunoglobin; foscarnet
What are the complications of ganciclovir?	Bone marrow suppression
What are the signs/ symptoms of HSV?	Herpetic lesions, shingles, fever, neutropenia, rejection of transplant
What is the treatment of HSV?	Acyclovir until patient is asymptomatic

MALIGNANCY

What are the most common types?	Skin/lip cancer (40%), B-cell cancer, cervical cancer in women, T-cell lymphoma, Kaposi's sarcoma

Which epithelial cancers are important after transplant?	Skin/lip cancer, especially basal cell and squamous cell
What is post-transplant lymphoma associated with?	Multiple doses of OKT3 EBV Young > elderly
What is the treatment for post-transplant lympho-proliferative disease (PTLD)?	1. Drastically reduce immunosuppression 2. ± Radiation 3. ± Chemotherapy

Chapter 74

Orthopaedic Surgery

ORTHOPAEDIC TERMS

What do the following abbreviations stand for:

ORIF?	**O**pen **R**eduction **I**nternal **F**ixation
ROM?	**R**ange **O**f **M**otion
FROM?	**F**ull **R**ange **O**f **M**otion
ACL?	**A**nterior **C**ruciate **L**igament
PCL?	**P**osterior **C**ruciate **L**igament
MCL?	**M**edial **C**ollateral **L**igament
PWB?	**P**artial **W**eight **B**earing
FWB?	**F**ull **W**eight **B**earing
WBAT?	**W**eight **B**earing **A**s **T**olerated

THA?	**T**otal **H**ip **A**rthroplasty
TKA?	**T**otal **K**nee **A**rthroplasty
THR?	**T**otal **H**ip **R**eplacement
TKR?	**T**otal **K**nee **R**eplacement
PROM?	**P**assive **R**ange **O**f **M**otion
AROM?	**A**ctive **R**ange **O**f **M**otion
AFO?	**A**nkle **F**oot **O**rthotic
AVN?	**AV**ascular **N**ecrosis

Define the following terms:

Supination	Palm up
Pronation	Palm down
Plantarflexion	Foot down at ankle joint (plant foot in ground)
Foot dorsiflexion	Foot up at ankle joint
Adduction	Movement toward the body (**ADD**uction = **ADD** to the body)
Abduction	Movement away from the body
Inversion	Foot sole faces midline
Eversion	Foot sole faces laterally
Volarflexion	Hand flexes at wrist joint toward flexor tendons
Wrist dorsiflexion	Hand flexes at wrist joint toward extensor tendons
Allograft bone	Bone from human donor other than patient

Reduction   Maneuver to restore proper alignment to fracture or joint

Closed reduction   Reduction done without surgery (e.g., casts, splints)

Open reduction   Surgical reduction

Fixation   Stabilization of a fracture after reduction by means of surgical placement of hardware that can be external or internal (e.g., pins, plates, screws)

Tibial pin   Pin placed in the tibia for treating femur or pelvic fractures by applying skeletal traction

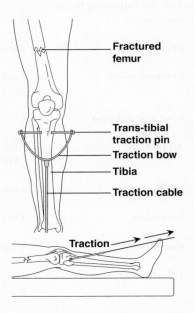

Unstable fracture or dislocation   Fracture or dislocation in which further deformation will occur if reduction is **not** performed

Varus   Extremity abnormality with apex of
                            defect pointed away from midline
                            (e.g., genu varum = bowlegged; with
                            valgus, this term can also be used to
                            describe fracture displacement)
                            (Think: knees are very **varied** apart)

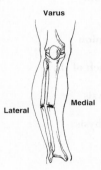

Valgus   Extremity abnormality with apex of
                            defect pointed toward the midline
                            (e.g., genu valgus = knock-kneed)

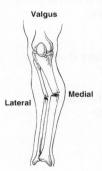

Dislocation   Total loss of congruity and contact
                            between articular surfaces of a joint

Subluxation   Loss of congruity between articular
                            surfaces of a joint; articular contact still
                            remains

Arthroplasty	Total joint replacement (most last 10 to 15 years)
Arthrodesis	Joint fusion with removal of articular surfaces
Osteotomy	Cutting bone (usually wedge resection) to help realigning of joint surfaces
Non-union	Failure of fractured bone ends to fuse

Define each of the following:

Diaphysis	Main shaft of long bone
Metaphysis	Flared end of long bone
Physis	Growth plate, found only in immature bone

TRAUMA GENERAL PRINCIPLES

Define extremity examination in fractured extremities.	1. Observe entire extremity (e.g., open, angulation, joint disruption) 2. Neurologic (sensation, movement) 3. Vascular (e.g., pulses, cap refill)
Which x-rays should be obtained?	Two views (also joint above and below fracture)
How are fractures described?	1. Skin status (open or closed) 2. Bone (by thirds: proximal/middle/distal) 3. Pattern of fracture (e.g., comminuted) 4. Alignment (displacement, angulation, rotation)
How do you define the degree of angulation, displacement, or both?	Define lateral/medial/anterior/posterior displacement and angulation of the distal fragment(s) in relation to the proximal bone

Identify each numbered structure:

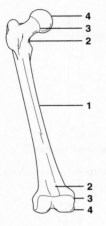

1. Diaphysis
2. Metaphysis
3. Physis
4. Epiphysis

FRACTURES

Define the following patterns of fracture:

Closed fracture

Intact skin over fracture/hematoma

Open fracture

Wound overlying fracture, through which fracture fragments are in continuity with outside environment; high risk of infection (***Note:*** Called "compound fracture" in the past)

Simple fracture

One fracture line, two bone fragments

Comminuted fracture

Results in more than two bone fragments; a.k.a. fragmentation

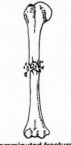

Comminuted fracture

Segmental fracture

Two complete fractures with a "segment" in between

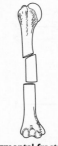

Segmental fracture

Transverse fracture

Fracture line perpendicular to long axis of bone

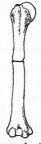

Transverse fracture

Oblique fracture

Fracture line creates an oblique angle with long axis of bone

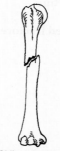

Oblique fracture

Spiral fracture Severe oblique fracture in which fracture plane rotates along the long axis of bone; caused by a twisting injury

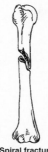

Spiral fracture

Longitudinal fracture Fracture line parallel to long axis of bone

Impacted fracture Fracture resulting from compressive force; end of bone is driven into contiguous metaphyseal region without displacement

Pathologic fracture Fracture through abnormal bone (e.g., tumor-laden or osteoporotic bone)

Stress fracture Fracture in normal bone from cyclic loading on bone

Greenstick fracture Incomplete fracture in which cortex on **only one side** is disrupted; seen in children

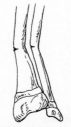

Greenstick fracture

Torus fracture

Impaction injury in children in which cortex is buckled but not disrupted (a.k.a. buckle fracture)

Avulsion fracture

Fracture in which tendon is pulled from bone, carrying with it a bone chip

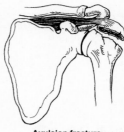

Avulsion fracture

Periarticular fracture

Fracture close to but not involving the joint

Intra-articular fracture

Fracture through the articular surface of a bone (usually requires ORIF)

Define the following specific fractures:
Colles' fracture

Distal radius fracture with dorsal displacement and angulation, usually from falling on an outstretched hand (a common fracture!)

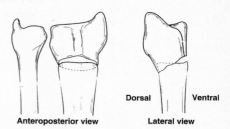

Dorsal | Ventral

Anteroposterior view | **Lateral view**

Smith's fracture

"Reverse Colles' fracture"—distal radial fracture with volar displacement and angulation, usually from falling on the **dorsum** of the hand (uncommon)

Jones' fracture

Fracture at the base of the fifth metatarsal diaphysis

Bennett's fracture

Fracture-dislocation of the base of the first metacarpal (thumb) with disruption of the carpometacarpal joint

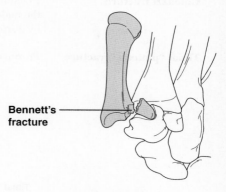

Boxer's fracture

Fracture of the metacarpal neck, "classically" of the small finger

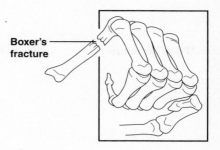

Nightstick fracture

Ulnar fracture

Clay shoveler's avulsion fracture

Fracture of spinous process of C6–C7

Hangman's fracture

Fracture of the pedicles of C2

Transcervical fracture

Fracture through the neck of the femur

Tibial plateau fracture

Intra-articular fracture of the proximal tibia (the plateau is the flared proximal end)

Monteggia fracture

Fracture of the proximal third of the ulna with dislocation of the radial head

Galeazzi fracture

Fracture of the radius at the junction of the middle and distal thirds accompanied by disruption of the distal radioulnar joint

Tibial "plateau" fracture

Proximal tibial fracture

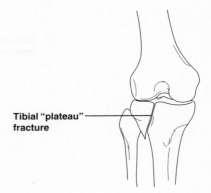

"Pilon" fracture

Distal tibial fracture

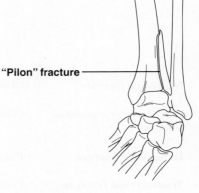

Pott's fracture

Fracture of distal fibula

Pott's disease

Tuberculosis of the spine

ORTHOPAEDIC TRAUMA

What are the major orthopaedic emergencies?

1. Open fractures/dislocations
2. Vascular injuries (e.g., knee dislocation)
3. Compartment syndromes
4. Neural compromise, especially spinal injury
5. Osteomyelitis/septic arthritis; acute, i.e., when aspiration is indicated
6. Hip dislocations—require immediate reduction or patient will develop avascular necrosis; "reduce on the x-ray table"
7. Exsanguinating pelvic fracture (binder, external fixator)

What is the main risk when dealing with an open fracture?

Infection

Which fracture has the highest mortality?

Pelvic fracture (up to 50% with open pelvic fractures)

What factors determine the extent of injury (3)?

1. Age: suggests susceptible point in musculoskeletal system:
   Child—growth plate
   Adolescent—ligaments
   Elderly—metaphyseal bone
2. Direction of forces
3. Magnitude of forces

What is the acronym for indications for OPEN reduction?

"NO CAST":
Nonunion
Open fracture

Compromise of blood supply
Articular surface malalignment
Salter-Harris grade III, IV fracture
Trauma patients who need early ambulation

Define open fractures by Gustilo-Anderson classification:
Grade I?

<1-cm laceration

Grade II?

>1 cm, minimal soft tissue damage

Grade IIIA?	Open fracture with massive tissue devitalization/loss, contamination
Grade IIIB?	Open fracture with massive tissue devitalization/loss and extensive periosteal stripping, contamination, inadequate tissue coverage
Grade IIIC?	Open fracture with major vascular injury requiring repair

What are the five steps in the initial treatment of an open fracture?	1. Prophylactic antibiotics to include IV gram-positive ± anaerobic coverage:
	    Grade I—cefazolin (Ancef ®)
	    Grade II or III—cefoxitin/gentamicin
	2. Surgical débridement
	3. Inoculation against tetanus
	4. Lavage wound <6 hours postincident with high-pressure sterile irrigation
	5. Open reduction of fracture and stabilization (e.g., use of external fixation)

What structures are at risk with a humeral fracture?	Radial nerve, brachial artery
What must be done when both forearm bones are broken?	Because precise movements are needed, open reduction and internal fixation are musts
How have femoral fractures been repaired traditionally?	Traction for 4 to 6 weeks
What is the newer technique?	Intramedullary rod placement
What are the advantages?	Nearly immediate mobility with decreased morbidity/mortality
What is the chief concern following tibial fractures?	Recognition of associated compartment syndrome
What is suggested by pain in the anatomic snuff-box?	Fracture of scaphoid bone (a.k.a. navicular fracture)
What is the most common cause of a "pathologic" fracture in adults?	Osteoporosis

COMPARTMENT SYNDROME

What is acute compartment syndrome?

Increased pressure within an osteofascial compartment that can lead to ischemic necrosis

How is it diagnosed?

Clinically; using intracompartmental pressures is also helpful (especially in unresponsive patients); fasciotomy is clearly indicated if pressure in the compartment is >40 mm Hg (30 to 40 mm Hg is a gray area)

What are the causes?

Fractures, vascular compromise, reperfusion injury, compressive dressings; can occur after any musculoskeletal injury

What are common causes of forearm compartment syndrome?

Supracondylar humerus fracture, brachial artery injury, radius/ulna fracture, crush injury

What is Volkmann's contracture?

Final sequela of forearm compartment syndrome; **contracture** of the forearm flexors from replacement of dead muscle with fibrous tissue

What is the most common site of compartment syndrome?

Calf (four compartments: anterior, lateral, deep posterior, superficial posterior compartments)

What situations should immediately alert one to be on the lookout for a developing compartment syndrome (4)?

1. Supracondylar elbow fractures in children
2. Proximal/midshaft tibial fractures
3. Electrical burns
4. Arterial/venous disruption

What are the symptoms of compartment syndrome?

Pain, paresthesias, paralysis

What are the signs of compartment syndrome?

Pain on passive movement (out of proportion to injury), cyanosis or pallor, hypoesthesia (decreased sensation, decreased two point discrimination), firm compartment

Can a patient have a compartment syndrome with a palpable or Doppler-detectable distal pulse?	YES!
What are the possible complications of compartment syndrome?	Muscle necrosis, nerve damage, contractures, myoglobinuria
What is the initial treatment of the orthopaedic patient developing compartment syndrome?	Bivalve and split casts, remove constricting clothes/dressings, place extremity at heart level
What is the definitive treatment of compartment syndrome?	Fasciotomy within 4 hours (6–8 hours maximum) if at all possible

MISCELLANEOUS TRAUMA INJURIES AND COMPLICATIONS

Name the motor and sensation tests used to assess the following peripheral nerves:	
Radial	Wrist extension; dorsal web space; sensation: between thumb and index finger
Ulnar	Little finger abduction; sensation: little finger-distal ulnar aspect
Median	Thumb opposition or thumb pinch sensation: index finger-distal radial aspect
Axillary	Arm abduction; sensation: deltoid patch on lateral aspect of upper arm
Musculocutaneous	Elbow (biceps) flexion; lateral forearm sensation
How is a peripheral nerve injury treated?	Controversial, although clean lacerations may be repaired primarily; most injuries are followed for 6 to 8 weeks (EMG)
What fracture is associated with a calcaneus fracture?	L-spine fracture (usually from a fall)

Name the nerves of the brachial plexus.	Think: "morning rum" or **"A.M. RUM"** = **A**xillary, **M**edian, then **R**adial, **U**lnar, and **M**usculocutaneous nerves
What are the two indications for operative exploration with a peripheral nerve injury?	1. Loss of nerve function *after* reduction of fracture 2. No EMG signs of nerve regeneration after 8 weeks (nerve graft)

DISLOCATIONS

SHOULDER

What is the most common type?	95% are anterior (posterior are associated with seizures or electrical shock)
Which two structures are at risk?	1. Axillary nerve 2. Axillary artery
How is it diagnosed?	Indentation of soft tissue beneath acromion
What are the three treatment steps?	1. Reduction via gradual traction 2. Immobilization for 3 weeks in internal rotation 3. ROM exercises

ELBOW

What is the most common type?	Posterior
Which three structures are at risk?	1. Brachial artery 2. Ulnar nerve 3. Median nerve
What is the treatment?	Reduce and splint for 7 to 10 days

HIP

When should hip dislocations be reduced?	Immediately, to decrease risk of avascular necrosis; "reduce on the x-ray table!"
What is the most common cause of a hip dislocation?	High velocity trauma (e.g., MVC)

What is the most common type?	Posterior—"dashboard dislocation"—often involves fracture of posterior lip of acetabulum
Which structures are at risk?	Sciatic nerve; blood supply to femoral head—avascular necrosis (AVN)
What is the treatment?	Closed or open reduction

KNEE

What are the common types?	Anterior or posterior
Which structures are at risk?	Popliteal artery and vein, peroneal nerve—especially with posterior dislocation, ACL, PCL (**Note:** need arteriogram)
What is the treatment?	Immediate attempt at relocation (do not wait to x-ray), arterial repair, and then ligamentous repair (delayed or primary)

THE KNEE

What are the five ligaments of the knee?	1. **A**nterior **C**ruciate **L**igament (**ACL**), 2. **P**osterior **C**ruciate **L**igament (**PCL**), 3. **M**edial **C**ollateral **L**igament (**MCL**), 4. **L**ateral **C**ollateral **L**igament (**LCL**), 5. Patellar Ligament

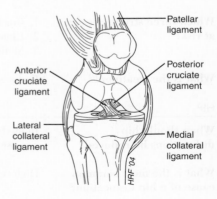

What is the Lachman test for a torn ACL?

Thigh is secured with one hand while the other hand pulls the tibia anteriorly

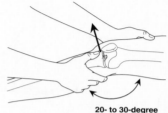

20- to 30-degree
knee flexion

What is the meniscus of the knee?

Cartilage surface of the tibia plateau (lateral and medial meniscus); tears are repaired usually by arthroscopy with removal of torn cartilage fragments

What is McMurray's sign?

Seen with a medial meniscus tear: medial tenderness of knee with flexion and internal rotation of the knee

What is the "unhappy triad"?

Lateral knee injury resulting in:
1. ACL tear
2. MCL tear
3. Medial meniscus injury

What is a "locked knee"?

Meniscal tear that displaces and interferes with the knee joint and prevents complete extension

What is a "bucket-handle tear"?

Meniscal tear longitudinally along contour of normal "C" shape of the meniscus

In collateral ligament and menisci injuries, which are more common, the medial or the lateral?

Medial

ACHILLES TENDON RUPTURE

What are the signs of an Achilles tendon rupture?

Severe calf pain, also bruised swollen calf, two ends of ruptured tendon may be felt, patient will have weak plantar flexion from great toe flexors that should be intact; patient often hears a "pop"

Name the test for an INTACT Achilles tendon.

Thompson's test: a squeeze of the gastrocnemius muscle results in plantar flexion of the foot

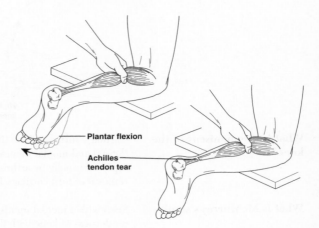

What is the treatment for an Achilles tendon rupture?

Young = surgical repair
Elderly = many can be treated with progressive splints

ROTATOR CUFF

What four muscles form the rotator cuff?

Think: **"SITS"**:
1. **S**upraspinatus, etc.
2. **I**nfraspinatus
3. **T**eres minor
4. **S**ubscapularis

When do tears usually occur?

Fifth decade

What is the usual history?

Intermittent shoulder pain especially with **overhead** activity, followed by an episode of acute pain corresponding to a tendon tear; weak abduction

What is the treatment?

Most tears: symptomatic pain relief
Later: if poor muscular function persists, surgical repair is indicated

What is Volkmann's contracture?

Contracture of forearm flexors secondary to **forearm compartment syndrome**

What is the usual cause of Volkmann's contracture?	Brachial artery injury, **supracondylar humerus fracture,** radius/ulnar fracture, crush injury, etc.

MISCELLANEOUS

Define the following terms:	
Dupuytren's contracture	Thickening and contracture of palmar fascia; incidence increases with age
Charcot's joint	Joint arthritis from peripheral neuropathy
Tennis elbow	Tendonitis of the lateral epicondyle of the humerus; classically seen in tennis players
Turf toe	Hyperextension of the great toe (tear of the tendon of the flexor hallucis brevis); classically seen in football players
Shin splints	Exercise-induced anterior compartment hypertension (compartment syndrome); seen in runners
Heel spur	Plantar fasciitis with abnormal bone growth in the plantar fascia; classically seen in runners and walkers
Nightstick fracture	Ulnar fracture
Kienbock's disease	Avascular necrosis of the lunate
What is traumatic myositis?	Abnormal bone deposit in a muscle after blunt trauma deep muscle contusion (benign)
How does a "cast saw" cut the cast but not the underlying skin?	It is an "oscillating" saw (designed by Dr. Homer Stryker in 1947) that goes back and forth cutting anything hard while moving the skin back and forth without injuring it

ORTHOPAEDIC INFECTIONS

OSTEOMYELITIS

What is osteomyelitis?	Inflammation/infection of bone marrow and adjacent bone
What are the most likely causative organisms?	Neonates: *Staphylococcus aureus*, gram-negative *streptococcus* Children: *S. aureus, Haemophilus influenzae*, streptococci Adults: *S. aureus* Immunocompromised/drug addicts: *S. aureus* gram-negative Sickle cell: *Salmonella*
What is the most common organism isolated in osteomyelitis in the general adult population?	*S. aureus*
What is the most common isolated organism in patients with sickle cell disease?	*Salmonella*
What is seen on physical examination?	Tenderness, decreased movement, swelling
What are the diagnostic steps?	History and physical examination, needle aspirate, blood cultures, CBC, ESR, bone scan
What are the treatment options?	Antibiotics with or without surgical drainage
What is a Marjolin's ulcer?	Squamous cell carcinoma that arises in a chronic sinus from osteomyelitis

SEPTIC ARTHRITIS

What is it?	Inflammation of a joint beginning as synovitis and ending with destruction of articular cartilage if left untreated

What are the causative agents?	Same as in osteomyelitis, except that gonococcus is a common agent in the adult population
What are the findings on physical examination?	Joint pain, decreased motion, joint swelling, joint warm to the touch
What are the diagnostic steps?	Needle aspirate (look for pus; culture plus Gram stain), x-ray, blood cultures, ESR
What is the treatment?	Decompression of the joint via needle aspiration and IV antibiotics; hip, shoulder, and spine must be surgically incised, débrided, and drained

ORTHOPAEDIC TUMORS

What is the most common type in adults?	Metastatic!
What are the common sources?	Breast, lung, prostate, kidney, thyroid, and multiple myeloma
What is the usual presentation?	Bone pain or as a pathologic fracture
What is the most common primary malignant bone tumor?	Multiple myeloma (45%)
What is the differential diagnosis of a possible bone tumor?	Metastatic disease Primary bone tumors Metabolic disorders (e.g., hyperparathyroidism) Infection
What are the benign bone tumors (8)?	1. Osteochondroma 2. Enchondroma 3. Unicameral/aneurysmal bone cysts 4. Osteoid osteoma 5. Chondroblastoma 6. Fibroxanthoma 7. Fibrous dysplasia 8. Nonossifying fibroma

What are the malignant bone tumors (7)?	1. Multiple myeloma 2. Osteosarcoma 3. Chondrosarcoma 4. Ewing's sarcoma 5. Giant cell tumor (locally malignant) 6. Malignant melanoma 7. Metastatic

Compare benign and malignant bone tumors in terms of:

Size	Benign—small; <1 cm Malignant— >1 cm
Bone reaction	Benign—sclerotic bone reaction Malignant—little reaction
Margins	Benign—sharp Malignant—poorly defined
Invasive	Benign—confined to bone Malignant—often extends to surrounding tissues

Are most pediatric bone tumors benign or malignant?	80% are benign (most common is osteochondroma)
Are most adult bone tumors benign or malignant?	66% are malignant (most commonly metastatic)
What are the four diagnostic steps?	1. PE/lab tests 2. Radiographs 3. CT scan, technetium scan, or both 4. Biopsy
What are the radiographic signs of malignant tumors?	Large size Aggressive bone destruction, poorly defined margins Ineffective bone reaction to tumor Extension to soft tissues
What are the radiographic signs of benign tumors?	Small Well circumscribed, sharp margins Effective bone reaction to the tumor (sclerotic periostitis) No extension—confined to bone

What are some specific radiographic findings of the following:

    Osteosarcoma?   "Sunburst" pattern

    Fibrous dysplasia   Bubbly lytic lesion, "ground glass"

    Ewing's sarcoma   "Onion skinning"

What is the mainstay of treatment for bone tumors?

Surgery (excision plus débridement) for both malignant and benign lesions; radiation therapy and chemotherapy as adjuvant therapy for many malignant tumors

OSTEOSARCOMA

What is the usual age at presentation?

10 to 20 years

What is the gender distribution?

Male > female

What is the most common location?

≈66% in the distal femur, proximal tibia

What is the radiographic sine qua non?

Bone formation somewhere within tumor

What is the treatment?

Resection (limb sparing if possible) plus chemotherapy

What is the 5-year survival rate?

≈70%

What is the most common site of metastasis?

Lungs

What is the most common benign bone tumor?

Osteochondroma; it is cartilaginous in origin and may undergo malignant degeneration

What is a chondrosarcoma?

Malignant tumor of cartilaginous origin; presents in middle-aged and older patients and is unresponsive to chemotherapy and radiotherapy

EWING'S SARCOMA

What is the usual presentation?	Pain, swelling in involved area
What is the most common location?	Around the knee (distal femur, proximal tibia)
What is the usual age at presentation?	Evenly spread among those younger than 20 years of age
What are the associated radiographic findings?	Lytic lesion with periosteal reaction termed "onion skinning," which is calcified layering Central areas of tumor can undergo liquefaction necrosis, which may be confused with purulent infection (particularly in a child with fever, leukocytosis, and bone pain)
What is a memory aid for Ewing's sarcoma?	"**TKO** Ewing": **T**wenty years old or younger **K**nee joint "**O**nion skinning"
What is the 5-year survival rate?	50%
How can Ewing's sarcoma mimic the appearance of osteomyelitis?	Bone cysts
What is a unicameral bone cyst?	Fluid-filled cyst most commonly found in the proximal humerus in children 5 to 15 years of age
What is the usual presentation?	Asymptomatic until pathologic fracture
What is the treatment?	Steroid injections
What is an aneurysmal bone cyst?	Hemorrhagic lesion that is locally destructive by expansile growth, but does not metastasize

What is the usual presentation?	Pain and swelling; pathologic fractures are rare
What is the treatment?	Curettage and bone grafting

ARTHRITIS

Which arthritides are classified as degenerative?	Osteoarthritis Post-traumatic arthritis
What signs characterize osteoarthritis?	Heberden's nodes/Bouchard's nodes **Symmetric** destruction, usually of the hip, knee, or spine
What are Bouchard's nodes?	Enlarged PIP joints of the hand from cartilage/bone growth
What are Heberden's nodes?	Enlarged DIP joints of the hand from cartilage/bone growth
What is post-traumatic arthritis?	Usually involves one joint of past trauma
What are the treatment options for degenerative arthritis (3)?	1. NSAIDS for acute flare-ups, **not** for long-term management 2. Local corticosteroid injections 3. Surgery
What are the characteristics of rheumatoid arthritis?	Autoimmune reaction in which invasive pannus attacks hyaline articular cartilage; rheumatoid factor (anti-IgG/IgM) in 80% of patients; 3× more common in women; skin nodules (e.g., rheumatoid nodule)
What is pannus?	Inflammatory exudate overlying synovial cells inside the joint
What are the classic hand findings with rheumatoid arthritis?	Wrist: radial deviation Fingers: ulnar deviation
What are the surgical management options for joint/bone diseases (3)?	1. Arthroplasty 2. Arthrodesis (fusion) 3. Osteotomy

What is the major difference between gout and pseudogout?	Gout: caused by urate deposition, negative birefringent, needle crystal Pseudogout: caused by calcium pyrophosphate positive birefringent square crystals (Think: **P**ositive **S**quare crystals = **PS**eudogout)
What is a Charcot's joint?	Arthritic joint from peripheral neuropathy

PEDIATRIC ORTHOPAEDICS

What are the major differences between pediatric and adult bones?	Children: increased bone flexibility and bone healing (thus, many fractures are treated closed, whereas an adult would require O.R.I.F.), physis (weak point)
What types of fractures are unique to children?	Greenstick fracture Torus fracture Fracture through physis

SALTER-HARRIS CLASSIFICATION

What does it describe?	Fractures in children involving physis
What does it indicate high risk of?	Potential growth arrest
Define the following terms: **Salter I**	Through physeal plate only
Salter II	Involves metaphysis and physis
Salter III	Involves physis and epiphysis
Salter IV	Extends from metaphysis through physis, into epiphysis
Salter V	Axial force crushes physeal plate

**Define the following fractures
by Salter-Harris grade:**

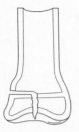

Salter III

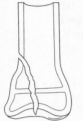

Salter IV

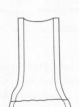

Salter I

Salter V

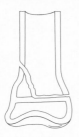

Salter II

What acronym can help you remember the Salter classifications?

"SALTR":
   Separated = type I
   Above = type II
   Lower = type III
   Through = type IV
   Ruined = type V

What is the simple numerical method for remembering the Salter-Harris classification?

(N = normal)

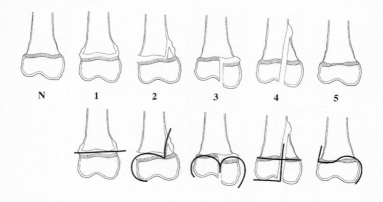

N   1   2   3   4   5

Why is the growth plate of concern in childhood fractures?

Growth plate represents the "weak link" in the child's musculoskeletal system; fractures involving the growth plate of long bones may compromise normal growth, so special attention should be given to them

What is a chief concern when oblique/spiral fractures of long bones are seen in children?	Child abuse is a possibility; other signs of abuse should be investigated
What is usually done during reduction of a femoral fracture?	Small amount of overlap is allowed because increased vascularity from injury may make the affected limb longer if overlap is not present; treatment after reduction is a spica cast
What is unique about ligamentous injury in children?	Most "ligamentous" injuries are actually fractures involving the growth plate!
What two fractures have a high incidence of associated compartment syndrome?	1. Tibial fractures 2. Supracondylar fractures of humerus (Volkmann's contracture)

CONGENITAL HIP DISLOCATION

What is the epidemiology?	Female > male, firstborn children, breech Presentation, 1 in 1000 births
What percentage are bilateral?	10%
How is the diagnosis made?	Barlow's maneuver, Ortolani's sign Radiographic confirmation is required
What is Barlow's maneuver?	Detects unstable hip: patient is placed in the supine position and attempt is made to push femurs posteriorly with knees at 90°/hip flexed and hip will dislocate (Think: push **B**ack = **B**arlow)
What is Ortolani's sign?	"Clunk" produced by relocation of a dislocated femoral head when the examiner abducts the flexed hip and lifts the greater trochanter anteriorly; detects a dislocated hip (Think: **O**ut = **O**rtolani's)
What is the treatment?	Pavlik harness—maintains hip reduction with hips flexed at 100° to 110°

SCOLIOSIS

What is the definition?	Lateral curvature of a portion of the spine Nonstructural: corrects with positional change Structural: does not correct
What are three treatment options?	1. Observation 2. Braces (Milwaukee brace) 3. Surgery
What are the indications for surgery for scoliosis?	Respiratory compromise Rapid progression Curves >40° Failure of brace

MISCELLANEOUS

Define the following terms: **Legg-Calvé-Perthes disease**	Idiopathic avascular necrosis of femoral head in children
Slipped capital femoral epiphysis	Migration of proximal femoral epiphysis on the metaphysis in children; the proximal femoral epiphysis externally rotates and displaces anteriorly from the capital femoral epiphysis, which stays reduced in the acetabulum (**Note:** Hip pain in children often presents as knee pain)
Blount's disease	Idiopathic varus bowing of tibia
Nursemaid's elbow	Dislocation of radial head (from pulling toddler's arm)
Little League elbow	Medial epicondylitis
Osgood-Schlatter's disease	Apophysitis of the tibial tubercle resulting from repeated powerful contractions of the quadriceps; seen in adolescents with an open physis Treatment of mild cases: activity restriction Treatment of severe cases: cast
What is the most common pediatric bone tumor?	Osteochondroma (Remember, 80% of bone tumors are benign in children)

Chapter 75 **Neurosurgery**

HEAD TRAUMA

What is the incidence?

70,000 fatal injuries/year in the United States, 500,000 head injuries per year

What percentage of trauma deaths result from head trauma?

50%

Identify the dermatomes:

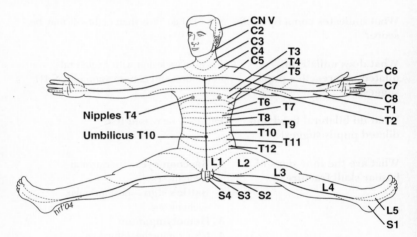

What is the Glasgow Coma Scale (GCS)?

GCS is an objective assessment of the level of consciousness after trauma

GCS SCORING SYSTEM

Eyes?

Eye Opening (E)
    4—opens spontaneously
    3—opens to voice (command)
    2—opens to painful stimulus
    1—does not open eyes
    (Think: **"4 eyes"**)

Motor?	**Motor Response (M)** 6—obeys commands 5—localizes painful stimulus 4—withdraws from pain 3—decorticate posture 2—decerebrate posture 1—no movement (Think: **6**-cylinder **motor**)
Verbal?	**Verbal Response (V)** 5—appropriate and oriented 4—confused 3—inappropriate words 2—incomprehensible sounds 1—no sounds (Think: Jackson **5** = **verbal 5**)
What indicates coma by GCS score?	**<8** (Think: "less than eight—it may be too late")
What does unilateral, dilated, nonreactive pupil suggest?	Focal mass lesion with ipsilateral herniation and compression of CN III
What do bilateral fixed and dilated pupils suggest?	Diffusely increased ICP
What are the four signs of basilar skull fracture?	1. **Raccoon eyes**—periorbital ecchymoses 2. **Battle's sign**—postauricular ecchymoses 3. **Hemotympanum** 4. **CSF** rhinorrhea/otorrhea
What is the initial radiographic neuroimaging in trauma?	1. Head CT scan (if LOC or GCS <15) 2. C-spine CT 3. T/L spine AP and lateral
Should the trauma head CT scan be with or without IV contrast?	**Without!**
What is normal ICP?	5 to 15 mm H_2O

What is the worrisome ICP?

>20 mm H_2O

What determines ICP (Monroe-Kelly hypothesis)?

1. Volume of brain
2. Volume of blood
3. Volume of CSF

What is the CPP?

Cerebral **P**erfusion **P**ressure = mean arterial pressure—ICP (normal CPP is >70)

What is Cushing's reflex?

Physiologic response to increased ICP:
1. Hypertension
2. Bradycardia
3. Decreased RR

What are the three general indications to monitor ICP after trauma?

1. GCS <9
2. Altered level of consciousness or unconsciousness with multiple system trauma
3. Decreased consciousness with focal neurologic examination abnormality

What is Kocher's point?

Landmark for placement of ICP monitor bolt:

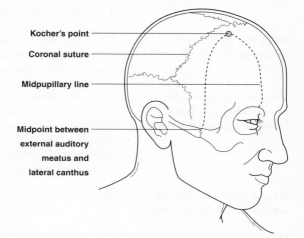

What nonoperative techniques are used to decrease ICP?

1. **Elevate** head of bed (HOB) 30° (if spine cleared)
2. Diuresis-mannitol (osmotic diuretic), Lasix®, limit fluids
3. Intubation (P_{CO_2} control)
4. Sedation
5. Pharmacologic paralysis
6. Ventriculostomy (CSF drainage)

What is the acronym for the treatment of elevated ICP?

"ICP HEAD":
INTUBATE
CALM (sedate)
PLACE DRAIN (ventriculostomy)/
    PARALYSIS

HYPERVENTILATE TO P_{CO_2} ≈35
ELEVATE head
ADEQUATE BLOOD PRESSURE
    (CPP >70)
DIURETIC (e.g., mannitol)

Can a tight c-collar increase the ICP?

Yes (it blocks venous drainage from brain!)

Why is prolonged hyperventilation dangerous?

It may result in severe vasoconstriction and ischemic brain necrosis!
Use only for very brief periods

What is a Kjellberg? (pronounced "shellberg")

Decompressive bifrontal craniectomy with removal of frontal bone frozen for possible later replacement

How does cranial nerve examination localize the injury in a comatose patient?

CNs proceed caudally in the brain stem as numbered: Presence of corneal reflex (CN 5 + 7) indicates intact pons; intact gag reflex (CN 9 + 10) shows functioning upper medulla (*Note:* CN 6 palsy is often a false localizing sign)

What is acute treatment of seizures after head trauma?

Benzodiazepines (Ativan®)

What is seizure prophylaxis after severe head injury?

Give phenytoin for 7 days

What is the significance of hyponatremia (low sodium level) after head injury?

SIADH must be ruled out; remember, **SIADH** = **S**odium **I**s **A**lways **D**own **H**ere

EPIDURAL HEMATOMA

What is an epidural hematoma?

Collection of blood between the skull and dura

What causes it?

Usually occurs in association with a skull fracture as bone fragments lacerate meningeal arteries

Which artery is associated with epidural hematomas?

Middle meningeal artery

What is the most common sign of an epidural hematoma?

>50% have ipsilateral blown pupil

What is the classic history with an epidural hematoma?

LOC followed by a "lucid interval" followed by neurologic deterioration

What are the classic CT scan findings with an epidural hematoma?

Lenticular (lens)-shaped hematoma (Think: **E**pidural = **LE**nticular)

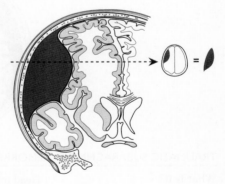

What is the surgical treatment for an epidural hematoma?

Surgical evacuation

What are the indications for surgery with an epidural hematoma?

Any symptomatic epidural hematoma; any epidural hematoma >1 cm

SUBDURAL HEMATOMA

What is it?   Blood collection under the dura

What causes it?   Tearing of "bridging" veins that pass
                                       through the space between the cortical
                                       surface and the dural venous sinuses or
                                       injury to the brain surface with resultant
                                       bleeding from cortical vessels

What are the three types of   1. Acute—symptoms within 48 hours of
subdurals?   injury
                                       2. Subacute—symptoms within 3 to 14 days
                                       3. Chronic—symptoms after 2 weeks or
                                          longer

What is the treatment of   Mass effect (pressure) must be reduced;
epidural and subdural   craniotomy with clot evacuation is usually
hematomas?   required

What classic findings appear   Curved, crescent-shaped hematoma
on head CT scan for a   (Think: sUbdural = cUrved)
subdural hematoma?

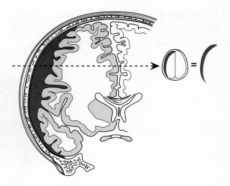

TRAUMATIC SUBARACHNOID HEMORRHAGE

What is it?   Head trauma resulting in blood below the
                                       arachnoid membrane and above the pia

What is the treatment?   Anticonvulsants and observation

CEREBRAL CONTUSION

What is it?   Hemorrhagic contusion of brain parenchyma

What are coup and contrecoup injuries?	Coup—injury at the site of impact Contrecoup—injury at the site opposite the point of impact
What is DAI?	**D**iffuse **A**xonal **I**njury (shear injury to brain parenchyma) from rapid deceleration injury; 33% mortality; long-term coma
What is the best diagnostic test for DAI?	MRI
What can present after blunt trauma with neurological deficits and a normal brain CT scan?	DAI, carotid artery injury

SKULL FRACTURE

What is a depressed skull fracture?	Fracture in which one or more fragments of the skull are forced below the inner table of the skull
What are the indications for surgery?	1. Contaminated wound requiring cleaning and débridement 2. Severe deformity 3. Impingement on cortex 4. Open fracture 5. CSF leak
What is the treatment for open skull fractures?	1. Antibiotics 2. Seizure prophylaxis (phenytoin) 3. Surgical therapy

SPINAL CORD TRAUMA

What are the two general types of injury?	1. Complete—no motor/sensory function below the level of injury 2. Incomplete—residual function below the level of injury
Define "spinal shock."	Loss of all reflexes and motor function, hypotension, bradycardia

Define "sacral sparing."

Sparing of sacral nerve level: anal sphincter intact, toe flexion, perianal sensation

What initial studies/ intervention are important?

1. ABCs—obtain airway and ventilate if needed
2. Maintain BP (IVF, pressors if refractory to fluids)
3. NG tube—prevents aspiration
4. Foley
5. High-dose steroids—proven to improve outcome if given <8 hours post injury
6. Complete cervical x-rays and those of lower levels as indicated by examination

What are the diagnostic studies?

Plain films, CT scan, MRI

What are the indications for emergent surgery with spinal cord injury?

Unstable vertebral fracture
Incomplete injury with extrinsic compression
Spinal epidural or subdural hematoma

What is the indication for IV high-dose steroids with spinal cord injury?

Controversial: Blunt spinal cord injury with neurologic deficit (methylprednisolone: high-dose bolus [30 mg/kg] followed by continuous infusion [5.4 mg/kg] for 23 hours)

Have steroids been proven to help after PENETRATING spine injury?

No

Describe the following conditions:
    Anterior cord syndrome

Affects corticospinal and lateral spinothalamic tracts, paraplegia, loss of pain/temperature sensation, preserved touch/vibration/proprioception

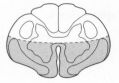

Central cord syndrome	Preservation of some lower extremity motor and sensory ability with upper extremity weakness

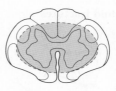

Brown-Séquard syndrome	Hemisection of cord resulting in ipsilateral motor weakness and touch/proprioception loss with contralateral pain/temperature loss

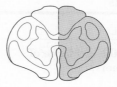

Posterior cord syndrome	Injury to posterior spinal cord with loss of proprioception distally
How can the findings associated with Brown-Séquard syndrome be remembered?	Think: **CAPTAIN** Brown-Séquard = "**CPT**": **C**ontralateral **P**ain **T**emperature loss
Define the following terms:	
Jefferson's fracture	Fracture through **C1** arches from axial loading (unstable fracture)
Hangman's fracture	Fracture through the pedicles of **C2** from hyperextension; usually stable Think: A hangman (C2) is below stature of President T. Jefferson (C1)
Odontoid fracture	Fracture of the odontoid process of C2 (view with open-mouth odontoid x-ray)
Priapism	Penile erection seen with spinal cord injury

Chance fracture   Transverse vertebral fracture

Clay shoveler's fracture   Fracture of spinous process of C7

Odontoid fractures   A: Type I—fracture through tip of dens
                                       B: Type II—fracture through base of
                                          dens
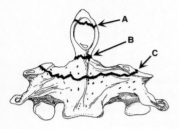   C: Type III—fracture through body
                                          of C2

TUMORS

GENERAL

What is the incidence of CNS tumors?
≈1% of all cancers; third leading cause of cancer deaths in people 15 to 34 years of age; second leading cause of cancer deaths in children

What is the usual location of primary tumors in adults/children?
In adults, ≈66% of tumors are supratentorial, ≈33% are infratentorial; the reverse is true in children (i.e., ≈66% infratentorial)

What is the differential diagnosis of a ring-enhancing brain lesion?
Metastatic carcinoma, abscess, GBM, lymphoma

What are the adverse effects of tumors on the brain?
1. Increased ICP
2. Mass effect on cranial nerves
3. Invasion of brain parenchyma, disrupting nuclei/tracts
4. Seizure foci
5. Hemorrhage into/around tumor mass

What are the signs/symptoms of brain tumors?
1. Neurologic deficit (66%)
2. Headache (50%)
3. Seizures (25%)
4. Vomiting (classically in the morning)

How is the diagnosis made?	CT scan or MRI is the standard diagnostic study
What are the surgical indications?	1. Establishing a tissue diagnosis 2. Relief of increased ICP 3. Relief of neurologic dysfunction caused by tissue compression 4. Attempt to cure in the setting of localized tumor
What are the most common intracranial tumors in adults?	Metastatic neoplasms are most common; among primaries, gliomas are #1 (50%) and meningiomas are #2 (25%)
What are the three most common in children?	1. Medulloblastomas (33%) 2. Astrocytomas (33%) 3. Ependymomas (10%)

GLIOMAS

What is a glioma?	General name for several tumors of neuroglial origin (e.g., astrocytes, ependymal, oligodendrocytes)
What are the characteristics of a LOW-grade astrocytoma?	Nuclear atypia, high mitotic rate, high signal on T2 weighted images, nonenhancing with contrast CT scan
What is the most common primary brain tumor in adults?	Glioblastoma multiforme (GBM) (Think: **GBM** = **G**reatest **B**rain **M**alignancy)
What are its characteristics?	Poorly defined, highly aggressive tumors occurring in the white matter of the cerebral hemispheres; spread extremely rapidly
What is the average age of onset?	Fifth decade
What is the treatment?	Surgical debulking followed by radiation
What is the prognosis?	Without treatment, >90% of patients die within 3 months of diagnosis; with treatment, 90% die within 2 years

MENINGIOMAS

What is the layer of origination?	Arachnoid cap cells
What are the risk factors?	Radiation exposure Neurofibromatosis type 2 Female gender
What are the associated histologic findings?	Psammoma bodies (concentric calcifications), whorl formations ("onion skin" pattern)
What is the histologic malignancy determination?	Brain parenchymal invasion
What is the peak age of occurrence?	40 to 50 years
What is the gender ratio?	Females predominate almost 2:1
What is the clinical presentation?	Variable depending on location; lateral cerebral convexity tumors can cause focal deficits or headache; sphenoid tumors can present with seizures; posterior fossa tumors with CN deficits; olfactory groove tumors with anosmia
What is the treatment?	Preoperative embolization and surgical resection

CEREBELLAR ASTROCYTOMAS

What is the peak age of occurrence?	5 to 9 years
What is the usual location?	Usually in the cerebellar hemispheres; less frequently in the vermis
What are the signs/symptoms?	Usually lateral cerebellar signs occur: ipsilateral incoordination or dysmetria (patient tends to fall to side of tumor) as well as nystagmus and ataxia; CN deficits are also frequently present, especially in CNs VI and VII

What are the treatment and prognosis?	Completely resectable in 75% of cases, which usually results in a cure; overall 5-year survival rate exceeds 90%

MEDULLOBLASTOMA

What is the peak age of occurrence?	First decade (3 to 7 years)
What is the cell of origin?	External granular cells of cerebellum
What is the most common location?	Cerebellar vermis in children; cerebellar hemispheres of adolescents and adults
What are the signs/ symptoms?	Headache, vomiting, and other signs of increased ICP; also usually truncal ataxia
What are the treatment and prognosis?	Best current treatment includes surgery to debulk the tumor, cranial and spinal radiation, and chemotherapy; 5-year survival rate is >50%

PITUITARY TUMORS

What is the most common pituitary tumor?	Prolactinoma
What is the most common presentation of a prolactinoma?	Bitemporal hemianopsia (lateral visual fields blind)

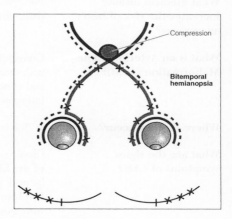

What are the blood prolactin levels with a prolactinoma?	>300 mg/L is diagnostic for prolactinoma (>100 mg/L is abnormal)
Medical treatment of a prolactinoma?	Bromocriptine
Surgical treatment for a prolactinoma?	Transsphenoidal resection of the pituitary tumor (in cases refractory to bromocriptine)
What is the treatment of a recurrent prolactinoma after surgical resection?	Radiation therapy

VASCULAR NEUROSURGERY

SUBARACHNOID HEMORRHAGE (SAH)

What are the usual causes?	Most cases are due to **trauma;** of nontraumatic SAH, the leading cause is ruptured **berry aneurysm,** followed by arteriovenous malformations
What is a berry aneurysm?	Saccular outpouching of vessels in the circle of Willis, usually at bifurcations
What is the usual location of a berry aneurysm?	Anterior communicating artery is #1 (30%), followed by posterior communicating artery and middle cerebral artery
What medical disease increases the risk of berry aneurysms?	Polycystic kidney disease and connective tissue disorders (e.g., Marfan's syndrome)
What is an Arterio-Venous Malformation (AVM)?	Congenital abnormality of the vasculature with connections between the **arterial** and **venous** circulations without interposed capillary network
Where do they occur?	>75% are supratentorial
What are the signs/ symptoms of SAH?	Classic symptom is **"the worst headache of my life";** meningismus is documented by neck pain and positive Kernig's and Brudzinski's signs; occasionally LOC, vomiting, nausea, photophobia

What comprises the workup of SAH?

If SAH is suspected, head CT should be the first test ordered to look for subarachnoid blood; LP may show xanthochromic CSF, but is not necessary if CT scan is definitive; this test should be followed by arteriogram to look for aneurysms or AVMs

What are the possible complications of SAH?

1. Brain edema leading to increased ICP
2. Rebleeding (most common in the first 24 to 48 hours posthemorrhage)
3. **Vasospasm** (most common cause of morbidity and mortality)

What is the treatment for vasospasm?

Nimodipine (calcium channel blocker)

What is the treatment of aneurysms?

Surgical treatment by placing a metal clip on the aneurysm is the mainstay of therapy; alternatives include balloon occlusion or coil embolization

What is the treatment of AVMs?

Many are on the brain surface and accessible operatively; preoperative embolization can reduce the size of the AVM; for surgically inaccessible lesions, radiosurgery (gamma knife) has been effective in treating AVMs <3 cm in diameter

INTRACEREBRAL HEMORRHAGE

What is it?

Bleeding into the brain parenchyma

What is the etiology?

#1 is hypertensive/atherosclerotic disease giving rise to Charcot-Bouchard aneurysms (small tubular aneurysms along smaller terminal arteries); other causes include coagulopathies, AVMs, amyloid angiopathy, bleeding into a tumor, and trauma

Where does it occur?

66% occur in the basal ganglia; putamen is the structure most commonly affected

How often does blood spread to the ventricular system?	66% of cases
What is the usual presentation?	66% present with coma; large putamen bleeding classically presents with contralateral hemiplegia and hemisensory deficits, lateral gaze preference, aphasia, and homonymous hemianopsia
What is the associated diagnostic study?	CT scan
What are the surgical indications?	CN III palsy, progressive alteration of consciousness
What is the prognosis?	Poor, especially with ventricular or diencephalons involvement

SPINE

LUMBAR DISC HERNIATION

What is it?	Extrusion of the inner portion of the intervertebral disc (nucleus pulposus) through the outer annulus fibrosis, causing impingement on nerve roots exiting the spinal canal
Which nerve is affected?	Nerve exiting at the level below (e.g., an L4–L5 disc impinges on the L5 nerve exiting between L5–S1)
Who is affected?	Middle-aged and older individuals
What is the usual cause?	Loss of elasticity of the posterior longitudinal ligaments and annulus fibrosis as a result of aging
What are the most common sites?	L5–S1 (45%) L4–L5 (40%)
What is the usual presenting symptom?	Low back pain

What are the signs:

L5–S1?

Decreased ankle jerk reflex
Weakness of plantar flexors in foot
Pain in back/midgluteal region to
    posterior calf to lateral foot
Ipsilateral radiculopathy on straight leg
    raise

L4–L5?

Decreased biceps femoris reflex
Weak extensors of foot

L3–L4?

Decrease or absence of knee jerks,
    weakness of the quadriceps femoris,
    pain in lower back/buttock, pain in
    lateral thigh and anterior thigh
Pain in hip/groin region to posterolateral
    thigh, lateral leg, and medial toes

How is the diagnosis made?

CT scan, CT myelogram, or MRI

What is the treatment?

Conservative—bed rest and analgesics
Surgical—partial hemilaminectomy and
    discectomy (removal of herniated disc)

**What are the indications for
emergent surgery?**

1. Cauda equina syndrome
2. Progressive motor deficits

**What is cauda equina
syndrome?**

Herniated disc compressing multiple
S1, S2, S3, S4 nerve roots, resulting in
bowel/bladder incontinence, "saddle
anesthesia" over buttocks/perineum, low
back pain, sciatica

What is "sciatica"?

Radicular or nerve root pain

CERVICAL DISC DISEASE

What is it?

Basically the same pathology as lumbar
disc herniation, except in the cervical
region; the disc impinges on the nerve
exiting the canal at the same level of the
disease (e.g., a C6–C7 disc impinges on
the C7 nerve root exiting at the C6–C7
foramen)

What are the most common sites?	C6–C7 (70%) C5–C6 (20%) C7–T1 (10%)
What are the signs/ symptoms: **C7?**	Decreased triceps reflex/strength, weakness of forearm extension Pain from neck, through triceps and into index and middle finger
C6?	Decreased biceps and brachioradialis reflex Weakness in forearm flexion Pain in neck, radial forearm, and thumb
C8?	Weakness in intrinsic hand muscles, pain in fourth/fifth fingers
How is the diagnosis made?	CT scan or MRI
What is the treatment?	Anterior or posterior discectomy with fusion PRN
What are the symptoms of central cervical cord compression from disc fragments?	Myelopathic syndrome with LMN signs at level of compression and UMN signs distally; e.g., C7 compression may cause bilateral loss of triceps reflex and bilateral hyperreflexia, clonus, and Babinski signs in lower extremities
What is Spurling's sign?	Reproduction of radicular pain by having the patient turn his head to the affected side and applying axial pressure to the top of the head

SPINAL EPIDURAL ABSCESS

What is the etiology?	Hematogenous spread from skin infections is most common; also, distant abscesses/ infections, UTIs, postoperative infections, spinal surgery, epidural anesthesia
What is the commonly associated medical condition?	Diabetes mellitus

What are the three most common sites?	1. Thoracic 2. Lumbar 3. Cervical
What is the most common organism?	*Staphylococcus aureus*
What are the signs/ symptoms?	Fever; severe pain over affected area and with flexion/extension of spine; weakness can develop, ultimately leading to paraplegia; 15% of patients have a back furuncle
How is the diagnosis made?	MRI = test of choice
Which test is contraindicated?	LP, because of the risk of seeding CSF with bacteria, causing meningitis
What is the treatment?	Surgical drainage and appropriate antibiotic coverage
What is the prognosis?	Depends on preop condition; severe neurologic deficits (e.g., paraplegia) show little recovery; 15% to 20% of cases are fatal

PEDIATRIC NEUROSURGERY

HYDROCEPHALUS

What is it?	Abnormal condition consisting of an increased volume of CSF along with distension of CSF spaces
What are the three general causes?	1. Increased production of CSF 2. Decreased absorption of CSF 3. Obstruction of normal flow of CSF (90% of cases)
What is the normal daily CSF production?	≈500 mL
What is the normal volume of CSF?	≈150 mL in the average adult

Define "communicating" versus "noncommunicating" hydrocephalus.

Communicating—unimpaired connection of CSF pathway from lateral ventricle to subarachnoid space

Noncommunicating—complete or incomplete obstruction of CSF flow within or at the exit of the ventricular system

What are the specific causes of hydrocephalus?

Congenital malformation
Aqueductal stenosis
Myelomeningocele
Tumors obstructing CSF flow
Inflammation causing impaired absorption of fluid
Subarachnoid hemorrhage
Meningitis
Choroid plexus papilloma causing ↑ production of CSF

What are the signs/symptoms?

Signs of increased ICP: HA, nausea, vomiting, ataxia, increasing head circumference exceeding norms for age

How is the diagnosis made?

CT scan, MRI, measurement of head circumference

What is the treatment?

1. Remove obvious offenders
2. Perform bypass obstruction with ventriculoperitoneal shunt or ventriculoatrial shunt

What is the prognosis if untreated?

50% mortality; survivors show decreased IQ (mean = 69); neurologic sequelae: ataxia, paraparesis, visual deficits

What are the possible complications of treatment?

1. Blockage/shunt malfunction
2. Infection

What is hydrocephalus ex vacuo?

Increased volume of CSF spaces from brain atrophy, not from any pathology in the amount of CSF absorbed or produced

What is a "shunt series"?

Series of x-rays covering the entire shunt length—looking for shunt disruption/kinking to explain malfunction of shunt

SPINAL DYSRAPHISM/NEURAL TUBE DEFECTS

What is the incidence?	≈1/1000 live births in the United States
What are the race/gender demographics?	More common in white patients and female patients
Define spina bifida occulta.	Defect in the development of the posterior portion of the vertebrae
What are the signs/symptoms?	Usually asymptomatic, though it may be associated with other spinal abnormalities; usually found incidentally on x-rays
What is the most common clinically significant defect?	Myelomeningocele: herniation of nerve roots and spinal cord through a defect in the posterior elements of the vertebra(e); the sac surrounding the neural tissue may be intact, but more commonly is ruptured and therefore exposes the CNS to the external environment
What are the three most common anatomic sites?	1. Lumbar region 2. Lower thoracic region 3. Upper sacral region
What are the signs/symptoms?	Variable from mild skeletal deformities to a complete motor/sensory loss; bowel/bladder function is difficult to evaluate, but often is affected and can adversely affect survival
What is the treatment?	With open myelomeningoceles, patients are operated on immediately to prevent infection
What is the prognosis?	≈95% survival for the first 2 years, compared with 25% in patients not undergoing surgical procedures
Which vitamin is thought to lower the rate of neural tube defects in utero?	Folic acid

CRANIOSYNOSTOSIS

What is it?	Premature closure of one or more of the sutures between the skull plates
What is the incidence?	1/200 live births in the United States
What are the types?	Named for the suture that is fused (e.g., sagittal, coronal, lambdoid); sagittal craniosynostosis accounts for >50% of all cases; more than one suture can be fused, and all or part of a suture may be affected
How is the diagnosis made?	Physical examination can reveal ridges along fused sutures and lessened suture mobility; plain x-rays can show a lack of lucency along the fused suture, but are rarely required
What are the indications for surgery?	Most often the reasons are cosmetic, as the cranial vault will continue to deform with growth; occasionally, a child will present with increased ICP secondary to restricted brain growth
What is the timing of surgery?	Usually 3 to 4 months of age; earlier surgery increases the risk of anesthesia; later surgeries are more difficult because of the worsening deformities and decreasing malleability of the skull
What is the operative mortality?	<1%

MISCELLANEOUS

What is the most common bacteria causing postneurosurgery meningitis?	*Staphylococcus aureus* (skin flora)
What classically presents as the "worst headache of my life"?	Spontaneous subarachnoid hemorrhage
What classically has a "lucid interval"?	Epidural hemorrhage

What is the most common location of a hypertensive intracerebral hemorrhage?	Putamen
What is Horner's syndrome?	Cervical sympathetic chain lesion; Think: **"MAP"**: **M**iosis **A**nhydrosis of ipsilateral face **P**tosis
What is a third-nerve palsy?	Think: **Third** nerve does **three** things: 1. Diplopia 2. Ptosis 3. Mydriasis
What is Millard-Gubler syndrome?	Pons infarction: 1. VI nerve palsy 2. VII nerve palsy 3. Contralateral hemiplegia
What is syringomyelia?	Central pathologic cavitations of the spinal cord

Chapter 76   Urology

Define the following terms: **Cystogram**	Contrast study of the bladder
Ureteral stents	Plastic tubes placed via cystoscope into the ureters for stenting, identification, etc.
Cystoscope	Scope placed into the urethra and into the bladder to visualize the bladder
Perc nephrostomy	Catheter placed through the skin into the kidney pelvis to drain urine with distal obstruction, etc.
Retrograde pyelogram	Dye injected into the ureter up into the kidney, and films taken

RUG

Retrograde **U**rethro**G**ram (dye injected into the urethra and films taken; rules out urethral injury, usually in trauma patients)

Gomco clamp

Clamp used for circumcision; protects penis glans

Bell clapper's deformity

Condition of congenital absence of gubernaculum attachment to scrotum

Fournier's gangrene

Extensive tissue necrosis/infection of the perineum in patients with diabetes

Foley catheter

Straight bladder catheter placed through the urethra

Coudé catheter

Basically, a Foley catheter with hook on the end to get around a large prostate

Suprapubic catheter

Bladder catheter placed through the skin above the pubic symphysis into the bladder

Posthitis

Foreskin infection

Hydrocele

Clear fluid in the processus vaginalis membrane

Communicating hydrocele

Hydrocele that communicates with peritoneal cavity and, thus, gets smaller and larger as fluid drains and then reaccumulates

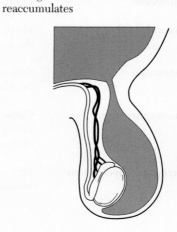

Noncommunicating hydrocele

Hydrocele that does not communicate with the peritoneal cavity; hydrocele remains the same size

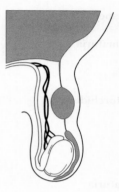

Varicocele

Abnormal dilation of the pampiniform plexus to the spermatic vein in the spermatic cord; described as a "bag of worms"

Spermatocele

Dilatation of epididymis or vas deferens

Epididymitis

Infection of the epididymis

Prehn's sign

Elevation of the painful testicle that reduces the pain of epididymitis

TRUS

Trans**R**ectal **U**ltra**S**ound

DRE

Digital **R**ectal **E**xamination

Orchitis

Inflammation/infection of the testicle

Pseudohermaphroditism

Genetically **one** sex; partial or complete opposite-sex genitalia

Urgency

Overwhelming sensation to void immediately

Dysuria

Painful urination (usually burning sensation)

Frequency

Urination more frequently than usual

Polyuria	Urination in larger amounts than usual
Nocturia	Awakening to urinate
Hesitancy	Delay in urination
Pneumaturia	Air passed with urine via the urethra
Pyuria	WBCs in urine; UTI >10 WBCs/HPF
Cryptorchidism	Undescended testicle
IVP	IntraVenous Pyelogram (dye is injected into the vein, collects in the renal collecting system, and an x-ray is taken)
Hematuria	RBCs in urine
Space of Retzius	Anatomic extraperitoneal space in front of the bladder
Enuresis	Involuntary urination while asleep
Incontinence	Involuntary urination
TURP	TransUrethral Resection of the Prostate
PVR	PostVoid Residual
Priapism	Prolonged, painful erection
Paraphimosis	Foreskin held (stuck) in the retracted position
Phimosis	Inability to retract the foreskin
Balanitis	Inflammation/infection of the glans penis
Balanoposthitis	Inflammation/infection of the glans and prepuce of the penis
UTI	Urinary Tract Infection
Peyronie's disease	Abnormal fibrosis of the penis shaft, resulting in a bend upon erection

BPH	**B**enign **P**rostatic **H**yperplasia
Epispadias	Abnormal urethral opening on the dorsal surface of the penis
Hypospadiasis	Abnormal urethral opening on the ventral surface of the penis; may occur in anterior, middle, or posterior of penis
Erectile dysfunction	Inability to achieve an erection
Sterility	Inability to reproduce
Appendix testis	Common redundant testicular tissue
VUR	**V**esico**U**reteral **R**eflux

SCROTAL ANATOMY

What are the layers of the scrotum?

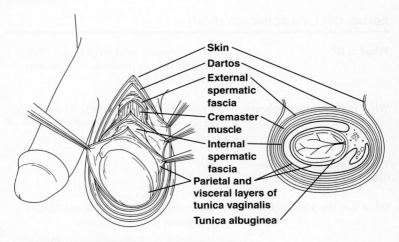

Skin
Dartos
External spermatic fascia
Cremaster muscle
Internal spermatic fascia
Parietal and visceral layers of tunica vaginalis
Tunica albuginea

UROLOGIC DIFFERENTIAL DIAGNOSIS

What is the differential diagnosis of scrotal mass?

Cancer, torsion, epididymitis, hydrocele, spermatocele, varicocele, inguinal hernia, testicular appendage, swollen testicle after trauma, nontesticular tumor (paratesticular tumor: e.g., rhabdomyosarcoma, leiomyosarcoma, liposarcoma)

What are the causes of hematuria?	Bladder cancer, trauma, UTI, cystitis from chemotherapy or radiation, stones, kidney lesion, BPH
What is the most common cause of severe gross hematuria without trauma or chemotherapy/radiation?	Bladder cancer
What is the differential diagnosis for bladder outlet obstruction?	BPH, stone, foreign body, urethral stricture, urethral valve
What is the differential diagnosis for ureteral obstruction?	Stone, tumor, iatrogenic (suture), stricture, gravid uterus, radiation injury, retroperitoneal fibrosis
What is the differential diagnosis for kidney tumor?	Renal cell carcinoma, sarcoma, adenoma, angiomyolipoma, hemangiopericytoma, oncocytoma

RENAL CELL CARCINOMA (RCC)

What is it?	Most common solid renal tumor (90%); originates from proximal renal tubular epithelium
What is the epidemiology?	Primarily a tumor of adults 40 to 60 years of age with a 3:1 male:female ratio; 5% of cancers overall in adults
What percentage of the tumors are bilateral?	1%
What are the risk factors?	Male sex, tobacco, von Hippel-Lindau syndrome, polycystic kidney
What are the symptoms?	Pain (40%), hematuria (35%), weight loss (35%), flank mass (25%), HTN (20%)
What is the classic TRIAD of renal cell carcinoma?	1. Flank pain 2. Hematuria 3. Palpable mass (**triad** occurs in only 10%–15% of cases)

How are most cases diagnosed these days?	Found incidentally on an imaging study (CT, MRI, U/S) for another reason
What radiologic tests are performed?	1. IVP 2. Abdominal CT scan with contrast
Define the stages (AJCC): **Stage I?**	Tumor <2.5 cm, no nodes, no metastases
Stage II?	Tumor >2.5 cm limited to kidney, no nodes, no metastases
Stage III?	Tumor extends into IVC or main renal vein; positive regional lymph nodes but <2 cm in diameter and no metastases
Stage IV?	Distant metastasis or positive lymph node >2 cm in diameter, or tumor extends past Gerota's fascia
What is the metastatic workup?	CXR, IVP, CT scan, LFTs, calcium
What are the sites of metastases?	Lung, liver, brain, bone; tumor thrombus entering renal vein or IVC is not uncommon
What is the unique route of spread?	Tumor thrombus into **IVC lumen**
What is the treatment of RCC?	Radical nephrectomy (excision of the kidney and adrenal, including Gerota's fascia) for stages I through IV
What gland is removed with a radical nephrectomy?	Adrenal gland
What is the unique treatment for metastatic spread?	1. α-interferon 2. LAK cells (lymphokine-activated killer) and IL-2 (interleukin-2)
What is a syndrome of RCC and liver disease?	Stauffer's syndrome

What is the concern in an adult with new onset left varicocele?	Left RCC—the left gonadal vein drains into the left renal vein

BLADDER CANCER

What is the incidence?	Second most common urologic malignancy Male:female ratio of 3:1 White patients are more commonly affected than are African American patients
What is the most common histology?	**T**ransitional **C**ell **C**arcinoma (**TCC**)—90%; remaining cases are squamous or adenocarcinomas
What are the risk factors?	**Smoking,** industrial carcinogens (aromatic amines), schistosomiasis, truck drivers, petroleum workers, cyclophosphamide
What are the symptoms?	**Hematuria,** with or without irritative symptoms (e.g., dysuria), frequency
What is the classic presentation of bladder cancer?	"Painless hematuria"
What tests are included in the workup?	Urinalysis and culture, IVP, cystoscopy with cytology and biopsy
Define the AJCC transitional cell bladder cancer stages:	
Stage 0?	Superficial, carcinoma in situ
Stage I?	Invades subepithelial connective tissue, no positive nodes, no metastases
Stage II?	Invades superficial or deep muscularis propria, no positive nodes, no metastases
Stage III?	Invades perivesical tissues, no positive nodes, no metastases
Stage IV?	Positive nodal spread with distant metastases and/or invades abdominal/pelvic wall

What is the treatment according to stage:

Stage 0? TURB and intravesical chemotherapy

Stage I? TURB

Stages II and III? Radical cystectomy, lymph node dissection, removal of prostate/uterus/ovaries/anterior vaginal wall, and urinary diversion (e.g., ileal conduit) +/− chemo

Stage IV? +/− Cystectomy and **systemic chemotherapy**

What are the indications for a partial cystectomy? Superficial, isolated tumor, apical with 3-cm margin from any orifices

What is TURB? **T**rans**U**rethral **R**esection of the **B**ladder

If after a TURB the tumor recurs, then what? Repeat TURB and intravesical chemotherapy (mitomycin C) or bacillus Calmette-Guérin

What is and how does bacillus Calmette-Guérin work? Attenuated TB vaccine—thought to work by immune response

PROSTATE CANCER

What is the incidence? **Most common** GU cancer (>100,000 new cases per year in the United States); most common carcinoma in men in the U.S.; second most common cause of death in men in the U.S.

What is the epidemiology? "Disease of elderly men" present in 33% of men 70 to 79 years of age and in 66% of men 80 to 89 years of age at autopsy; African American patients have a 50% higher incidence than do white patients

What is the histology? Adenocarcinoma (95%)

What are the symptoms?	Often asymptomatic; usually presents as a nodule found on routine rectal examination; in 70% of cases, cancer begins in the periphery of the gland and moves centrally; thus, obstructive symptoms occur late
What percentage of patients have metastasis at diagnosis?	40% of patients have metastatic disease at presentation, with symptoms of bone pain and weight loss
What are the common sites of metastasis?	Osteoblastic bony lesions, lung, liver, adrenal
What provides lymphatic drainage?	Obturator and hypogastric nodes
What is the significance of Batson's plexus?	Spinal cord venous plexus; route of isolated skull/brain metastasis
What are the steps in early detection?	1. Prostate-specific antigen (PSA)—most sensitive and specific marker 2. Digital rectal examination (DRE)

When should men get a PSA-level check?	Controversial:
	    1. All men >50 years old
	    2. >40 years old if first-degree family history or African American patient

What percentage of patients with prostate cancer will have an elevated PSA?	≈60%
What is the imaging test for bladder cancer?	**T**rans**R**ectal **U**ltra**S**ound (**TRUS**)
How is the diagnosis made?	Transrectal biopsy

What is the Gleason score?	Histologic grades 2–10:
	    Low score = well differentiated
	    High score = poorly differentiated

What are the indications for transrectal biopsy with normal rectal examination?	PSA >10 or abnormal transrectal ultrasound

Staging (AJCC):

Stage I? | Tumor involves <50% of 1 lobe, no nodes, no metastases, PSA <10, Gleason ≤6

Stage II? | Tumor within prostate; lobe <50% but PSA >10, or Gleason >6; or >50% of 1 lobe, no nodes, no metastases

Stage III? | Tumor through prostate capsule or into seminal vesicles, no nodes, no metastases

Stage IV? | Tumor extends into adjacent structures (other than seminal vesicles) or + nodes or + metastases

What does a "radical prostatectomy" remove?
1. Prostate gland
2. Seminal vesicles
3. Ampullae of the vasa deferentia

What is "androgen ablation" therapy?
1. Bilateral orchiectomy or
2. **L**uteinizing **H**ormone-**R**eleasing **H**ormone (**LHRH**) agonists

How do LHRH agonists work?
Decrease LH release from pituitary, which then decreases testosterone production in the testes

What are the generalized treatment options according to stage:

Stage I? | Radical prostatectomy

Stage II? | Radical prostatectomy, +/− lymph node dissection

Stage III? | Radiation therapy, +/− androgen ablation

Stage IV? | Androgen ablation, radiation therapy

What is the medical treatment for systemic metastatic disease?
Androgen ablation

What is the option for treatment in the early stage prostate cancer patient >70 years old with comorbidity?	XRT

BENIGN PROSTATIC HYPERPLASIA

What is it also known as?	BPH
What is it?	Disease of elderly men (average age is 60 to 65 years); prostate gradually enlarges, creating symptoms of urinary outflow obstruction
What is the size of a normal prostate?	20 to 25 gm
Where does BPH occur?	Periurethrally (*Note:* prostate cancer occurs in the periphery of the gland)
What are the symptoms?	Obstructive-type symptoms: hesitancy, weak stream, nocturia, intermittency, UTI, urinary retention
How is the diagnosis made?	History, DRE, elevated **P**ost**V**oid **R**esidual (**PVR**), urinalysis, cystoscopy, U/S
What lab tests should be performed?	Urinalysis, PSA, BUN, CR
What is the differential diagnosis?	**Prostate cancer** (e.g., nodular)—biopsy Neurogenic bladder—history of neurologic disease Acute prostatitis—hot, tender gland Urethral stricture—RUG, history of STD Stone UTI
What are the treatment options?	Pharmacologic—α-1 blockade Hormonal—antiandrogens Surgical—TURP, TUIP, open prostate resection Transurethral balloon dilation

Why do α-adrenergic blockers work?

1. Relax sphincter
2. Relax prostate capsule

What is Proscar®?

Finasteride: 5-α-reductase inhibitor; blocks transformation of testosterone to dihydrotestosterone; may shrink and slow progression of BPH

What is Hytrin®?

Terazosin: α-blocker; may increase urine outflow by relaxing prostatic smooth muscles

What are the indications for surgery in BPH?

Due to obstruction:
Urinary retention
Hydronephrosis
UTIs
Severe symptoms

What is TURP?

TransUrethral Resection of Prostate: resection of prostate tissue via a scope

What is TUIP?

TransUrethral Incision of Prostate

What percentage of tissue removed for BPH will have malignant tissue on histology?

Up to 10%!

What are the possible complications of TURP?

Immediate:
Failure to void
Bleeding
Clot retention
UTI
Incontinence

TESTICULAR CANCER

What is the incidence?

Rare; 2 to 3 new cases per 100,000 men per year in the United States

What is its claim to fame?

Most common solid tumor of young adult males (20 to 40 years)

What are the risk factors?

Cryptorchidism (6% of testicular tumors develop in patients with a history of cryptorchidism)

What is cryptorchidism? Failure of the testicle to descend into the scrotum

Does orchiopexy as an adult remove the risk of testicular cancer? NO

What are the symptoms? Most patients present with a painless lump, swelling, or firmness of the testicle; they often notice it after incidental trauma to the groin

What percentage of patients present with an acute hydrocele? 10%

What percentage present with symptoms of metastatic disease (back pain, anorexia)? ≈10%

What are the classifications? Germ cell tumors (95%):
Seminomatous (≈35%)
Nonseminomatous (≈65%)
Embryonal cell carcinoma
Teratoma
Mixed cell
Choriocarcinoma
Nongerminal (5%):
Leydig cell
Sertoli cell
Gonadoblastoma

What is the major classification based on therapy? Seminomatous and nonseminomatous tumors

What are the tumor markers for testicular tumors? 1. Beta-human chorionic gonadotropin (β-HCG)
2. Alpha-fetoprotein (AFP)

What are the tumor markers by tumor type? β-HCG—↑ in choriocarcinoma (100%), embryonal carcinoma (50%), and rarely in pure seminomas (10%); nonseminomatous tumors (50%)
AFP—↑ in embryonal carcinoma and yolk sac tumors; nonseminomatous tumors (50%)

Define the difference between seminomatous and NONseminomatous germ cell testicular tumor markers.	NONseminomatous **common** = 90% have a positive AFP and/or β-HCG Seminomatous **rare** = **only** 10% are AFP positive
Which tumors almost *never* have an elevated AFP?	Choriocarcinoma and seminoma
In which tumor is β-HCG almost always found elevated?	Choriocarcinoma
How often is β-HCG elevated in patients with pure seminoma?	Only about 10% of the time!
How often is β-HCG elevated with nonseminoma?	≈65%
What other tumor markers may be elevated and useful for recurrence surveillance?	LDH, CEA, **H**uman **C**horionic **S**omatomammotropic (**HCS**), **G**amma-**G**lutamyl **T**ranspeptidase (**GGT**), **PL**acental **A**lkaline **P**hosphate (**PLAP**)
What are the steps in workup?	PE, scrotal U/S, check tumor markers, CXR, CT (chest/pelvis/abd)
Define the stages according to TMN staging (AJCC):	
Stage I?	Any tumor size, no nodes, no metastases
Stage II?	**Positive** nodes, no metastases, any tumor
Stage III?	Distant **metastases** (any nodal status, any size tumor)
What is the initial treatment for all testicular tumors?	**Inguinal** orchiectomy (removal of testicle through a groin incision)
What is the treatment of *seminoma* at the various stages:	
Stage I and II?	Inguinal orchiectomy and **radiation** to retroperitoneal nodal basins
Stage III?	Orchiectomy and chemotherapy

What is the treatment of NONseminomatous disease at the various stages:

    Stages I and II?

Orchiectomy and retroperitoneal lymph node **dissection** versus close follow-up for retroperitoneal nodal involvement

    Stage III?

Orchiectomy and chemotherapy

What percentage of stage I seminomas are cured after treatment?

95%

Which type is most radiosensitive?

Seminoma (Think: **S**eminoma = **S**ensitive to radiation)

Why not remove testis with cancer through a scrotal incision?

It could result in tumor seeding of the scrotum

What is the major side effect of retroperitoneal lymph node dissection?

Erectile dysfunction

TESTICULAR TORSION

What is it?

Torsion (twist) of the spermatic cord, resulting in venous outflow obstruction, and subsequent arterial occlusion → infarction of the testicle

What is the classic history?

Acute onset of scrotal pain usually after vigorous activity or minor trauma

What is a "bell clapper" deformity?

Bilateral nonattachment of the testicles by the gubernaculum to the scrotum (free like the clappers of a bell)

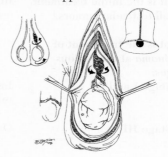

What are the symptoms?	Pain in the scrotum, suprapubic pain
What are the signs?	Very tender, swollen, elevated testicle; nonillumination; absence of cremasteric reflex
What is the differential diagnosis?	Testicular trauma, inguinal hernia, epididymitis, appendage torsion
How is the diagnosis made?	Surgical exploration, U/S (solid mass) and Doppler flow study, cold Tc-99m scan (nuclear study)
What is the treatment?	Surgical detorsion and bilateral orchiopexy to the scrotum
How much time is available from the onset of symptoms to detorse the testicle?	<6 hours will bring about the best results; >90% salvage rate
What are the chances of testicle salvage after 24 hours?	<10%

EPIDIDYMITIS

What is it?	Infection of the epididymis
What are the signs/symptoms?	Swollen, tender testicle; dysuria; scrotal ache/pain; fever; chills; scrotal mass
What is the cause?	Bacteria from the urethra
What are the common bugs in the following types of patients:	
Elderly patients/children?	*Escherichia coli*
Young men?	STD bacteria: Gonorrhea, chlamydia
What is the major differential diagnosis?	Testicular torsion
What is the workup?	U/A, urine culture, swab if STD suspected, +/− U/S with Doppler or nuclear study to rule out torsion
What is the treatment?	Antibiotics

PRIAPISM

What is priapism?	Persistent penile erection
What are its causes?	Low flow: leukemia, drugs (e.g., prazosin), sickle-cell disease, erectile dysfunction treatment gone wrong High flow: pudendal artery fistula, usually from trauma
What is first-line treatment?	1. Aspiration of blood from corporus cavernosum 2. α-Adrenergic agent

ERECTILE DYSFUNCTION

What is it?	Inability to achieve an erection
What are the six major causes?	1. **Vascular:** decreased blood flow or leak of blood from the corpus cavernosus (most common cause) 2. **Endocrine:** low testosterone 3. **Anatomic:** structural abnormality of the erectile apparatus (e.g., Peyronie's disease) 4. **Neurologic:** damage to nerves (e.g., postoperative, IDDM) 5. **Medications** (e.g., clonidine) 6. **Psychologic:** performance anxiety, etc. (very rare)
What lab tests should be performed?	Fasting GLC (rule out diabetes and thus diabetic neuropathy) Serum testosterone Serum prolactin

CALCULUS DISEASE

What is the incidence?	1 in 10 people will have stones
What are the risk factors?	Poor fluid intake, IBD, hypercalcemia ("CHIMPANZEES"), renal tubular acidosis, small bowel bypass

What are the four types of stones?

1. Calcium oxalate/calcium PO_4 (75%)—secondary to hypercalciuria ($\uparrow$ intestinal absorption, $\downarrow$ renal reabsorption, $\uparrow$ bone reabsorption)
2. Struvite (MgAmPh)(15%)—infection stones; seen in UTI with urea-splitting bacteria (*Proteus*); may cause staghorn calculi; high urine pH
3. Uric acid (7%)—stones are radiolucent (Think: **U**ric = **U**nseen); seen in gout, Lesch-Nyhan, chronic diarrhea, cancer; low urine pH
4. Cystine (1%)—genetic predisposition

What type of stones are not seen on AXR?

Uric acid (Think: **U**ric = **U**nseen)

What stone is associated with UTIs?

Struvite stones (Think: **S**truvite = **S**epsis)

What stones are seen in IBD/bowel bypass?

Calcium oxalate

What are the symptoms of calculus disease?

Severe pain; patient cannot sit still: renal colic (typically pain in the kidney/ureter that radiates to the testis or penis), hematuria (remember, patients with peritoneal signs are motionless)

What are the classic findings/symptoms?

Flank pain, stone on AXR, hematuria

Diagnosis?

KUB (90% radiopaque), IVP, urinalysis and culture, BUN/Cr, CBC

What is the significance of hematuria and pyuria?

Stone with concomitant infection

Treatment?

Narcotics for pain, vigorous hydration, observation
Further options: ESWL (lithotripsy), ureteroscopy, percutaneous lithotripsy, open surgery; metabolic workup for recurrence

What are the indications for intervention?	Urinary tract obstruction Persistent infection Impaired renal function
What are the contraindications of outpatient treatment?	Pregnancy, diabetes, obstruction, severe dehydration, severe pain, urosepsis/fever, pyelonephritis, previous urologic surgery, only one functioning kidney
What are the three common sites of obstruction?	1. UreteroPelvic Junction (**UPJ**) 2. UreteroVesicular Junction (**UVJ**) 3. Intersection of the ureter and the iliac vessels

INCONTINENCE

What are the common types of incontinence?	Stress incontinence, overflow incontinence, urge incontinence
Define the following terms: **Stress incontinence**	Loss of urine associated with coughing, lifting, exercise, etc.; seen most often in women, secondary to relaxation of pelvic floor following multiple deliveries
Overflow incontinence	Failure of the bladder to empty properly; may be caused by bladder outlet obstruction (BPH or stricture) or detrusor hypotonicity
Urge incontinence	Loss of urine secondary to detrusor instability in patients with stroke, dementia, Parkinson's disease, etc.
Mixed incontinence	Stress **and** urge incontinence combined
Enuresis	Bedwetting in children
How is the diagnosis made?	History (including meds), physical examination (including pelvic/rectal examination), urinalysis, postvoid residual (PR), urodynamics, cystoscopy/vesicocystourethrogram (VCUG) may be necessary

What is the "Marshall test"?	Woman with urinary stress incontinence placed in the lithotomy position with a full bladder leaks urine when asked to cough
What is the treatment of the following disorders:	
Stress incontinence?	Bladder neck suspension
Urge incontinence?	Pharmacotherapy (anticholinergics, α-agonists)
Overflow incontinence?	Self-catheterization, surgical relief of obstruction, α-blockers

URINARY TRACT INFECTION (UTI)

What is the etiology?	Ascending infection, instrumentation, coitus in females
What are the three common organisms?	1. *E. coli* (90%) 2. *Proteus* 3. *Klebsiella, Pseudomonas*
What are the predisposing factors?	Stones, obstruction, reflux, diabetes mellitus, pregnancy, indwelling catheter/stent
What are the symptoms?	Lower UTI—frequency, urgency, dysuria, nocturia Upper UTI—back/flank pain, fever, chills
How is the diagnosis made?	Symptoms, urinalysis (>10 WBCs/HPF, >10^5 CFU)
When should workup be performed?	After first infection in male patients (unless Foley is in place) After first pyelonephritis in prepubescent female patients
What is the treatment?	Lower: 1 to 4 days of oral antibiotics Upper: 3 to 7 days of IV antibiotics

MISCELLANEOUS UROLOGY QUESTIONS

Why should orchiopexy be performed?	↓ the susceptibility to blunt trauma ↑ the ease of follow-up examinations
In which area of the prostate does BPH arise?	Periurethral
In which area of the prostate does prostate cancer arise?	Periphery
What type of bony lesions is seen in metastatic prostate cancer?	Osteoblastic (radiopaque)
What percentage of renal cell carcinoma show evidence of metastatic disease at presentation?	≈33%
What is the most common site of distant metastasis in renal cell carcinoma?	Lung
What is the most common solid renal tumor of childhood?	Wilms' tumor
What type of renal stone is radiolucent?	Uric acid (Think: **U**ric = **U**nseen)
What are posterior urethral valves?	Most common obstructive urethral lesion in infants and newborns; occurs only in males; found at the distal prostatic urethra
What is the most common intraoperative bladder tumor?	Foley catheter—don't fall victim!
What provides drainage of the left gonadal (e.g., testicular) vein?	Left renal vein

What provides drainage of the right gonadal vein?	IVC
What are the signs of urethral injury in the trauma patient?	"High-riding, ballottable" prostate, blood at the urethral meatus, severe pelvic fracture, ecchymosis of scrotum
What is the evaluation for urethral injury in the trauma patient?	**RUG** (**R**etrograde **U**rethro**G**ram)
What is the evaluation for a transected ureter intraoperatively?	IV indigo carmine and then look for leak of blue urine in the operative field
What aid is used to help identify the ureters in a previously radiated retroperitoneum?	Ureteral stents
How can a small traumatic EXTRAperitoneal bladder rupture be treated?	Foley catheter
How should a traumatic INTRAperitoneal bladder rupture be treated?	Operative repair
What percentage of patients with an injured ureter will have no blood on urinalysis?	33%
What is the classic history for papillary necrosis?	Patient with diabetes taking NSAIDs or patient with sickle cell trait
What is Fournier's gangrene?	Necrotizing fasciitis of perineum, polymicrobial, diabetes = major risk factor
What unique bleeding problem can be seen with prostate surgery?	Release of TPA and urokinase (treat with ε-aminocaproic acid)
What is the scrotal "blue dot" sign?	Torsed appendix testis

What is Peyronie's disease?   Curved penile orientation with erection
                                    due to fibrosis of corpora cavernosa

What is a ureterocele?   Dilation of the ureter—treat with
                                    endoscopic incision or operative excision

What is a "three-way"   Foley catheter that irrigates and then
irrigating Foley catheter?   drains

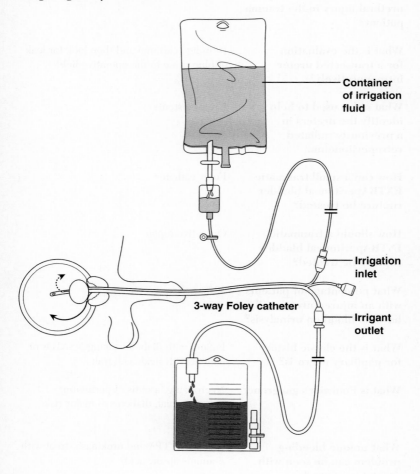

Rapid Fire Power Review

TOP 100 CLINICAL SURGICAL MICROVIGNETTES

1. **Elderly woman, SBO, and air in biliary tract** — Gallstone ileus

2. **Elderly woman with pain down inner aspect of thigh** — Obturator hernia (Howship-Romberg sign)

3. **Abdominal pain, hypotension, and abdominal pulsatile mass** — Ruptured abdominal aortic aneurysm (AAA)

4. **Abdominal pain "out of proportion" to abdominal exam** — Mesenteric ischemia

5. **Arm pain and syncope with arm movement** — Subclavian steal syndrome

6. **Increasing creatinine on ACE inhibitor** — Renal artery stenosis

7. **Child with MIDLINE neck mass** — Thyroglossal duct cyst

8. **Child with LATERAL neck mass** — Branchial cleft cyst

9. **Crush injury and dark urine** — Myoglobinuria

10. **Emesis, chest pain radiating to back, and mediastinal air** — Boerhaave's

11. **Lower GI bleed + technetium pertechnetate scan** — Meckel's diverticulum

12.	Flushing, diarrhea, and right-sided heart failure	Carcinoid
13.	Pneumaturia and LLQ pain	Colovesicular fistula
14.	Desmoid tumor, osteoma, and colon cancer	Gardner's syndrome
15.	Epigastric pain radiating to back and flank ecchymosis	Hemorrhagic pancreatitis
16.	Pancreatitis and palpable epigastric mass	Pancreatic pseudocyst
17.	Liver abscess with "anchovy paste"	Amebic abscess
18.	RUQ pain, travel, and exposure to sheep	Hydatid cyst
19.	Caput medusa	Portal hypertension
20.	45-year-old woman with RUQ pain for 12 hours, fever, and leukocytosis	Acute cholecystitis
21.	Elderly man with large nontender palpable gallbladder	Pancreatic cancer (Courvoisier's sign)
22.	Female taking birth control pills with liver mass	Hepatic adenoma
23.	Liver tumor with "central scar"	Focal nodular hyperplasia
24.	Pancreatic mass, gallstones, diabetes, and diarrhea	Somatostatinoma
25.	RUQ bruit and CHF in young adult	Liver hemangioma

26. **Excruciating pain with bowel movement** — Anal fissure

27. **Abdominal pain, diarrhea, and anal fistulae** — Crohn's disease

28. **EKG with "peaked" T waves** — Hyperkalemia

29. **Buccal mucosa with pigmentation** — Peutz-Jeghers syndrome

30. **LLQ pain, fever, and change in bowel habits** — Diverticulitis

31. **Elevated urine 5-HIAA** — Carcinoid

32. **Institutionalized, abdominal pain, vomiting, and distention, with proximal colonic dilation** — Sigmoid volvulus

33. **Infant with projectile vomiting** — Pyloric stenosis

34. **Newborn with failure to pass meconium in first 24 hours** — Hirschsprung's

35. **Infant with bilious vomiting** — Malrotation

36. **Newborn with abdominal defect and umbilical cord on sac** — Omphalocele

37. **Teenager with knee pain and "onion skinning" on x-ray** — Ewing's sarcoma

38. **Pulmonary capillary wedge pressure <18, CXR with bilateral pulmonary infiltrates, and PaO$_2$:FiO$_2$ ratio <200** — Acute respiratory distress syndrome (ARDS)

39. **Increased peak airway pressure, low urine output, and urinary bladder >25 mmHg** — Abdominal compartment syndrome

40. **Newborn with inability to "pass an NGT"** — Esophageal atresia

41. **Traumatic blinding in one eye followed by blindness in the contralateral eye 2 weeks later** — Sympathetic ophthalmia

42. **Mitotic pupil, ptosis, and anhydrosis** — Horner's syndrome

43. **Traumatic head injury, conscious in ER followed by unconsciousness** — Epidural hematoma ("lucid interval")

44. **"Worst headache of my life"** — Subarachnoid hemorrhage

45. **Hematuria, flank pain, and abdominal mass (palpable)** — Renal cell carcinoma

46. **60-year-old white man with painless hematuria** — Bladder cancer

47. **RUQ pain, jaundice, and fever** — Cholangitis

48. **Epigastric pain radiating to back, with nausea and vomiting** — Pancreatitis

49. **Chest pain radiating to back and described as a "tearing" pain** — Aortic dissection

50. **40-year-old man with tachycardia/ hypertension and confusion on postoperative day #2** — Alcohol withdrawal

51. **Marfanoid body habitus and mucosal neuromas** — MEN II-b

52. **Psammoma bodies** — Papillary thyroid cancer

53. **Sulphur granules** — Actinomyces infection

54. **Thyroid tumor with AMYLOID tissue** — Thyroid medullary cancer

55. **PALPABLE neck tumor and hypercalcemia** — Parathyroid cancer

56. **Hypertension, diaphoresis (episodic), and palpitations** — Pheochromocytoma

57. **Jejunal ulcers** — Zollinger-Ellison syndrome

58. **Pituitary tumor, pancreatic tumor, and parathyroid tumor** — MEN- I

59. **Necrotizing migratory erythema** — Glucagonoma

60. **Medullary thyroid cancer, pheochro- mocytoma, and hyperparathyroidism** — MEN-IIa

61. **Hypokalemia refractory to IV potassium supplementation** — Hypomagnesemia

62. **Newborn with pneumatosis** — Necrotizing enterocolitis (NEC)

63. **Child with abdominal mass that crosses midline** — Neuroblastoma

64. **Child <4 years of age with abdominal tumor that does NOT cross midline** — Wilms' tumor

65. **"Currant jelly" stools and abdominal colic** — Intussusception

66. **Femur fracture, respiratory failure, petechiae, and mental status changes** — Fat embolism

67. **Hearing loss, tinnitus, and vertigo** — Ménière's disease

68. **Adolescent boy with nasal obstruction and recurrent epistaxis** — Juvenile nasopharyngeal angiofibroma

69. **Child <5 years of age sitting upright and drooling, with "hot-potato" voice** — Epiglottitis

70. **Angina, syncope, and CHF** — Aortic stenosis

71. **Tobacco use, asbestos exposure, and pleuritic chest pain** — Mesothelioma

72. **Supracondylar fracture and contracture of forearm flexors** — Volkmann's contracture

73. **Tibia fracture, "pain out of proportion," pain on passive foot movement, and palpable pulses** — Compartment syndrome

74. **25-year-old man with liver mass with fibrous septae and NO history of cirrhosis or hepatitis** — **Fibrolamellar** hepatocellular carcinoma

75. **EKG with flattening of T waves and U waves**	Hypokalemia
76. **Central pontine myelinosis**	Too-rapid correction of hyponatremia
77. **Polydipsia, polyuria, and constipation**	Hypercalcemia
78. **Factor VIII deficiency**	Hemophilia A
79. **Abdominal pain, fever, hypotension, HYPERkalemia, and HYPOnatremia**	Adrenal insufficiency (Addisonian crisis)
80. **Massive urine output and HYPERnatremia**	Diabetes insipidus
81. **Increased urine osmolality, HYPOnatremia, and low serum osmolality**	SIADH
82. **IV antibiotics, fever, diarrhea**	*Clostridium difficile* pseudomembranous colitis
83. **Bleeding gums and wound dehiscence**	Vitamin C deficiency
84. **Fever, central line, and HYPERglycemia**	Central line infection
85. **Appendectomy followed by fever and abdominal pain on post-operative day #7**	Peritoneal abscess
86. **Advancing crepitus, fever, and blood blisters**	Necrotizing fasciitis
87. **High INTRAoperative fever**	Malignant hyperthermia
88. **Confusion, ataxia, and ophthalmoplegia**	Wernicke's encephalopathy

89. Tracheal deviation, decreased breath sounds, and hyperresonance — Tension pneumothorax

90. Hypotension, decreased heart sounds, and JVD — Pericardial tamponade

91. Four ribs broken in two places and pulmonary contusion — Flail chest

92. Otorrhea (clear) and Battle's sign — Basilar skull fracture

93. Ulcer and decreased pain with food — Duodenal ulcer

94. Vomiting, retching, and epigastric pain — Mallory-Weiss tear

95. Fever on postoperative day #1, with "bronze" weeping, tender wound — Clostridial wound infection

96. Hematochezia and tenesmus — Rectal cancer

97. Upper GI bleed, jaundice, and RUQ pain — Hemobilia

98. Gallstones, epigastric pain radiating to back, and nausea — Gallstone pancreatitis

99. 18-year-old woman with bloody nipple discharge — Ductal papilloma

100. Irritability, diaphoresis, weakness, tremulousness, and palpitations — Insulinoma

Figure Credits

Chapter 6 (Poole sucker)
Blackbourne, LH. *Advanced Surgical Recall,* 3rd ed. Baltimore, MD: Lippincott Williams & Wilkins; 2007:55.

Chapter 6 (Gigli saw)
Blackbourne, LH. *Advanced Surgical Recall,* 3rd ed. Baltimore, MD: Lippincott Williams & Wilkins; 2007:51.

Chapter 10 (carotid endarterectomy)
Lawrence PF, Bell RM, Dayton MT. *Essentials of General Surgery.* 3rd ed. Philadelphia, PA: Lippincott Williams & Wilkins; 2000:545.

Chapter 14 (Pringle maneuver)
Blackbourne, LH. *Advanced Surgical Recall,* 3rd ed. Baltimore, MD: Lippincott Williams & Wilkins; 2007:93.

Chapter 14 (percutaneous endoscopic gastrostomy)
Blackbourne, LH. *Advanced Surgical Recall,* 3rd ed. Baltimore, MD: Lippincott Williams & Wilkins; 2007:55.

Chapter 30 (craniocaudal view and MLO view mammograms)
Gay SB, Woodcock RJ Jr. *Radiology Recall.* Philadelphia, PA: Lippincott Williams & Wilkins; 2000:522.

Chapter 30 (free air seen on chest radiograph)
Lawrence PF, Bell RM, Dayton MT. *Essentials of General Surgery.* 3rd ed. Philadelphia, PA: Lippincott Williams & Wilkins; 2000:267, Fig 7-19A.

Chapter 38 (anatomy of the larynx)
Doherty GM, Meko JB, Olson JA, et al. *The Washington Manual of Surgery,* 2nd ed. Philadelphia, PA: Lippincott Williams & Wilkins; 1999:635, Fig 42-6.

Chapter 38 (pneumothorax)
Daffner RH. *Clinical Radiology. The Essentials.* 2nd ed. Baltimore, MD: Williams & Wilkins; 1999:154, Fig 4-91B.

Chapter 38 (widened mediastinum)
Greenfield LJ, Mulholland MW, Oldham KT, et al. *Surgery: Scientific Principles and Practice.* 3rd ed. Philadelphia, PA: Lippincott Williams & Wilkins; 2001:330, Fig 11-40.

Chapter 56 (rectus abdominis flap reconstruction)
Greenfield LJ, Mulholland M, Oldham KT, et al. *Surgery: Scientific Principles and Practice.* 2nd ed. Philadelphia, PA: Lippincott-Raven; 1997:2238, Fig 114-4.

Chapter 40 (Sengstaken-Blakemore balloon)
Lawrence PF, Bell RM, Dayton MT. *Essentials of General Surgery.* 3rd ed. Philadelphia, PA: Lippincott Williams & Wilkins; 2000:353, Fig 18-8.

Chapter 42 (lap-band)
Blackbourne, LH. *Advanced Surgical Recall,* 3rd ed. Baltimore, MD: Lippincott Williams & Wilkins; 2007:329.

Chapter 52 (French system)
Blackbourne, LH. *Advanced Surgical Recall,* 3rd ed. Baltimore, MD: Lippincott Williams & Wilkins; 2007:137.

Chapter 52 (liver segments)
Blackbourne, LH. *Advanced Surgical Recall,* 3rd ed. Baltimore, MD: Lippincott Williams & Wilkins; 2007:137.

Chapter 57 (gastrinoma triangle)
Greenfield LJ, Mulholland M, Oldham KT, et al. *Surgery: Scientific Principles and Practice.* 2nd ed. Philadelphia, PA: Lippincott-Raven; 1997:924, Fig 34-8.

Chapter 56 (mammogram showing breast cancer)
Daffner RH. *Clinical Radiology: The Essentials.* 2nd ed. Baltimore, MD: Williams & Wilkins; 1999:245, Fig 6-9A.

Chapter 66 (endovascular repair)
Zelenock GB, Huber TS, Messina LM, et al. *Mastery of Vascular and Endovas-cular Surgery.* Philadelphia, PA: Lippincott Williams & Wilkins; 2005.

Chapter 74 (Colles' fracture)
McKenney MG, Mangonon PC, Moylan JA. *Understanding Surgical Disease: The Miami Manual of Surgery.* Philadelphia PA: Lippincott-Raven; 1998:355, Fig 4.

Chapter 74 (Lachman test)
Redrawn from Spindler KP, Wright RW. "Anterior Cruciate Ligament Tear." *N Engl J Med* November 13, 2008; 359:2135, Fig 2.

Chapter 75 (Kocher's point)
Spector SA. *Clinical Companion in Surgery.* Philadelphia, PA: Lippincott Williams & Wilkins; 1999:430, Fig 33-1.

Chapter 75 (bitemporal hemianopsia)
Blackbourne, LH. *Advanced Surgical Recall,* 3rd ed. Baltimore, MD: Lippincott Williams & Wilkins; 2007:747.

Index